MASS VACCINATION

Studies of the Weatherhead East Asian Institute, Columbia University

The Studies of the Weatherhead East Asian Institute of Columbia University were inaugurated in 1962 to bring to a wider public the results of significant new research on modern and contemporary East Asia.

MASS VACCINATION

Citizens' Bodies and State Power in Modern China

Mary Augusta Brazelton

CORNELL UNIVERSITY PRESS   **ITHACA AND LONDON**

Publication of this book was made possible, in part, by a generous grant from the Chiang Ching-kuo Foundation for International Scholarly Exchange.

First published 2019 by Cornell University Press

Library of Congress Cataloging-in-Publication Data

Names: Brazelton, Mary Augusta, 1986– author.
Title: Mass vaccination : citizens' bodies and state power in modern China / Mary Augusta Brazelton.
Description: Ithaca : Cornell University Press, 2019. | Series: Studies of the Weatherhead East Asian Institute, Columbia University | Includes bibliographical references and index.
Identifiers: LCCN 2019008045 (print) | LCCN 2019009149 (ebook) | ISBN 9781501739996 (pdf) | ISBN 9781501740008 (epub/mobi) | ISBN 9781501739989 (cloth : alk. paper)
Subjects: LCSH: Vaccination—China—History—20th century. | Vaccination—China—Yunnan Sheng—History—20th century. | Immunology—Research—China—History—20th century. | Medical policy—China—History—20th century.
Classification: LCC RA638 (ebook) | LCC RA638 .B698 2019 (print) | DDC 614.4/7095135—dc23
LC record available at https://lccn.loc.gov/2019008045

For Hallet, Maria, and Let

Contents

Illustrations

Figures

Map

Acknowledgments

The evening before I left for a year's research in China in 2011, I met the late H. T. Huang and his wife, Rita, at their home. Dr. Huang was Joseph Needham's secretary in China during the Second Sino-Japanese War, and I am grateful for the chance to have met him.

This book benefited tremendously from the advice and encouragement of John Harley Warner, Peter Perdue, Marta Hanson, and Valerie Hansen. Whether providing letters of introduction to archives on short notice or giving meticulously detailed and insightful feedback on each chapter, John's guidance made this book possible. Peter provided characteristically brilliant insights that continue to shape my understanding of modern Chinese history—not least the importance of studying Manchu. I am grateful to Valerie for her advice throughout the writing process and especially for reminding me of the need for common sense and occasional skepticism in analyzing sources. The example that Marta has set with her own scholarship has been genuinely inspiring. Her guidance has made me a better researcher and writer.

Over the course of my research, many archivists and librarians spent considerable time helping me access materials, making copies for me, and (in China) urging me to drink more hot water for the sake of my health. I give heartfelt thanks to the staff at the Yunnan Provincial Archives, the Yunnan Provincial Library, and the Kunming Municipal Archives in Kunming; the Shanghai Library Modern Historical Materials Reading Room and the Shanghai Municipal Archives; the Chongqing Library and the Chongqing Municipal Archives; the National Library of China in Beijing; the Institute of Modern History at Academia Sinica, the Kuomintang Archives, and Academia Historica in Taipei; the League of Nations Archives in Geneva; the Centre des Archives diplomatiques de Nantes; the archives of the Pasteur Institute in Paris; the Archives nationales d'outre-mer in Aix-en-Provence; the Center for the History of Medicine at Harvard University; the Columbia Rare Books and Manuscripts Library; and the Cambridge University Archives. Special thanks go to John Moffett at the Needham Research Institute in Cambridge, Charles Aylmer at the Cambridge University Library, and Tang Li at Yale University's East Asia Library. I also thank Wu Xiaoliang and the graduate students of the History Department at Yunnan University, especially Huang Hanxin, Ding Qiong, and Qian Bingqi. They generously and patiently showed me how to find materials in the Yunnan Provincial Library, as well as how to play mah-jongg. Wang Wencheng of the Yunnan Academy of Social Sciences offered valuable advice, and Kevin Chang was a very kind host in Taiwan. Li Li and Zhang Sen at the Shanghai Academy of Social Sciences provided critical aid. Iris Borowy and Florence Bretelle-Establet were extremely generous with their time and resources.

At Cornell University Press, it was my great fortune to work with Emily Andrew, Susan Specter, and Don McKeon. At the Weatherhead Institute for East Asian Studies, Ross Yelsey was fantastically helpful. I am especially grateful to the anonymous reviewers of the manuscript. Thanks also go to the Chiang Ching-kuo Foundation, the National Science Foundation, the Yale University Council on East Asian Studies, and the McMillan Center for International Studies at Yale for their generous support.

This book had its very beginnings in a seminar with Leon Rocha; I benefited greatly from his guidance. Toby Lincoln introduced me to Duxiu and the vagaries of archival research in China. Many people at Yale provided encouragement, especially Naomi Rogers, as well as Paola Bertucci, Mariola Espinosa, Daniel Kevles, Helen Siu, Frank Snowden, Bruno Strasser, Bill Summers, and Michele Thompson.

I have been profoundly lucky to finish this book while teaching at the Department of History and Philosophy of Science at the University of Cambridge. Helen Anne Curry, Nick Hopwood, Jim Secord, and Wu Huiyi very kindly read and commented on parts of the manuscript. I have learned much from Simon Schaffer, Hans van de Ven, Simon Szreter, Liba Taub, Richard Staley, Lauren Kassell, Marta Halina, Hasok Chang, Dániel Margócsy, Tim Lewens, Steve John, and Jacob Stegenga. Conversations with Salim Al-Gailani, Toby Bryant, Sarah Bull, Andrew Buskell, Jenny Bulstrode, Lukas Engelmann, Tamara Hug, Steve Kruse, James Livesey, Dmitry Myelnikov, James Poskett, Louisa Russell, Susanne Schmidt, Kathryn Schoefert, and Yu Jia were extremely helpful throughout the writing process. Chris Cullen, Sir Geoffrey Lloyd, Jianjun Mei, John Moffett, and Wu Huiyi warmly welcomed me to the Needham Research Institute, for which I am grateful.

Yi-li Wu provided thoughtful feedback on an early chapter. Thomas Mullaney offered helpful suggestions at a crucial juncture, as did Fa-ti Fan. Bridie Andrews, Gao Xi, Sean Lei, Micah Muscolino, and Zhang Daqing all provided important advice. In addition, Nicole Barnes, Emily Baum, Bian He, Howard Chiang, Arunabh Ghosh, Miriam Gross, Seung-joon Lee, Jiang Lijing, Chien-ling Liu, David Luesink, Shen Yubin, Malcolm Thompson, Margaret Tillman, Wayne Soon, Xiao Shellen Wu, and Shirley Ye have been wonderful colleagues and friends. I thank Justin Barr, Robin Scheffler, Tan Ying Jia, and Courtney Thompson for their helpful input as well as Deborah Doroshow, David Koppstein, Tom Reznick, and Rachel Rothschild. Special thanks go to Virginia Anderson, Jonathan Chow, Yinliang He, Winnie Nip, Utpal Sandesara, Monica Thanawala, Laura Togut, Zachary Widbin, Thomas Wooten, and Jingshing Wu for their steadfast support and friendship. It was in our undergraduate years together that I first learned from Anne Harrington, Shigehisa Kuriyama, Everett Mendelsohn, and Steve Shapin, and I remain grateful to these teachers.

Three people were absolutely necessary to the completion of this book. Joy Rankin, Emily Wanderer, and David Singerman provided brilliant, thoughtful feedback on every chapter, and our writing group (later joined by Amy Johnson) was an essential source of cheer and commiseration. I came to know Boris Jardine and Jenny Bangham much later in the writing process; this book is the richer for both their friendship and their critical readings. And the podcast of Elis James and John Robins made long days of writing far more enjoyable.

Joshua Nall was this book's first reader and its best. One of the greatest joys of writing this book has been sharing it with him.

My brother Hallet has long provided a model for two skills critical to the craft of the historian: how to tell stories and how to argue convincingly. Let, Katie, Lia, and now the youngest Hallet have filled my life with humor, warmth, and happiness. My parents, Hallet and Maria, fostered in me curiosity about the world, a respect for knowledge in all its forms, and a love of books. For these things, and much more, I am deeply grateful. Recalling the life and sacrifices of my grandmother, Mildred, reminded me to keep thinking, reading, and writing, wherever I found myself.

Many documents cited in this book were hand-copied from archives and libraries. All faults are my own.

Abbreviations

ABMAC	American Bureau for Medical Aid to China
BCG	Bacille Calmette-Guérin (antituberculosis vaccine)
CCP	Chinese Communist Party
CRCMRC	Chinese Red Cross Medical Relief Corps
EMSTS	Emergency Medical Service Training School
IMCS	Imperial Maritime Customs Service
LNHO	League of Nations Health Organization
NEPB	National Epidemic Prevention Bureau
NHA	National Health Administration
NIH	National Institutes of Health
PLA	People's Liberation Army
PUMC	Peking Union Medical College
SBSCO	Sino-British Scientific Cooperation Office
WHO	World Health Organization

Note on Transliteration

Following standard practice, I use pinyin to denote romanized Chinese names (for example, Beijing), except in cases where Wade-Giles or alternative romanizations are very commonly used (for example, Chiang Kaishek). In the bibliography, for cases where primary source materials were published under names using alternative romanizations, I have included the original in parentheses following the pinyin name. Please consult the glossary for lists of key terms, names, and organizations using traditional Chinese characters. All translations are my own except when otherwise noted.

MASS VACCINATION

Introduction

In 1942, in a village in Yunnan Province, at the far southwestern reaches of war-torn China, a woman turned away from a group of missionaries offering injections that would, they claimed, protect her against the cholera invading her community.

In 1952, a group of schoolchildren in northeastern China—an explicitly "new China," the Communist People's Republic of China (PRC)—queued, their sleeves rolled up, holding out their arms to get jabbed by young women in nurses' uniforms holding needles.

And in 1954, an old man named Lin living in one small neighborhood of Kunming, the capital of Yunnan, turned to face a smallpox vaccination team, at last acquiescing to their demand that he be vaccinated after years of refusing to submit to their ministrations.

Both the spectacle and the mundanity of these individual encounters suggest the significance of vaccination as a means of political control as well as a measure of public health. This book argues that mass immunization programs made vaccination a cornerstone of Chinese public health and China a site of consummate biopower, or power over life. Over the twentieth century, through processes of increasing force, vaccines became medical technologies of governance that bound together the individual and the collective, authorities and citizens, and experts and the uneducated. These programs did not just transform public health in China—they helped shape the history of global health. Take the case of smallpox: The universal eradication of this disease in the 1970s depended on its elimination in the PRC, then the most populous nation in the world. In 1979, the World Health Organization (WHO) announced that the last cases of smallpox had occurred in China in 1960—just eleven years after the 1949 establishment of the PRC under Mao Zedong. Through a series of health campaigns in the 1950s that are only peripherally mentioned, if at all, in histories of public and global health, health workers had vaccinated approximately five hundred million people against the disease.

Yet the health campaigns that did so much to eliminate this one infectious pathogen had not, in fact, taken smallpox as their sole target. They had mandated vaccination against tuberculosis and typhoid fever too. Moreover, the material and administrative systems of mass immunization on which these campaigns relied had a longer history than the PRC itself. The Chinese Communist Party (CCP) championed as its own invention and dramatically expanded immunization systems that largely predated 1949 and had originated with public health programs developed in southwestern China during the Second Sino-Japanese War from 1937 to 1945. The nationwide implementation of these systems in the 1950s relied on transformations in research, pharmaceutical manufacturing, and concepts of disease that had begun in the first decades of the twentieth century. These processes spanned multiple regime changes, decades of war, and diverse forms of foreign intervention. Most important, they brought with them new ideas about what it meant to be a citizen of China.

What Happened at the Needle's Point

The vaccination programs that this book describes directly touched the lives of millions of Chinese people. How, exactly, did immunization transform their bodies? Put simply, the process of immunization usually employs a vaccine or serum to make an organism develop resistance, or immunity, to disease. This resistance often takes the form of producing antibodies, proteins that target disease-causing pathogens within the body. Vaccines, which typically contain an attenuated or killed form of the pathogen in question, are usually administered via injection, but they can also be given orally and in one or several doses, depending on the particular vaccine and the logistical capabilities of the vaccinators. Since the mid-twentieth century, epidemiologists have used vaccination programs to seek the condition of herd immunity in target populations, relying on the principle that when most people in a group receive vaccines against a disease, an epidemic is much less likely to occur—thus making immunization a question of managing populations as well as individual bodies.[1]

In the early twentieth century, infectious diseases such as smallpox, malaria, plague, and cholera had been responsible for much of the mortality of the Chinese population. In 1900, the average life expectancy in the Qing Empire was thirty years of age. The one form of vaccination established in China, against smallpox, had been practiced among only select groups in the largest cities of the vast but faltering empire. In 1905, a *New York Times* article deemed China the "sick man of the Far East," comparing it to the Ottoman Empire and reinforcing the metaphor of epidemic disease as political weakness.[2] When the Qing dynasty fell in 1911, the revolutionary and physician Sun Yatsen became president of a new Republic of China. But within a few years, China tumbled headlong into political and social chaos. Warlords seized power across the former provinces of the empire and established regional autonomy until 1927, when Chiang Kai-shek wrested control of the Nationalist Party from competitors and used military force to reunite much of southern and eastern China.

Throughout this period, little health infrastructure persisted outside major cities such as Beijing, Shanghai, and Guangzhou. In these and other municipalities, urban administrations first implemented hygienic activities of street sweeping, latrine building, and water sanitation. Drawing on terms of traditional Chinese medicine to describe Japanese adaptations of European hygiene, these practices were collectively termed *weisheng*. Yet they were just one of several approaches to epidemic control and prevention. So many medical traditions flourished and competed during this period as to make neat dichotomies between Chinese and Western medicine impossible. Controversy over epidemic management created conflict between local traditional physicians and advocates of newer practices. In so doing, the former sought to make their traditional knowledge modern and professional, even as contemporaneous discourses of modernity constructed science and Chinese medicine as fundamentally opposed. All the while, infectious diseases remained a major cause of mortality throughout the early twentieth century. Alongside periodic outbreaks of long-feared diseases such as smallpox and plague, tuberculosis and other new epidemiological dangers emerged; tuberculosis alone caused approximately four hundred of every hundred thousand deaths per year by 1935.[3]

If the recent past offered such a dismal view of health in China, then how did so many millions of people get vaccinated against smallpox and undergo a regular schedule of measles, polio, pertussis-diphtheria-tetanus, and tuberculosis immunizations by 1960? In considering mass immunization in China, I follow one practice in one national territory ruled by multiple regimes over the twentieth century. This method reflects the diverse sources that contribute to this narrative, drawn from archives and libraries in the PRC, Taiwan, France, Switzerland, the United Kingdom, and the United States. The following chapters explore the social and political impact of a single governmental practice—vaccination—by analyzing the research, personnel, finances, and politics shaping its implementation. This approach permits an articulation of the ways in which mass immunization was distinct from other health interventions of the time. It also suggests the particular significance that vaccination assumed in the relationship between regimes of governance and the bodies they sought to rule.

Although it fell under the rubric of *weisheng*, immunization was distinctive among practices of public health in China. Unlike street sweeping or sewer construction, the introduction of new vaccines clearly articulated the mutually constitutive relationships between Chinese and foreign medical traditions. For instance, the nineteenth-century promotion of Jennerian vaccination against smallpox replaced but also coexisted alongside older methods of variolation—using attenuated strains of smallpox rather than cowpox—that had been common since the eighteenth century.[4] However, the acceptance of Jennerian methods in many places depended upon their resemblance to traditional practices and physicians therefore typically scheduled vaccine drives to coincide with the traditionally auspicious season for variolation. Furthermore, many practices of *weisheng* aimed to transform individual behaviors, such as those encouraging people to use latrines, swat flies, and properly dispose of waste. Vaccination, by contrast, brought the power of the state to bear on individual bodies in a way that other hygienic infrastructures did not. The goals of immunization programs against cholera, typhoid, plague, and other diseases were not necessarily to change attitudes or individual actions in target populations. They simply sought to produce immunity in the bodies of the members of those populations. Whether those bodies were willing or not did not necessarily matter.

This book begins, therefore, with the development of technological systems that could support the large-scale production of immunizations. In the early twentieth century, microbiology emerged in China as a discipline whose researchers found institutional homes at medical schools and institutes in Beijing, Shanghai, Guangzhou, and other cities. Yet their work did not necessarily result in immediate public health measures. Outside urban environments, in largely rural provinces such as Yunnan, the politics of medicine and especially vaccination against smallpox reflected the struggles of foreign powers for influence. Throughout this period, microbiology and vaccine development depended crucially on the global circulation of standard bacterial and viral cultures as well as the containers, vehicles, and syringes that carried them.

The importance of these systems became clear when war threatened to destroy them. When the Japanese army invaded in 1937, Chiang Kaishek moved the national capital to Chongqing, in Sichuan Province. An influx of refugees to the southwestern borderlands facilitated the spread of disease; as a critical tool of epidemic control, vaccination became a central focus for research, manufacturing, and clinical testing during wartime outbreaks of cholera, typhoid fever, and plague. Contrary to narratives that present the wartime southwest as a chaotic, insignificant space where Western medicine and public health were virtually unknown, I suggest that the people, materials, and systems that contributed to mass vaccination in China actually first came together in the wartime southwest.[5] This endeavor involved a variety of actors who included refugee medical students, European researchers, foreign aid workers, and local health administrators. Most immunization campaigns sought to inject as many people as possible with vaccines specified and manufactured by the state and so to produce an official form of collective biological protection for the whole population. In at least some cases, these programs resorted to coercive measures. Still, immunizations for infectious diseases—smallpox, cholera, typhoid, or tuberculosis—reached only a small fraction of the Chinese population until the 1950s—in Yunnan, probably less than 5 percent.

The immunization systems established in war persisted across multiple medical regimes, as the final chapters show. Scholarship on the early PRC has emphasized the continuities, as well as radical breaks, in focus that characterized health policy and practice during the transition between Nationalist and Communist rule in China.[6] What difference did the establishment of the PRC make to mass immunization and epidemic control? After the Japanese surrendered in 1945, the same researchers and administrators who had championed wartime immunization under Chiang Kaishek assumed administrative roles in national public health, with the goal of the total eradication of major infectious diseases. After 1949, the CCP preserved much of Nationalist health policy but expanded provision of care to rural areas and primary health care. Immunization during this period reflects intensified attention to preventive health in rural areas, but it also calls attention to changing scales of policymaking and implementation. After 1949, vaccination programs expanded to a nationwide scope, reaching many local city and county administrations for the first time and immunizing as much as 90 percent of the population against smallpox and typhoid fever.

Although the scale of mass immunization programs expanded greatly during the early PRC, this quantitative change matters most because it reflected the qualitative transformations that had taken place in the capacity of the state to exert power over individual bodies and meanings of citizenship. Presenting mass vaccination as a project of the CCP helped establish the authority of the Chinese state to intervene in the daily lives and health of its residents. This is perhaps most clearly evident in the efforts of the PRC to publicize its medical accomplishments on an international stage. Mass immunization provided a basis on which the Communist government, especially, promoted its commitment to modern science and its legitimacy—and thus its development as a thoroughly biopolitical state.

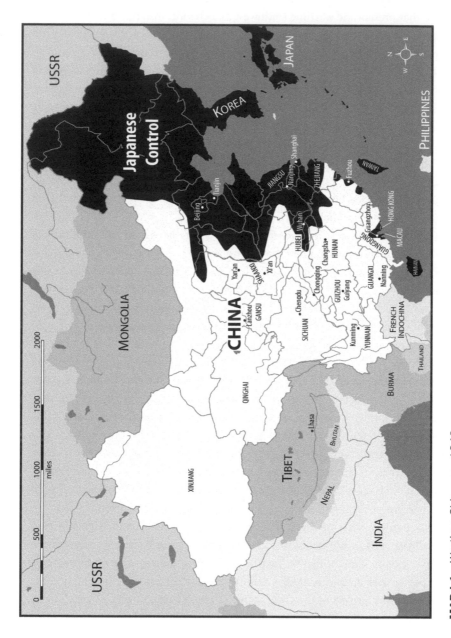

MAP I.1 Wartime China, ca. 1940.

Biotechnological Systems of Political Control

Biopolitics is a messy, unclear concept. It interrogates the relationship between politics and life, yet most scholars ultimately conclude that there is no coherent set of such relationships—only a "series of non-relations," as Timothy Campbell and Adam Sitze put it.[7] Some key features, though, can be identified: the emergence of the population as an object of study and governmental control, the rise of biopower as a set of "techniques for achieving the subjugation of bodies and the control of populations" in the words of Michel Foucault, and the significance of biomedicine and hygiene as providing a connection between scientific knowledge of the body and that of populations. Such a connection also gives rise to a means of political intervention that establishes a basis for norms of discipline and regulation.[8]

Within discourses of biopolitics, immunity has played a special role because it provides a metaphor for distinctions between self and other. Conversely, the long history of immunity as a legal and social concept throughout the early modern period shaped its adoption in microbiology. By the twentieth century, immunologists drew upon interwar and Cold War social theories—as well as longstanding military metaphors—in framing their field as a "science of the self," even as social theorists and philosophers drew upon immunology to naturalize claims about self and identity.[9] Roberto Esposito suggests that the "paradigm" of immunization provides a fundamental link between the Foucauldian anatomo-politics of the individual body and the biopolitics of populations. When the metaphor of the body politic was materially realized in the bodies of individual members of a national population, public health became "the pivot around which the entire economic, administrative, and political affairs of the state revolved," resulting in the expansion of medicine into new spheres through processes of medicalization. The administration of public health produced a "continuous passage—and mutual reinforcement—between sanitary measures, such as compulsory vaccination, and inclusionary/exclusionary ones of a socio-economic nature." Immunization thus exemplifies the symbiotic relationship between hygiene and social control.[10]

What happens when we consider these questions of politics, power, and immunity outside the contexts in which they originated? Although the overwhelming majority of scholarship on biopolitics focuses on the European and American contexts that inspired Foucault to develop these ideas, anthropologists and political scientists have recently begun to consider biopolitics and the emergence of the population as a focus of governance in non-Western contexts, giving special attention to China. Much of this work focuses on the mechanisms for reproductive control that arose in the postsocialist period, after the 1976 death of Mao and the 1978 launch of economic reforms. Anthropologist Susan Greenhalgh has claimed that especially after the restrictive and coercive one-child policy was instituted in 1979, the PRC became "the world's most striking contemporary case" of power over life. Studies also focus on the ways in which both state and market have shaped the relationships between politics and life in the PRC, as seen in postsocialist hospitals, blood banking, and patenting of biotechnology. The contemporary PRC has apparently developed systems of data banking, including fingerprinting, blood typing, DNA collection, and facial recognition, that are currently unmatched by any other nation in radically comprehensive programs of state surveillance.[11]

The postsocialist government of China was able to exert such power over the bodies of individuals and especially women—surveilling their behavior and their health, asserting control over their bodies and bodily products, mandating direct medical interventions through persuasion and force—in part because it had already done all of these things before under Mao and in some cases before his rule. Historians have investigated the schistosomiasis campaigns that made reluctant villagers go out to their fields to chase disease-carrying snails with chopsticks, the "barefoot doctor" programs that brought semiprofessional health workers to large swaths of the Chinese countryside, and the mass campaigns that ordered workers to destroy pests, clean drainage canals, and remove garbage.[12] Yet large-scale immunization, sitting at the nexus of individual bodily politics and the governance of populations, was one of the earliest and most important programs that laid the foundations for the extensive state control over individual bodies that made postsocialist programs such as the one-child policy possible. Mandatory public vaccination contributed to the construction of state power in twentieth-century China because it bound more and more people into increasingly strong obligations to submit to the orders of the central government.

Immunization programs were able to generate such processes of medical intensification in part because they relied upon large-scale technological systems of cultivation, preservation, and distribution. Historians of technology have shown that such systems engage with the social values and cultural priorities of their actors as well as the technical conditions of their operation.[13] It was only once health professionals and administrators treated mass immunization as a set of interconnected technological systems of cultivation, preservation, and distribution that it functionally succeeded as a public health strategy in China's wartime hinterlands.[14] Both the Nationalist and Communist governments focused their efforts on overcoming practical obstacles to producing, packaging, and transporting vaccines across the country not only because these products could stop epidemics but also because mass immunization indicated the establishment of a new, modern medical infrastructure that could contribute to the power of the state over life. Immunization systems thus became technologies of governance and administration. In this function, they were not alone. Tong Lam, for instance, has demonstrated that social surveys in Republican China were part of a broader nation-building effort to construct new organizing principles for social and cultural production.[15]

If vaccination programs in China were state-building processes that targeted all individuals in a population, their implementation also involved new ideas of citizenship and national belonging that sought to shape this population at the same time. Citizens of modern nation-states can be defined, or define themselves and their rights, in biological terms—as in European cases where meeting medical and legal criteria for disability has determined citizens' abilities to access social welfare programs as well as their membership in activist groups.[16] State-sponsored vaccination contributed to constructions of biological citizenship in twentieth-century China. Receiving vaccines mandated by the government and thereby possessing bodily immunity against a variety of infectious diseases came to define Chinese citizens, and some of their rights, before and after 1949.

Vaccination, citizenship, and the exertion of state power formed connections at many sites across the modern world. For instance, in Tokugawa Japan the enforcement of smallpox vaccination among the Ainu minority people assimilated them as modern Japanese citizens.[17] Yet in twentieth-century China—where legal, political, and social meanings of citizenship were especially unstable—the biological took on particular significance. After the 1911 Xinhai Revolution, the former subjects of the Qing dynasty became citizens of the new Republic of China in part by participating in civics education and other rituals of statehood.[18] Through processes such as adopting a unified solar calendar and participating in national day celebrations, they acquired national identities, civic rights, and social membership.[19] Immunization campaigns also entailed collective participation as a means of identity building in the Republic of China but went further in establishing the expectation that one subject his or her body physically to the dictates of the state. Biological assumptions underlay associated ideas of national belonging, and the Republican government—which had stressed the Han ethnic identity in promoting Chinese nationalism—presented vaccination as contributing to racial, as well as national, health.[20] In the calamitous environment of Japanese invasion and the Nationalist flight to the southwest, the promotion and enforcement of immunization policies by the National Health Administration (NHA), or Weishengshu, attempted to mandate that the residents of what had been remote borderlands participate in an act that, medical administrators claimed, would support the collective health of the central state.

The association of ideas about citizenship and national belonging with the act of immunization gained force during and after the establishment of the PRC.

After 1949, ideas of citizenship encountered those of class, collectivism, and the party. At this transformative moment, as theoretical and political definitions of "the citizen" (*guomin* or *gongmin*) and the people became mutable and multiple, other meanings—among them the biological—took on practical weight.[21] Throughout the Maoist era, almost everyone had to get immunized, except those in high-risk groups such as pregnant women and the very elderly. One's vaccination record partially dictated the ability to travel outside his or her work unit, enforcing connections between vaccination status and individual rights. Throughout the 1950s, the party's promotion of immunization programs in radio broadcasts, posters, and other propaganda portrayed model citizens and comrades as those who willingly received vaccines against smallpox, cholera, and typhoid fever.

And yet most people were not models. While the work of medical teams did often involve persuading people to comply with state orders, these orders also included provisions for compelling vaccination by force, regardless of individual objections. While the state's commitment to public health strained national coffers and capabilities, popular resistance impeded the implementation of immunization programs. During and after the Second Sino-Japanese War, this dynamic changed to reflect the growing power of the Nationalist and Communist states as both regimes enforced increasingly broad mandates for public vaccination and as official capacities to manufacture vaccines expanded. The normalization of state-provided vaccinations during the 1930s and 1940s afforded a wealth of new opportunities for individuals to embrace or resist the application of national policies to their own bodies. Although people continued to refuse and avoid vaccination throughout the early 1950s, the PRC's growing capacities for surveillance meant that those who resisted were liable to the increased scrutiny—and force—of local health administrations. A history of mass immunization during this period therefore offers an opportunity to partially reconstruct genealogies of the state's capability to control, as well as protect, life.

Sites of Vaccination: China in Global Histories of Science and Medicine

The processes of medical intensification that increasingly bound individuals into compliance with state vaccination policies also connected them to global networks of immunity and biology. The history of immunology has always been a global one. At its inception during the late nineteenth and early twentieth centuries, as researchers in European institutes investigated bodily immunity, antibody formation, and allergy, colonial regimes provided sites and test subjects for knowledge production in tropical environments where many infectious diseases were endemic.[22] In this respect, histories of microbiology, bacteriology, and immunology are part of familiar narratives of science and empire. More broadly, the history of science and medicine has tended to view the production of knowledge in non-Western spaces through a colonial prism. What mattered, if not the imperial metropoles of the West itself, were its colonial holdings as sites of innovation and research—British India, the American-occupied Philippines, French North Africa—so that much of what is now termed the "global history of science" is the study of colonial science and medicine by another name.[23]

There is very good reason to pursue such an approach. The global economic and intellectual systems that Western empires engineered reached around the world, even in places not directly under colonial rule. The emerging nineteenth-century disciplines of science and medicine were intrinsic to these enterprises and fundamentally supported them. China, under the influence of multiple Western powers by the mid-nineteenth century, was no exception. And yet Europe and the United States, and their colonies, were of course not the only places where knowledge about the natural world was made. A long tradition of research has made this point definitively for the case of China.[24] Amid such a wealth of scholarship, what the history of public health (and especially mass immunization) shows distinctively is that China was not just a site for the production of knowledge that ultimately contributed to the rise of a hegemonic Western science. Nor did it simply present an alternative to Western models of modernity and development. In the twentieth century, through the processes outlined above, China became an exemplar of the modern biopolitical state: the model against which we might measure others.

China assumed such a status in part through consistent engagement in global networks of knowledge and biomedical economies. In the nascent Republic of China, scientists and physicians translated texts on immunity from German, French, and English, often via Japanese, and corresponded with colleagues in Copenhagen, London, and Bombay to obtain samples of standard cultures by post. Students embarked on long journeys to study with European, American, and Japanese researchers and published their work in internationally distributed journals. It was these researchers who directed institutes for the manufacture of biological products, who developed new vaccines and sera for diseases endemic to China, and who worked with health administrators to distribute them domestically and regionally.

Global conflict afforded new opportunities for Chinese microbiologists to connect with foreign colleagues. After Japan's invasion, wartime aid from abroad reinforced a position China had long held in the sphere of international health: that of an impoverished non-Western polity subject to humanitarian but ultimately self-interested interventions by European and American organizations and experts. Since the late nineteenth century, sanitary conferences had identified China as a fearsome site of disease.[25] Throughout the early twentieth century and continuing into the 1940s, piteous narratives of the plight of epidemic-stricken Chinese peasants were the stock-in-trade of missionary and philanthropic organizations sponsoring medical projects there and seeking to raise funds in the United States and Europe. Continuing during the war, international organizations such as the League of Nations reinforced the traditional role of China as a vulnerable population in need of charitable medical aid and intervention.

Yet the wartime development of mass vaccination systems ultimately helped transform China into a nation that itself dispensed, and did not receive, medical aid. The Maoist period from 1949 to 1976 is commonly seen as an era of Chinese isolation from international health, in which the PRC largely withdrew from the WHO and retreated from participation in global research networks.[26] But in the socialist and nonaligned worlds, Chinese models of public health grew in influence. In the early 1950s, they benefited from cooperation with the Soviet Union, where coercive mass immunization campaigns were also emerging, with the aim as well of both ensuring preventive health and consolidating political legitimacy. By the early 1960s, the PRC was well on its way to assuming a prominent role in public health outside the West. Dora Vargha's work on polio vaccination in Cold War Hungary shows that technologies of, and support for, immunization played a key role in diplomatic relations for socialist states.[27] Certainly they were a part of the medical aid that the PRC sent to the governments of nonaligned states in Africa, Asia, and Latin America. In 1978, the WHO held a landmark meeting in Alma-Ata (now Almaty), capital of the Kazakh Soviet Socialist Republic (now Kazakhstan) that would establish a new strategic priority of "health for all." This new direction was the partial result of Chinese advocacy for models of primary health care along the lines of its barefoot doctor programs to train large corps of rural medical workers.[28] The eradication of smallpox in the PRC had supported Chinese claims for the success of these models in the socialist world. It also indicated the significance of China in the history of global health.

The Significance of the Southwest

For all its global import, the history of mass immunization in modern China relied on research and public health programs in what is now a relatively obscure part of the country. The remote province of Yunnan was the site of the final official case of smallpox infection in China when a local man named Hu Xiaofa contracted and recovered from the disease in 1960. But it was also the place where, decades earlier, Chinese researchers and health administrators had *begun* developing many of the systems necessary to establish nationwide immunization programs. In examining one discipline in the life sciences and its applications in public health, I also consider the importance of one province in the southwestern frontier. Why and how did the development of immunology and mass immunization programs depend upon wartime work in Yunnan, a borderland far from the cosmopolitan intellectual centers of prewar China?

Yunnan was, and remains, an exceptional place. Bordering contemporary Vietnam, Laos, and Myanmar, its uplands have traditionally been dominated by non-Han ethnic groups.[29] Until the early eighteenth century, when Yunnan became a province of the Qing Empire, its high mountains, subtropical climate, and thick vegetation made it an inhospitable place for Han soldiers and settlers. Imperial officials frequently fell prey to *zhangqi*, a set of endemic illnesses now identified with malaria.[30] Throughout the rise of the Nationalist Party, independent-minded powers lingered in many borderlands, including Yunnan. Despite the efforts of French and British agents to establish imperial influence in the 1910s and 1920s, warlords ruled the province with virtual autonomy from 1911 until the onset of war with Japan.

The place of Yunnan has gone largely unremarked in wartime narratives of medicine and society. Scholars have considered the Second Sino-Japanese War in terms of collaboration with and resistance to Japanese occupation, the rise of the CCP, and the rule of the Nationalist regime at Chongqing.[31] Yunnan is distinct from all of these contexts. It was an intellectual center for Chinese academics and researchers during the war, in part because a strong Allied military presence facilitated an unusual degree of academic, military, and material exchange with the world outside wartime China. Kunming became a key site for medical researchers and physicians because it was both a center of communications and, they believed, remote enough to escape major bombing. The singular environment and epidemiology of Yunnan had created this perceived seclusion. It also challenged and daunted researchers and administrators in ways that forced them to cooperate in developing comprehensive systems of immunization.

The end of the war might have signaled a relegation of southwestern China to its old status as a distant backwater. The retreat of the Japanese in 1945 is understood to have occasioned a return of power to coastal regions, and many biomedical experts and workers traveled back to their prewar homes in Shanghai, Guangzhou, and other urban centers.[32] But in terms of public health, the integration of the southwestern hinterland into the national government of mainland China endured through a tumultuous period of war, regime change, and diaspora.

Before these narratives of war and revolution, I turn first to the emergence of research communities in microbiology during the 1920s and 1930s, which were focused largely in the cosmopolitan cities of Beijing and Nanjing. These former imperial metropoles were the centers of a young republic, founded on principles of democracy and internationalism, which promised the development of a new Chinese modernity on the global stage—not least in terms of health and biomedicine. These ambitions proved fatal for many—they would come crashing down in war and destruction and diaspora—but the enduring drive to realize them gripped individuals, institutions, and governments.

JOURNEY TO THE SOUTHWEST

In September 1938, a short, bespectacled man named Tang Feifan drove into the city of Kunming, capital of Yunnan Province. He was at the head of an unusual convoy: six trucks that carried rabbits, guinea pigs, and a variety of scientific equipment. The rabbits were test animals for standardizing sera, and Tang was the new chief of the National Epidemic Prevention Bureau (Zhongyang fangyi chu), a Nationalist government agency that oversaw the development and manufacture of vaccines.[1] Originally based in Beijing and Nanjing, Tang and his staff fled these cities when the Japanese army invaded in 1937 and traveled over a thousand miles to the southwest.

Tang could scarcely have imagined that the misfortunes of war would take him to a place like Yunnan. Since leaving his home village in Hunan Province for the city of Changsha to begin medical studies at the Yale-Xiangya Medical College in the late 1910s, Tang's career had taken him to many new environs: postdoctoral research in Cambridge, Massachusetts, a visiting fellowship in London, and then a comfortable home in Shanghai's French concession. To Tang and other scientific researchers who came to the southwest from the fallen cities of Beijing, Shanghai, and Nanjing, Kunming was a barely civilized backwater. These specialists had come to Yunnan *because* it was a hinterland, ostensibly far from the war front. Yet they disparaged the city's remoteness and poverty, a far cry from their own elite backgrounds.

A substantial number of people with advanced training in medicine and biology traveled to China's wartime southwest after the Nationalist government moved its capital to Chongqing in 1937. They came for many reasons: in some cases, under orders to accompany the transfer of government institutions; in others, out of a patriotic desire to support the war effort. Others were seeking opportunities for professional advancement. They all had already lived through a remarkable period of political upheaval. After the 1911 collapse of the Qing dynasty and the subsequent establishment of the Republic of China, warlords quickly assumed control over most regions of the new nation. After 1915, the republic survived in the weakened form of the Beiyang government at Beijing (known as Beiping from 1928 to 1949) until Chiang Kaishek and the Nationalist Party consolidated power in 1927.

Contrary to typical narratives focusing on events and actors in Western Europe and North America, archival materials, published materials, and personal accounts show clearly that Chinese doctors and biologists were an active part of a global research community in microbiology before the Second World War. Trained primarily in Europe and the United States and frequently supervising colleagues educated domestically and in Japan, they published the results of their experimental work, occupied research chairs in private and public institutes, and advised local governments. Yet the financial and logistical limitations of public health administration, as well as widespread resistance to immunization efforts in rural and nonelite communities, meant that clinical applications of microbiology via vaccines, sera, or other tools often failed to immediately result in significant transformations of health in China—at least until the outbreak of the Second World War created conditions conducive to change via the reconfiguration of professional communities.

At the conclusion of the First World War, microbiology was a field in flux around the globe. The emergence of the germ theory of disease in the late nineteenth century had given rise to new sciences of bacteriology and immunology. Much activity in the European centers of Paris and Berlin focused on the microscopic identification of agents of disease. Following the work of Patrick Manson and Ronald Ross in Hong Kong and India, the emerging discipline of tropical medicine had revealed more complex mechanisms by which microorganisms infected humans with malaria, elephantiasis, and other parasitic diseases. From the late 1910s on, research priorities and outcomes in immunology underwent a sea change away from such dramatic events and toward the slow development of new techniques and tools via chemical investigations. Several influential achievements occurred during this period—for instance, the 1921 production of the Bacille Calmette-Guérin (BCG) vaccine against tuberculosis by Albert Calmette and Camille Guérin—but in general, fewer techniques and tools were developed, and they took longer to produce. Immunology became a realm of chemical inquiries about antibodies and antigens, in which principal activities included establishing serotypes for various bacteria and developing serodiagnostics such as the Dick test for scarlet fever.[2]

While the pace of research slowed over the 1920s and 1930s, microbiology grew as a profession around the world. Many nations established organizations in bacteriology, immunology, and virology, with attendant publications. In 1927, the International Society for Microbiology was established, with its first meeting of representatives from thirty member nations being held three years later. Yet the work done in these fields varied tremendously across national and regional borders, and consequently the society sought to establish universal standards and classifications.[3] The international network of Pasteur Institutes, largely established in sites of French colonial power and influence during the late nineteenth century, continued to expand and establish new laboratories as part of the imperial "civilizing mission," especially in Southeast Asia and North Africa. During this period, major research projects in bacteriology continued to develop in colonial and postcolonial environments, notably British India and Cuba, relying on the labor and leadership of indigenous researchers and administrators.[4]

In contrast to these narratives, the emergence of microbiology as a discipline in China during the early twentieth century did not rely on any single organization, charismatic leader, or colonial influence. Instead, multiple institutes and universities in Beijing, Nanjing, Shanghai, and other cities emerged as centers for research, and a small group of highly educated physicians and scientists participated in global research networks, even as they trained Chinese students and advised local health administrations. In the 1920s and 1930s, emerging fields such as immunology, virology, and bacteriology were identified with broader categories of inquiry, such as the medical sciences (*yike*) or microbiology (*weishengwu xue*). Chinese researchers interested in studying the causes of disease found institutional homes at medical schools in Beijing, Shanghai, Guangzhou, and other large cities. In addition to laboratory research, they translated new terms into Chinese and established professional organizations. Although research programs in microbiology were productive, their applications to public health were limited to specific projects in major cities. One important urban institution was the National Epidemic Prevention Bureau. After its 1919 establishment in Beijing, the bureau became a center for vaccine production and sponsored limited urban immunization campaigns. The outbreak of formal war with Japan in 1937 and the subsequent move of many researchers to the southwest disrupted the development of microbiology in China. Yet it also created opportunities for new cooperative relationships to form in the field of public health.

Microbiology in China's Early Twentieth Century

Very few of the scientists, doctors, and students who ended up producing vaccines in wartime Kunming would have seen themselves as immunologists from the beginning. In the 1920s and 1930s, most professionals in this field held the title of "microbiologist" (*weishengwu xuejia*). Since the end of the First World War, Chinese scholars had translated texts about and begun their own research on bacteria, viruses, and parasites.[5] By the 1930s, researchers in microbiology included the faculty, students, and staff of some of China's top medical schools and research institutes, who used institutional resources to support the construction of specialized laboratories. Before the war broke out, these researchers focused their work on experimentation, translation, and disciplinary formation through the establishment of professional organizations and journals.

A 1933 textbook, *Mianyixue yuanli* (Principles of immunology), gives a representative overview of knowledge about the human immune system in China before the war. Author Long Yuying distinguished between congenital immunity and immunity acquired after birth and outlined debates between theories of humoral immunity (caused by bodily fluids) and cellular immunity (caused by particular kinds of cells) that had evolved in France and Germany in the late nineteenth century.[6] Comparison to the topics covered by a contemporary American textbook, William W. C. Topley and Graham S. Wilson's *Principles of Bacteriology and Immunity*, shows the authors' shared concern with antitoxic and antibacterial immunities and indicates that medical students in China and the United States were engaging with broadly comparable bodies of knowledge.[7]

As a graduate of the prominent Yale-Xiangya Medical College and head of the Hunan Provincial Health Laboratory, Long Yuying was part of an exclusive group. The world of microbiology in 1920s and 1930s China was a small community whose members had gone to the same schools and worked in the same places. Their backgrounds reveal ties to key institutions that supported research in microbiology. Take the case of Tang Feifan. Born in 1897 in Hunan's Liling County, in 1921 he ranked at the top of the first class to graduate from the Yale-Xiangya Medical School. After postdoctoral training at the Peking Union Medical College (PUMC), he traveled to the Harvard Medical School to work under Hans Zinsser, the bacteriologist famous for his work on the etiology of typhus. Before taking up the leadership of the bureau in 1938, Tang had served as head of the Department of Bacteriology at the Henry Lester Institute of Medical Research and as a faculty member of the medical college at the prestigious National Central University, both in Shanghai. In 1936, he was invited to visit London's National Institute for Medical Research, where he collaborated with Sir Henry Dale, the joint winner of the 1936 Nobel Prize in Physiology or Medicine, who specialized in studies of ergot alkaloids, acetylcholine, and histamines.[8] Tang was well known and even notorious for his dedication to laboratory research. Early in his career, he was preoccupied with attempts to isolate the pathogen that caused trachoma. In 1933, he tested a trachoma bacillus that Japanese researcher Hideyo Noguchi had claimed to discover by injecting it into his own eyes, staking his vision and career on the conviction that Noguchi was wrong. Tang did not contract the disease, thereby powerfully discrediting Noguchi's work. Several decades later, in 1955, Tang would become the first to isolate successfully the small bacterium that causes trachoma, *Chlamydia trachomatis*.[9]

Tang was captivated by a single question: What was the causative agent of trachoma? Similar questions drove his colleagues at other institutions of Western medicine, especially the Rockefeller Foundation–managed PUMC in Beijing. How did the presence of antibodies in the blood lead the human body to resist disease? What were the causative agents for the viral and bacterial diseases that most affected Chinese people, and how did the body's immune system react to their introduction?

A number of researchers spent their prewar careers attempting to answer these questions. In Beijing, Liu Sizhi and Wu Xian—both professors of biochemistry at PUMC—researched antigen-antibody reactions, which provide the basis of antibody-mediated immunity to infectious diseases. Liu's research focused on the effect that hormones had upon metabolism of antibodies.[10] Xie Shaowen, a professor of bacteriology at PUMC who had also undertaken postdoctoral studies at the Harvard Medical School with Zinsser, studied the bacteriology of typhus. In 1932, he identified the bacterium responsible for causing an epidemic of brucellosis in northern China. (Brucellosis, also known as undulant fever, is a chronic disease that induces profuse sweating, joint pain, and muscle ache.) Two years later, Xie became the first to cultivate *Rickettsia prowazekii*, the bacterium that causes epidemic typhus, using the membranes of developing chicken eggs.[11] A colleague of Xie in bacteriology, Chen Zongxian (Edgar Tsung-Hsien Tsen), received an MD from the Harvard Medical School of China in Shanghai in 1914. Upon his graduation, Chen moved to the United States and worked with Zinsser at Columbia University, specializing in the etiology of poliomyelitis and efforts to develop antisera for the disease, before returning to China to take up a position at PUMC.[12]

Beijing was not the only Chinese center of research into the human immune system. Yu He and Lin Feiqing were early forces in immunological research in Shanghai. A member of the serology department at the Pasteur Institute of Shanghai, Yu investigated cholera, typhoid fever, diphtheria, and other infectious diseases. In 1933, Yu was the first to propose that the pathogenesis of rheumatic fever was allergy-mediated, implying that the disease is caused by autoimmune reactions. Lin, a rare woman in the field, studied immune responses to bacterial infection. After receiving her PhD from PUMC in 1932, she taught in the Department of Bacteriology at the medical college of the National Central University.[13]

The work of researchers such as Liu Sizhi and Tang Feifan required the development of a vocabulary to articulate novel microbiological concepts in Chinese. Translation of biomedical terminologies in early twentieth-century China was much more than a mundane technical exercise. David Luesink has suggested that it was in fact a means of institutionalizing particular concepts of Western science and medicine in China, not least because the Ministry of Education only approved medical textbooks for publication if they used the terms stipulated by official dictionaries. In 1918, a Medical Terminology Investigation Committee (Yixue mingci shenchahui) convened, publishing its first draft of medical terms relating to bacteriology and immunology two years later. In addition to individual terms, longer works were translated into Chinese from English, German, French, Japanese, and other languages. In 1930, Yu He worked with researchers Li Tao and Tang Feifan to produce the first Chinese translation of a classic bacteriological text, *Zinsser's Bacteriology*. More editions followed, and the 1930s saw a proliferation of Chinese translations and articles about immunology, bacteriology, microbiology, and related fields.[14]

Tang Feifan was one such translator as a member of a committee of experts in the National Institute for Compilation and Translation, which identified key terms in immunology and bacteriology. They published a book titled *Xijunxue mianyixue mingci* (Dictionary of immunology and bacteriology) in 1937 that included the German, English, French, Japanese, and new Chinese translations of these terms. Comparison with a similar dictionary produced in 1918 suggests a growing scholarly interest in the immune system. By 1937, immunology (*mianyixue*) had its own section, comprising forty-nine words. While the 1918 text had included such terms as "immune agglutinin" and "immune opsonin," the 1937 dictionary dispensed with these now-outdated names in favor of a focus on types and principles of immunity.[15] Terms that fell under the domain of "immunology" in the 1937 book made up just one section alongside the vocabularies of many other subdivisions in the life sciences, such as toxicology, serology, bacteriology, and microbiology. The new dictionary thus reflected changing disciplinary structures as well as new areas of research. More people were getting more interested, and more knowledgeable, about how the human body could repel disease.

Translations and dictionaries were not the only forms in which knowledge about immunology was transmitted to medical spheres in Republican China. Magazines for professional and popular audiences offered introductions to the field at varying levels of specialized knowledge. For example, a 1931 article in *Yiyao pinglun* (Medical review), a medical journal published in Shanghai with the aim of "scientizing the thoughts of the masses" (*minzhong sixiang kexuehua*), outlined Paul Ehrlich's side-chain theory of immunity. The theory suggested that all cells have special receptors, or "side-chains"—unique structures that permit the introduction of external nutrients to the nucleus. When these receptors combined with nonnutritious foreign matter, or antigens, the cell would overproduce the receptors, or antibodies, and secrete them into tissue fluids. The piece devoted some space to discussing the practical implications of the side-chain theory for individual adverse reactions to vaccination. It also explained Ehrlich's theory that vaccination produced immunity by creating antibodies that circulated in the blood. These were not cutting-edge concepts—Ehrlich had first published on the side-chain theory in 1897.[16] But their discussion in Chinese medical journals indicated that physicians of the early 1930s found principles of immunology relevant to clinical practice insofar as they could explain complications of and negative reactions to the process of immunization.

Another article, published in 1936 by Xie Shaowen in the journal *Yiyu* (Medical education), discussed the significance of bacteriology and immunology to medical training. Xie outlined the scope, kinds of teachers, curriculum, and practical instruction that a thorough education in bacteriology and immunology ought to include, writing that those who completed such a course would hopefully aid "provincial and county authorities in popularizing the establishment of public health." He claimed that this was essential knowledge for doctors to diagnose and treat communicable diseases as well as for public health officials to carry out preventive work.[17]

The establishment of new professional institutions further reflected the disciplinary development of microbiology in China. The earliest medical organization in the country was the National Medical Association (Zhonghua yixue hui), which was founded in 1915 and began publishing the *National Medical Journal of China* (Zhonghua yixue zazhi) in the same year. In 1922, Lin Kesheng (also known as Robert "Bobby" Lim) and others at PUMC founded a Beijing branch of the Society for Experimental Biology and Medicine, and in 1928, Wu Liande and colleagues established the Chinese Society for Microbiology.

The members of these organizations translated texts, published articles in Chinese and English periodicals, and gave presentations at international conferences.[18] Yet no one figure stood out as a galvanizing leader of microbiology in China. A number of prominent figures, laboratories, and institutions provided spaces and opportunities for research.

Prewar Relationships between Medical Research and Public Health

Among these different institutional homes, researchers began to assume positions in the health administration of the Republic of China from 1911 onwards. Yet research in microbiology did not have a strong direct impact on public health in prewar China. Ruth Rogaski has shown that the establishment of hygiene (*weisheng*) in late nineteenth-century and early twentieth-century China largely occurred in the treaty ports of the eastern and southern coasts. The case of Tianjin demonstrates that a variety of colonial administrations, local elites, and the emergent Chinese state established "hygienic modernity" via urban sanitary reforms such as water treatment and quarantine that were Western in origin but typically transferred from the Japanese context. Most accounts of the history of public health in Republican China focus on the introduction of sanitary practices to cities and the rural demonstration stations that existed outside Nanjing, Shanghai, and in Hebei Province at Dingxian.[19]

Vaccination was among these activities of *weisheng*, but the application of bacteriology and related disciplines to clinical medicine via the development and manufacturing of vaccines, sera, and other "biological products" (*shengwu zhipin*) was generally confined to the major cities of Beijing, Shanghai, Nanjing, and Guangzhou. Individual researchers were consulted as advisers by health departments in these urban areas and rural health demonstration counties, and in national institutes they developed new vaccines using particular local strains of bacteria and viruses. However, their efforts did not give rise to systematic programs of mass immunization or national public health.

The circumscription of public health to the urban sphere was partly a consequence of the financial inability of the Republican government to fund rural health reforms and partly a reflection of global trends. By the early twentieth century, research in microbiology—and, later, the fields of virology and immunology—had generally failed to fulfill the early promise of halting epidemics with better therapies or the widespread dissemination of new vaccines.

Although epidemics slowed in progression and killed fewer people by the early twentieth century, the cause lay in sanitary reforms rooted in older theories of contagion and miasma as well as in emerging germ theories.

An apt demonstration of this point in the Chinese context lies in an important moment for sanitary reform, the 1910 outbreak of pneumonic plague in Manchuria. The emergence of pneumonic plague at the very end of the Qing dynasty made northeastern China a vulnerable political target. The Russian army's expansive construction of railroads across Manchuria had facilitated the spread of the disease, and it was Russian and Japanese agents of empire who competed to build plague hospitals and provide medical aid to the region, with the aim of establishing bases of political influence. With the sponsorship of the Qing government, the famous physician Wu Liande and his colleagues sought to stop the epidemic using harsh isolation measures and enshrined themselves in popular memory as doctors who conclusively demonstrated the superiority of Western biomedicine over practitioners of Chinese medicine in the eyes of the media and state. Although they cast their work as a watershed moment for the application of microscopic methods to diagnosis and management of epidemic disease in the country, historians have pointed out that it was a strict quarantine, not newly developed therapeutics or prophylactics, that apparently succeeded in quelling the epidemic.[20]

The draconian measures of isolation that Wu Liande and his team took may well have been the decisive factor in ending the epidemic, but they terrified local populations in Manchuria, who sought to escape and avoid them. A similar ambiguity in attitudes and responses applied to other practices of public health, notably immunization. The first clear records of coercive vaccination in China dated to the end of the Qing dynasty, when police regulations mandated compulsory smallpox immunization. These regulations remained in place through the early Republic of China (1911–28), although the extent to which local governments implemented them remains unclear. While some educated, elite social groups in major cities such as Canton welcomed inoculation against smallpox and plague, these interventions had a limited reach, and reports suggested that many populations tended to avoid inoculation.[21]

Despite the limited applications of microbiology to public health, by 1920 the Republican government had established an institute that would employ experts in microbiology and bacteriology to produce vaccines and sera. The National Epidemic Prevention Bureau was originally local to Beijing. In 1918, Qian Nengxun, then minister of the interior of the Republic of China, had authorized the establishment of this organization following an outbreak of plague in northern Suiyuan and Shanxi Provinces in December 1917.[22] The bureau was given facilities at a highly symbolic location in central Beijing: the outer buildings of the Temple of Heaven, where the Ming and Qing emperors had historically led prayers for good harvests (see fig. 1.1). This placement indicated the central role intended for the bureau, not only in preventing epidemics but also in health administration. It also suggested that the Beiyang government then in place had decisively rejected the imperial era and embraced modernity, replacing religion with a symbol of science in service of national interests. The bureau's work quickly grew to include biomedical research on infectious diseases, epidemiological data gathering, and urban vaccination programs as well as manufacturing of sera and vaccines. By 1924, it had established sales agencies in the cities of Hankou, Shenyang, Nanjing, Beijing, Shanghai, and Tianjin, indicating the nationwide (albeit urban) scope of its ambitions.[23]

After 1927, the Nationalist Party under Chiang Kaishek gained authority over the republic and across much of mainland China. During the ensuing Nanjing Decade, the growing central government enacted policies and programs that attempted to establish modern health practices and education across the nation. However, these programs were primarily urban in scope and perniciously underfunded. Difficult directive questions also troubled the fledgling administration: Should the government focus on widespread public health or concentrate its energies and funds? Should the state support modern biomedicine to

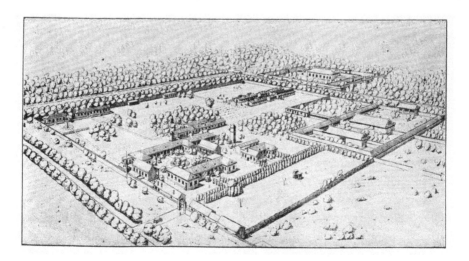

FIGURE 1.1   "Bird's Eye View of National Epidemic Prevention Bureau," 1934. NHA and Central Field Health Station, *National Epidemic Prevention Bureau*. Reproduced courtesy of the Center for the History of Medicine, Harvard University.

the exclusion of traditional Chinese medicine? Founded in 1927 and reorganized under the Ministry of the Interior in 1931, the NHA articulated an administrative logic for provincial and municipal health organizations; established numerous national centers for health activities including a Central Hygienic Laboratory (Zhongyang weisheng shiyan suo); and brought the National Epidemic Prevention Bureau under its jurisdiction. The NHA also legislated mandatory smallpox vaccination in 1928. It encouraged local governments to sponsor mass inoculation campaigns against cholera, typhoid, and other diseases and also distributed smallpox vaccines across the nation—but vaccination figures for cholera, typhoid, and diphtheria remained low.[24]

In its new institutional home, the National Epidemic Prevention Bureau grew in scope over the 1930s, establishing a branch laboratory at Lanzhou (capital of Gansu Province) and a cooperative relationship with the Suiyuan Epidemic Prevention Bureau in what is now Inner Mongolia, an institute that dealt primarily with identifying and producing vaccines for epizootic (animal-borne) diseases. Throughout the 1920s and 1930s, the bureau intervened in epidemic outbreaks from Beijing by sending personnel, vaccines, and sera to regions struck by cholera, plague, smallpox, diphtheria, and other infectious diseases. When cholera broke out in Shanghai and Nanjing in 1925, for instance, it sent stocks of cholera vaccines to these cities, held free inoculations in Beijing, and produced posters and newspaper items advertising anticholera measures.[25]

Although the bureau described its involvement in epidemics as generally working to quell disease incidence, this work was not without its risks and difficulties. In March 1921, one staffer, Yu Shufen, died at age thirty-five when he contracted pneumonic plague while trying to control an outbreak of the disease in Shandong Province. Moreover, people continued to resist or avoid immunization. For instance, a 1934 report of the bureau notes that even in the metropolis of Beijing, where from 1919 to 1928 free inoculations against smallpox, cholera, and typhoid were offered to the public, "the people showed very little response except in the case of smallpox vaccination," and even then "so few persons availed themselves of the opportunity of free vaccination" against smallpox that the bureau did not bother to keep records of these visits until 1922.[26] A 1930 report on vaccine and sera production in the *National Medical Journal of China* noted the widespread lack of interest in immunization, even among individuals who had studied abroad in Europe and the United States. The author, Lin Zongyang, did not elaborate further on why either educated elites or regular citizens did not endorse vaccination, although he did argue that local health administrators should prioritize immunization as a means of preventing disease.[27] Nevertheless, the piece suggested that by 1930, many people in China still did not see mass immunization as a necessary or relevant practice.

Despite these limitations, by the mid-1930s the National Epidemic Prevention Bureau was considered "the primary agent" in efforts to control and eradicate communicable diseases in China. After Chen Zongxian was appointed director in 1930, he involved the bureau in attempts to create national vaccination schemes. Under the authority of the NHA, it mounted a smallpox vaccination campaign that prepared smallpox vaccines for municipal and district health administrations at heavily subsidized prices of a half cent per dose. The campaigns were largely confined to cities but included training classes for vaccinators and in 1935 distributed 1,013,032 tubes of smallpox vaccine. In the same year, the headquarters of the bureau transferred to new offices in the national capital, Nanjing. The generously provisioned facilities at this site suggested the organization's rise in prominence, with modern equipment that included cold storage rooms, incubating chambers, air conditioners, and steam radiators.[28]

During the 1930s, the rise of factory-style production and commodification of vaccines brought up new concerns over the standardization, replication, and reliability of medical materials. The National Epidemic Prevention Bureau was a primary authority in arbitrating these conflicts. For example, its staff mediated a crisis of counterfeit vaccines in the city of Hankou that demonstrated the importance of trustworthy replicability. In July 1933, a letter from bureau staffers to J. Heng Liu, the minister of health, read, "There have appeared on the Hankou market cholera vaccines of unknown origin bearing this bureau's labels. The outside appearance is exactly like our product, but the glass bottle, stopper and sealing material are totally different. We do not know yet what is contained inside." The unnamed author called for an investigation, noting, "It is not at all impossible that similar products have appeared in other cities." A telegraph appended to the letter, dated a few days later from Liu, noted that the mayor of Hankou had made two arrests in the case and advised the bureau to dispatch a representative to Hankou to investigate the case. Because of this episode, the bureau bought a new inking machine to print information directly on glass ampoules and its packaging staff began to use a "special kind of paper" instead of ordinary white cardboard, "in order to prevent imitations."[29]

The Hankou affair highlighted the perceived threat that counterfeit vaccines and medicines posed as well as the limits of the prewar Nationalist public health administration in ensuring the safety of its biological products. It also suggested the role of the bureau as an increasingly major part of Nationalist health infrastructure in collecting information about these threats and actively policing them. By the 1937 outbreak of war, its offices produced over forty different types of sera, vaccines, and antitoxins against human and animal diseases (notably cholera, plague, dysentery, tetanus, pertussis, and diphtheria in addition to smallpox) and exported these goods to Taiwan, Korea, and Hong Kong.[30] Yet despite the role that this central institute played, the purchase and use of vaccines, sera, and other biological products continued to vary regionally, and immunization programs remained largely limited to urban areas.

The Japanese Invasion and the Flight to the Southwest

On July 7, 1937, Japanese soldiers stationed near the town of Wanping, southwest of Beijing, began firing their weapons at Chinese troops. Since 1931, the Japanese had occupied northeastern China, where they had established the puppet state of Manchukuo. These hostilities, known today as the Marco Polo Bridge Incident, represented a fresh aggression. They triggered a precipitous decline in relations between China and Japan, and on July 26, the Japanese army attacked Beijing and Tianjin. A few days later, both cities fell to the invaders. Chiang Kaishek formed a hasty, reluctant alliance with the CCP and prepared to defend central and southern China. In August, the Japanese army cut a bloody swath southward, embroiling Shanghai in months of armed conflict before its eventual occupation by the Japanese at the end of November. Nanjing followed quickly, and by December the Japanese controlled a wide band of territory from Shanghai north to Manchuria. Millions fled the occupied east, and Chiang retreated to the southwest, moving the seat of the Nationalist government to Chongqing.[31]

Biomedical researchers in immunology and bacteriology constituted a significant group among wartime refugees. Transferring to the southwestern hinterlands would not have been the first long-distance move for many of the Chinese scholars and professionals who fled there in the late 1930s. As discussed above, many had undertaken advanced training in microbiology at universities abroad. But whereas the previous journeys of these scholars and administrators to Japan and the West had generally kept them within elite intellectual circles, the move to Kunming was in character quite different.[32] It was borne of exigency, not ambition. To the students and staff newly arriving there, Yunnan and its environs posed new medical, logistical, and social issues that evoked considerable trepidation and created logistical barriers to the reestablishment of research and manufacturing facilities. These challenges brought medical personnel and researchers together in Kunming and forced them to connect across disciplines, regions, and national borders—and in some cases, despite their own predilections.

The wartime flight of Chinese scientists and physicians to the southwest was also unusual because it remained almost entirely domestic. Most biomedical experts in wartime China did not emigrate during the war, whether for patriotic reasons or because they lacked the opportunity or means. Some did not leave home at all, remaining in territory occupied by the Japanese army. For instance, Xie Shaowen spent the war years working at a hospital in Tianjin. They were not the only medical researchers and physicians in occupied zones. In the northeast, Japanese personnel established new institutions and programs of mass immunization, which implemented smallpox inoculation as early as 1906, plague vaccination in 1911, and semicompulsory vaccination against scarlet fever for students in 1931.[33]

Microbiologists who had occupied elite positions in prewar cities generally decided to flee only under extreme duress. Many saw their journeys to the hinterlands as patriotic sacrifices for the sake of the Nationalist wartime effort. However, the flight to the southwest also produced a dilemma for researchers who sought to retain their status as elite, highly trained scientists but without any of the laboratories, equipment, or institutions that had once provided defining markers of such an identity.

For those who did go to southwestern China, the arduous journey vividly illustrated the contrast between prewar positions of relative privilege and the impoverished hinterlands. To get there, students and researchers traversed difficult sub-tropical terrain and adjusted to an elevation of approximately nineteen hundred meters. Along the way, they survived air raids, fires, and disease. One associate of the National Tongji University Medical College (Guoli tongji daxue yixueyuan) described the overland journey of its faculty and students from Shanghai to Ganzhou, through Yunnan, and then to southern Sichuan, finally concluding, "During these events, we experienced untold hardships" (literally qianxin wanku, "a thousand labors and ten thousand bitternesses").[34]

Given the difficulties most researchers faced in simply getting to Kunming, much less reestablishing their work there, it was a strange choice of destination. Why not go to the wartime capital at Chongqing or the military base of operations emerging in Guiyang? In contrast to these alternatives, the capital of Yunnan Province was an academic hub that offered relative distance from Japanese forces and strong communication networks. Long Yun, the warlord who had effectively ruled the province with autonomy before the war brought the central government to his doorstep, welcomed intellectuals, especially those who might be critical of the central government and Chiang Kaishek's Nationalist Party.[35] Moreover, Yunnan's capital had good connections to the world outside China. The Kunming-Hanoi Railroad supplied one communication link, and the Burma Road project from 1937 to 1945, which sought to connect Kunming to Lashio in Burma, provided another. Although the road itself was constantly under construction and reconstruction, it ensured a substantial American military presence in Yunnan. And Kunming did not provide the obvious target that the wartime capital of Chongqing did, although Yunnan certainly did not escape Japanese air raids.

Not all the research institutes that came to Yunnan were biomedical in nature, but they shaped the character of academic life there. The most prominent of these was the National Southwest Associated University, or Lianda, a wartime conglomeration of students and staff from Peking, Tsinghua, and Nankai Universities—many of whom had marched on foot from Changsha to Kunming in 1938. The establishment of Lianda made Kunming an intellectual center for refugee academics and fostered a scholarly climate in the city that made Yunnan attractive to researchers. Indeed, several leading medical schools from China's largest cities established temporary facilities in wartime Yunnan, most notably the National Zhongshan University Medical School (Guoli zhongshan daxue yixueyuan) from Guangzhou, the National Tongji University Medical College and the National Shanghai Medical College (Guoli Shanghai yixueyuan), both from Shanghai, and the new National Zhongzheng Medical College (Guoli zhongzheng yixueyuan) from Nanchang, capital of Jiangxi Province.[36] The spectrum of medical migrants in wartime Kunming also included physicians who practiced independently. Local newspapers carried advertisements for individual physicians who had migrated from larger cities to set up private clinics. By 1939, a Kunming city government census counted eighty-three physicians with medical degrees, fifty-six male and twenty-seven female. While nineteen were native to Yunnan, fifty-seven were from elsewhere in China, mostly Guangdong, and seven were foreign.[37]

The National Epidemic Prevention Bureau was the most important of these groups for vaccine research and development. Yet its transfer to Kunming was contingent on wartime circumstance, and Tang Feifan assumed leadership over the bureau at a precarious moment in its history. In 1938, Yan Fuqing, head of the NHA, decreed that the bureau should move to Changsha in order to assist the Nationalist government in addressing epidemic crises. At around the same time, Yan asked Tang, then in Shanghai, to accept the chairmanship of the wartime bureau.[38] Almost immediately after Tang accepted, the NHA ordered the bureau to move to Kunming. Tang therefore sold off the remaining smallpox vaccines, antitoxins for diphtheria and tetanus, and unnecessary equipment that bureau staff had brought to Changsha.

While Tang could dispense with extra vaccines and supplies, the living organisms used to produce immunizations were too valuable to discard. According to British pharmacologist John Cameron, Tang oversaw the transport of what remained—six trucks' worth of rabbits, guinea pigs, and other experimental materials—to Kunming, approximately eleven hundred kilometers away. Shortly after their September departure, the Japanese army besieged Changsha. On November 13, fires erupted across the capital of Hunan in accordance with Chiang Kaishek's scorched-earth strategy of retreat.[39] For the bureau, there was no turning back.

The Challenges of the Hinterlands

In addition to the basic threat of bombardment, the move to Kunming presented logistical problems for many scientific and educational institutes. Some found themselves moving into old temples amid a shortage of facilities. In 1940, a Tongji Medical School affiliate specifically pointed to the challenge of finding adequate accommodations. He wrote, "It was very difficult to find a suitable place for the school building, and every structure, classroom, etc. was set up separately."[40] His words spoke to a general lack of space available in wartime Kunming. Moving entire universities to a relatively small city, which had a limited infrastructure and at this point was already playing host to a number of other refugee institutions such as factories and administrative offices, virtually mandated the dissemination of students and faculty to all corners of Yunnan's capital.

Moreover, the impoverished southwestern frontier impeded supply networks for biomedical research and development. In summarizing the many migrations that Chinese research institutions made during the early years of the war, Zhu Hengbi, director of the National Shanghai Medical College, wrote, "During the exodus some of these schools managed to bring a few pieces of their more valuable apparata and equipments [sic] along with them, while others, starting out with full loads, lost much of what they had during the long journey." Even when schools and institutes were able to rebuild laboratories and operating rooms, their facilities were not necessarily usable. Zhu noted of his own medical school, "Some of our operating rooms, like these students' quarters, leaked when it rained, and many a doctor have had to work under opened umbrellas when operating during a storm."[41]

The dispersal of medical staff and students across Kunming led to new exchanges among biomedical students and researchers from different organizations. The alumni of the Tongji Medical College joined other physicians, nurses, and students at the provincial Kunhua and Red Cross Hospitals. A student at the Zhongzheng Medical College explained, "Because Kunming was in the hinterland, and people of ability had gathered there, engaging professors was relatively easy." For instance, Tang Feifan taught microbiology in addition to overseeing the National Epidemic Prevention Bureau, and his colleague Wei Xi lectured medical students on his area of specialty, *Rickettsia* (a genus of bacteria that cause typhus, scrub typhus, and a variety of spotted fevers).[42]

Medical researchers faced the ironic danger of contracting illnesses themselves. The southwestern environment was infamously unhealthy. The tropical diseases associated with Yunnan's geography had made the region an enduring borderland, inhospitable to Chinese settlement and governance since the Qing dynasty. The fear of getting sick persisted with good reason among wartime migrants. Many Lianda students, for instance, contracted trachoma, typhoid fever, scarlet fever, and malaria within two years of their arrival. In addition to incurring the dangers of endemic disease, wartime migrations also themselves changed the epidemiological map of China. The movements of soldiers and refugees into China's interior allowed contagious diseases to spread with alarming speed. This was particularly true in Kunming, which had become a key transportation hub for communication between Nationalist China and the West as the eastern terminus of the Burma Road. One discussion of antimalaria efforts in southern Yunnan by the journalist Dorothy Borg noted, "The situation has been aggravated by the construction of the Yunnan-Burma Road which greatly increases the opportunities for spreading the disease." The longstanding role of western Yunnan as a "disease well" for endemic plague also meant that increased travel through the region carried risks of spreading the disease across provincial and national borders.[43]

Although researchers from Beijing and Shanghai worried about the exceptional health risks that Yunnan posed, some of the dangers they perceived in this southwestern province (and even in the city of Kunming) were actually common across China. In Yunnan, many of these researchers were simply experiencing rural health conditions for the first time. For example, malaria and other parasitic diseases were endemic in many areas of southern China. Most rural populations were totally lacking in basic Western health care, which amplified the impact of a variety of chronic and infectious diseases. The use of human feces as fertilizer facilitated the spread of parasitic and infectious diseases such as schistosomiasis, typhoid, and cholera. People in these regions generally relied on religious healing and traditional drugs to remedy their illnesses.[44]

To some extent, the concerns of researchers newly arrived in Kunming simply reflected their new exposure to rural health conditions, but the epidemiology of wartime Yunnan *was* exceptional. The province held particular dangers of malaria, scarlet fever, plague, cholera, and other infectious pathogens. But Yunnan was also unusual in that at least some of its population had previously been exposed to Western public health administration, and specifically to Jennerian vaccination against smallpox, in one form or another. Since the late nineteenth century, French and British colonial physicians had vied with local warlords to establish health infrastructures in Kunming and other Yunnanese settlements. The next chapter will discuss the development of these infrastructures and their significance to the research community that emerged in wartime Yunnan.

To the students, staff, and researchers who traveled there in 1937, Kunming was a hinterland far removed from the comfortable and relatively well-financed work environments they had known previously. Their investigations into the microscopic agents of disease, the human immune system's workings, and other topics had been abruptly interrupted—as had their efforts at professional organization and publication. The hardships of the impoverished southwest suggested that any biomedical projects there faced a variety of logistical, structural, and financial trials. For refugee students, doctors, and researchers, these challenges entailed new interactions with local patients who held very different attitudes toward disease and health as well as with other medical migrants and local medical professionals. They also led to a focus on one particular type of public health intervention: mass vaccination.

LEGACIES OF WARLORDS AND EMPIRES

When Tang Feifan arrived in Kunming in 1937, he found himself in a city whose residents needed protection against many diseases. Bubonic plague, cholera, malaria, and typhoid fever were prevalent and could easily spread outside the province without preventive measures. Moreover, smallpox was still a major scourge of the area. As wartime physicians and scientists prepared to diagnose, treat, and prevent local infectious diseases, they decried what they considered a lack of modern medical structures and resources in wartime Yunnan.

Although the hardships that refugee scientists faced in southwestern China were real, archival sources from China and Europe show that wartime claims of a total absence of hygiene in Yunnan, often made in the course of funding applications to the central government or foreign aid bodies, were at least partly exaggerated. This chapter argues that by 1937, a medical infrastructure of Western hospitals and clinics already existed in Yunnan—many of which promoted Jennerian vaccination against smallpox, if not immunization against other diseases. This organization had hybrid origins in the efforts of French, British, and Chinese empires during the early twentieth century, although the province remained on the fringes of the emergent Nationalist medical administration until the late 1930s. Wartime biomedical experts in Kunming relied upon this limited but significant infrastructure to build a new vaccination scheme that sought universal coverage of urban and rural populations for the first time.

While China's Nationalist government nominally governed the southwest, local people had long exerted varying degrees of autonomy. The warlords who ruled the province from 1913 to 1937, Marshal Tang Jiyao and Gen. Long Yun, continued this tradition. The politics of medicine—and especially vaccination against smallpox—in prewar Yunnan therefore reflected power struggles between empires for influence in the region. Like the Russian, Japanese, and local forces that battled for controlling interests in Manchuria, French and British imperial powers in Yunnan competed with each other as they engaged with local warlords, sought to build economic and transportation networks in the region, and used medicine, especially epidemic control, as a means of establishing influence.

Ultimately, however, the politics of vaccination reflected the endurance of Yunnanese warlords' power. The efforts of Tang Jiyao and Long Yun to support public health clarify historical questions of warlord involvement in civil society. Most studies of the period from 1911 to 1927 prioritize the regional rise of military powers. Yet as Alfred Lin has shown, some warlords also pursued social welfare projects, not least because these projects were a strategic means of stabilizing their authority.[1] Yunnan was one such region, as the militarists Tang and Long both sought to administrate civilian health and welfare there. The patronage of vaccination work by Tang and Long, despite attempts by both British and French doctors to assert power over the medical administration of Yunnan, demonstrated their preservation of political and military sovereignty. Yet the limited scale of these programs also helps show why a comprehensive immunization scheme against cholera, plague, and the other diseases that ravaged Yunnan did not take root until the Second Sino-Japanese War.

The persistence of Yunnanese autonomy in public health reveals an alternative to narratives of colonial medicine that emphasize immunization as a tool of imperial domination and resistance in binary relationships of colonizer and colonized.[2] It suggests that public health could provide an important sphere for political relationships to develop and evolve at the edges of empires. In the colonial borderland of Yunnan, caught between French, British, and Chinese domains, no one power was willing or able to assert authoritative control. But competition for the favor of warlords and the custom of local patients produced a complex set of social and economic relationships defined primarily by efforts to build trust between locals and outsiders, government and populace, and physicians and patients. In this environment, South and Southeast Asian doctors often played crucial roles as intermediaries whose authority was both extensive and contested.

These issues of trust and confidence shaped the engagement of local Yunnanese with smallpox vaccination. The early twentieth century was marked by the growth of a provincial market and audience for immunization. Early descriptions by French and British authors of a lack of local interest gave way to discussions of the uneasy coexistence of traditional variolation and novel, Jennerian methods. A rise in receptivity to immunization brought with it alarming vulnerabilities as instances of misdiagnosis and malpractice threw the effectiveness and safety of vaccination into question. Throughout the 1910s and 1920s, as the free vaccinations offered by French and British physicians and local authorities rose and fell in popularity, Yunnanese households employed a calculus of risk, avoiding smallpox vaccination at certain strategic times but embracing it at others. By the early 1930s, the decision to seek out a vaccination at a foreign clinic or accept the ministrations of a county vaccinator who had attended a training course in Kunming was the result of highly contingent, individual considerations that did not necessarily reject novel methods of disease prevention—but also no longer necessarily saw Jennerian vaccination as new or foreign.

Yunnan as a Chinese Borderland

Both warlords and foreign agents of empire in prewar Yunnan understood it as a place that arguably had more in common with nearby French Indochina and Burma than with the rest of mainland China. The wealth of historical connections between Yunnan and contemporary Southeast Asia involved shared ethnic identities, commercial ties, and political structures. Understandings and practices of health also connected Yunnan to its southern and western neighbors. Before the twentieth century, medicine in the region relied on social and material networks based in present-day Myanmar and Vietnam. As political and military ties between Yunnan and the rest of China weakened during the early 1900s, shared medical practices demonstrated the enduring connections between the province and its non-Chinese neighbors.

Although Yunnan was technically a province of the Qing Empire until its collapse in 1911, the region maintained longstanding social, political, and cultural ties with neighboring states. Mountainous, tropical terrain posed significant geographical barriers between Yunnan and "China proper." Starting from the twelfth century, a distinctive Tai culture had developed in the uplands connecting Burma, Thailand, Laos, and Yunnan. Its inhabitants spoke closely related dialects, practiced Buddhism, developed their own writing systems, and operated within social structures based on irrigated rice farming in river valleys. The concept of zomia describes traditional political culture in these Southeast Asian uplands, where local inhabitants traditionally employed cultural pluralism, political decentralization, and indigenous leadership. Yunnan's geography, complex trade networks, and multiethnic population demonstrated these traits and had strong connections to neighboring *zomia* uplands in modern Burma (present-day Myanmar), Thailand, Laos, and Vietnam. This shared culture endured through the Qing conquest of Yunnan and into the late imperial period.[3]

Medical traditions also bound Yunnan to its non-Chinese neighbors. The history of medicine in Southeast Asia has stressed the diffusion of Chinese medical traditions to the region via South China Sea networks of exchange. Although standard narratives treat Vietnamese medicine as derivative of Chinese tradition, recent textual evidence suggests that materia medica also flowed north from Vietnam to China during the Tang and Song dynasties, indicating a bidirectional exchange.[4] In the case of smallpox prevention in Yunnan, the Chinese tradition of variolation—using attenuated smallpox virus, rather than cowpox as in Jennerian vaccination, to induce immunity—was interwoven with medical practices and materials native to neighboring Southeast Asian polities. Even though Chinese methods of grinding up smallpox scabs and inhaling them through the nostrils were widespread and the predominant means of smallpox prevention in pre-twentieth-century Yunnan, materials for variolation often came from Burma. And when Jennerian vaccination entered Asia during the nineteenth century via British, French, Spanish, and Portuguese agents, Hanoi, Macau, and Canton (now Guangzhou) became important distribution centers for cowpox lymph as key nodes of the South China Sea trading network.[5]

While connections between Yunnan and neighboring states remained stable, central Chinese control over the provincial administration eroded during the late nineteenth and early twentieth centuries. The tropical diseases associated with Yunnan helped make the province an enduring borderland in China. It was so famously inhospitable to Han settlement and governance that officials saw assignment to Yunnan as exile. From 1856 to 1873, the Panthay Rebellion, an uprising led by Yunnan's Hui Muslim people, caused social and political upheaval as well as population decline. Furthermore, the *tusi* (native official) relationships upon which the Qing had traditionally drawn in rural Yunnan left much power in the hands of local chieftains.[6]

Despite the recession of imperial power, the Qing provincial administration did arrange for local immunization against smallpox. Government-run programs existed as early as 1890, when the governor-general of Yunnan and Guizhou established an office in Kunming called the Bureau for the Management of Smallpox (Guan dou ju). The doctor who staffed the office offered Jennerian vaccinations to the children of the local populace. Private individuals could also go to two local Chinese medicine shops to vaccinate their children. By the late nineteenth century, then, vaccination against smallpox was one possible pediatric preventive health measure available in the provincial capital. As Angela Leung has shown in her study of smallpox vaccination in nineteenth-century Canton,

Kunming was not unusual in this mixture of private and public sponsorship of smallpox prevention, although such offerings were limited to cities and generally still left large rural populations untouched.[7]

The Establishment of French and British Influence in Yunnan, 1900–11

At the end of the nineteenth century, the rise of foreign empires brought Europeans and their medical traditions to Yunnan. British and French imperial agents alike moved into the region, dazzled by the economic potential they saw in establishing commercial trade routes into China, and attempted to use hygienic interventions to curry favor and influence with local governments. During this time, doctors from French Indochina left a much stronger imprint upon health infrastructure in Yunnan than the British or even representatives of the weakening Qing dynasty. France had slowly but steadily developed territorial holdings on the eastern Indochina Peninsula during the late nineteenth century. The 1884–85 Sino-French War ended in the establishment of French imperial domination over northern Vietnam, or Cochinchina.[8] From this position, French agents sought to extend their sphere of influence north into Yunnan to gain territorial dominance and control of trading routes into central China. One of the earliest health-related projects that the French government undertook in the region was to send state-employed physicians to Kunming (or Yunnanfou, as it was known in French) and the town of Mengzi in 1900. This action provided the basis of a novel medical infrastructure in Yunnan.

The work of French military doctors in Yunnan provided medical care to locals at a time when state health services provided by the Qing were extremely limited. As Florence Bretelle-Establet has demonstrated, these physicians established medical dispensaries across southern China as part of state efforts to institute a regional sphere of political influence. They quickly perceived a need to control epidemic outbreaks in the region.[9] Although the governor-general of French Indochina allocated a consular medical post at Kunming in 1899, it took one year—after the widely publicized antiforeign Boxer Rebellion of 1900 subsided in northern China—to staff the post. A Dr. Barbezieux occupied it from November 1904 to May 1907 and founded a short-lived medical school that accepted about a half dozen Chinese students for two years.[10] Outside Kunming, in 1900, a doctor in the colonial service named Ortholan took up a post at the consulate in Simao, now the city of Pu'er in southern Yunnan.

In Simao, Ortholan noted that smallpox was prevalent in the area, although the predominant strain was not very deadly. He wrote, "No precaution is taken and it is not uncommon to see in the streets, carried by their mothers, children still covered with smallpox scabs."[11] Over several months in the year 1900, he vaccinated about forty children using two-month old lymph from the Pasteur Institute in Saigon (now Ho Chi Minh City). Ortholan noted the comparative wealth of those who chose to vaccinate their children, writing, "Almost all children were vaccinated in families with a relatively high social status in general and which were rich. Quite the opposite is true for regular consultations." Ortholan gave no reason for this disparity, also saying, "Given the success of the vaccination, I have no doubt that in the years following, one may vaccinate many more children, but it depends on the routine and indolence of the Chinese."[12]

Ortholan's comment suggested the extent of the French commitment to establishing influence in Yunnan and the prominent role of medicine in that work. It also indicated, with its racialist comment on Chinese "indolence," the limited receptivity of Yunnanese to French vaccination efforts as well as the limits of French power. The goal of Ortholan and other French physicians was not to impose sanitary order but to gain favor among Yunnanese. Indeed, the inspector-general of the sanitation and medical boards of French Indochina wrote in 1910, "When the hospitals of Canton [Guangzhou], Hoihao [Haikou], Yunnansen [Yunnan] . . . were created, we were looking for a peaceful way of penetrating this country." Their desire, he added, had been "to gain the confidence and the sympathy of the indigenous population."[13]

British Incursions: Physicians in the Imperial Maritime Customs Service, 1900–11

While French doctors were beginning to operate in Yunnan in the early 1900s, their British counterparts were not far behind. In the nineteenth century, the British Empire had expanded its South Asian holdings eastward to encompass northern Burma and established itself as a ruling power along China's western borderlands. Yet British diplomatic agents and physicians remained wary of entering the province itself well into the 1900s, with good reason. In 1875, the British vice-consul Augustus Margary had made an ill-advised journey into its interior and was killed by locals. British diplomats used the Margary affair as leverage in negotiating the "unequal treaties" that granted the United Kingdom greater trading and legal privileges in China. Despite this disastrous history, they continued to see Yunnan as a space for expansion. Since the 1830s, the prospect of an overland route to China had been the subject of speculation and excitement on the part of British merchants in Burma who believed that Chinese markets could prove spectacularly lucrative.[14]

While British military forces ranged along the Yunnan frontier, in the 1900s consular agents and doctors ventured into the province and attempted to establish influence there. Physicians in Yunnan filed reports with the Imperial Maritime Customs Service (IMCS), a British-run customs system that regulated the treaty ports established in China after the Opium Wars. It also oversaw quarantine measures in China's ports and tracked epidemic diseases throughout the country.[15] Since Yunnan was a particular focus of British ambitions, the doctors there who reported to the IMCS actively sought to gain the trust of local Yunnanese, often by introducing Jennerian vaccination to them.

In 1903, the Bengali doctor Ram Loll Sircar was appointed as the medical officer for Great Britain's consulate at Tengyueh (now Tengchong), a town in western Yunnan.[16] In 1908, he wrote a report for the IMCS that discussed local smallpox vaccination practices, which he found insufficient, suspect, and outdated. Sircar condemned the persistence of traditional forms of variolation, saying, "This method of inoculation is followed by an attack of small-pox within a week's time." He noted the dangers of variolation, writing, "Not a few of the unfortunate children succumb every year as a result of this malpractice; many have disfigured faces, [and] some get partially or completely blind." Additionally, he found that many "vaccinators" in Tengyueh who claimed to use Jennerian methods were "quacks" who sought to take advantage of local unfamiliarity with the new practices. Sircar noted that during a severe smallpox epidemic in the past year, those afflicted by the disease had been completely unprotected, variolated, or "vaccinated by Chinese vaccinators." He claimed with pride that the one hundred children he himself vaccinated, by contrast, had been completely spared the ravages of smallpox that year.[17]

Sircar also noted that although local Chinese were adopting vaccination that used the cowpox virus instead of smallpox, they continued to procure materials from Southeast Asian neighbors. He wrote, "The Chinese vaccinators, on account of the scantiness of the supply of their lymph, which they receive from Burma, collect scales from the vesicles of successful vaccination cases and store them carefully." Sircar explained that the local method of preparation, in which vaccinators mixed these scales in powdered form with human milk immediately before vaccination, was less successful because the lymph was so attenuated.[18] A few years later, physician Wihal Chand observed the continued use of this method in Tengyueh, writing, "There are some native vaccinators who use the foreign vaccine paste, and vaccinate a good number of children in the city and in the adjacent villages." The "foreign" paste that Chand referred to is ambiguous, but given Sircar's earlier description, it could mean the continued use of Burmese materials—which would indicate the sustained reliance of Yunnanese on local Southeast Asian medical networks.[19]

The new Jennerian vaccination had its dangers. Sircar observed that the Qing administration of Tengyueh had set up a vaccination depot that had served over five hundred people free of charge. But the doctor whom the local authorities had hired was increasingly unpopular. Sircar wrote, "One woman brought to me a child who had lost one eye and the other was to be shortly blind. . . . She told me that she had another boy at home who had gone entirely blind." He explained that a botched vaccination was to blame, saying, "Both these boys were successfully vaccinated [i.e., the procedure produced a pustule on the skin, indicating that it had induced an immune reaction] at the government depot and they both were attacked with small-pox about fifteen days after vaccination." Sircar attributed the failings of the government-sponsored vaccination to common issues of contamination and identified a much greater danger in the fear this failed initiative might inspire in the public. He wrote, "I gather that either the lymph or scales, whatever it may have been, must have been infected with septic matter, or the lancet must have been dirty. These and other similar cases have brought discredit on vaccination and have prejudiced the minds of the people."[20] Sircar thus considered early state-sponsored vaccination work dangerous and ineffective.

IMCS physicians saw their vaccination work in Tengyueh as not only preventing smallpox epidemics but also restoring the faith of locals in vaccination and Western medicine more broadly. Chand, who visited Tengyueh after Sircar in 1909, praised Sircar's efforts to promote vaccination. He wrote, "I am glad to note that vaccination is now taking the place of inoculation [variolation] here, as the people have come to know about the dangerous effects of inoculation, and at the same time have learned to trust in vaccination."[21] In a second report one year later, Chand noted that Yunnanese vaccinated their children only during a few months of the year in accordance with the older Chinese practice of limiting variolation to a few months in the late winter or early spring.[22] That Yunnanese also applied this time limit to the new methods of Jennerian vaccination indicated both the active accommodations that Yunnanese made to new medical practices of Western provenance and the conditional acceptance that foreign physicians such as Chand faced in attempting to introduce these practices wholesale.

As physicians of South Asian background, Sircar and Chand faced challenges not just from their local patients but also from the racialist assumptions of the imperial structures in which they worked. In 1910, both physicians were the objects of defamation in the pages of the *China Medical Journal*, then the only English-language medical journal in China. W. T. Clark, a Protestant missionary doctor stationed with the China Inland Mission in Yunnan, announced that Chand and Sircar were unqualified to practice medicine. "They are low caste fellows, who will do any low trick for money," claimed Clark.[23] In the introduction to the next issue, however, the journal's editors issued a retraction of Clark's piece. "His remarks were quite uncalled for," they wrote, "and should never have been printed in our pages." They cited the correspondence of "one who knows," an anonymous imperial official, who explained that the title Sircar and Chand held, that of "hospital assistant," was a formal rank of the Indian Medical Service that required five years' training in medical school. "I have known many of them and have had them serving under me in India and Africa for years, and have invariably found them a reliable and intelligent type of man," wrote the informant. "They are, by no means, low caste."[24]

That this debate erupted in the pages of China's primary medical journal speaks to the contested, liminal roles of South Asian medical officers such as Chand and Sircar as well as a lack of clear medical authority in early twentieth-century China. At the very edges of formal empire, these two men— themselves part of the colonial subaltern—faced challenges to their authority from Clark, who himself would have been subject to criticisms of the incompetence and outmoded nature of missionary medicine in China.[25] The unnamed writer who defended the reputations of Chand and Sircar was writing from within the imperial hierarchy, defending the educational, socioeconomic, and governmental structures that Britain had established in India. Yet in the frontier space of Yunnan, a missionary doctor was able to challenge the authority of these imperial structures using inequitable language of race and caste that was itself enshrined by the British Empire.

Yunnan in Revolt and the Expansion of French Medicine, 1911–21

While the French and British were slowly establishing spheres of influence in Yunnan, a much more decisive political change loomed for the regional Chinese administration—one that would shape the character of public health there. When the Xinhai Revolution felled the Qing dynasty in 1911, Cai E (1882–1916) seized power in Yunnan and quickly formed an independent government. Educational reforms had shaped the provincial military into a cohesive, independent unit well placed to supplant the local Qing administration. Within six months, Cai unified Yunnan and southern Sichuan under his rule and, by December 1912, expanded the domain of the Yunnan provincial army to cover most of Guizhou and the Tibetan border region. Cai was widely admired because he denounced factional politics and called for a strong central government, but as his political star rose, local powers replaced him in Yunnan. In 1913, Cai and Yuan Shikai, president of the nascent Republic of China, appointed Tang Jiyao as the new provincial governor. The scion of a prominent Yunnanese family who had studied in Tokyo, Tang quickly consolidated power and in 1915 led his troops in revolt against Yuan, who had declared himself emperor. Yuan died a year later, and Tang independently ruled over Yunnan until 1927, with a brief interruption from 1920 to 1922 when his forces overreached themselves in Sichuan.[26]

Tang Jiyao and the ruling "Yunnan clique" were militarist warlords. The brunt of their ruling energies went toward building and maintaining the Yunnan provincial army, not matters of civil administration. Unlike many other warlords of the time, however, Tang oversaw limited social welfare programs during his time in power. For instance, he oversaw a project that reformed police-run brothels into state-controlled institutions whose profits financed various city services in Kunming, such as the local Hongji Hospital (Hongji yiyuan) and a women's reformatory.[27] Local materials provide more details on public health under Tang, noting that in 1913, the Yunnan provincial police department established a subsidiary provincial public health office (weishengke). This office's work included epidemic prevention alongside other clinical and pharmaceutical activities.[28]

Yet not everyone in Yunnan welcomed Jennerian immunization. In 1914, a cowpox inoculation seminar (niudou chuanxi suo) was established in Kunming's Hongji Hospital to train health workers to administer Jennerian immunizations.[29] A provincial gazetteer noted that after the seminar had already graduated a thousand vaccinators, older methods of variolation persisted: "Still many passed down old habits, and they rejected vaccination; those in charge of variolation [chuihua] harmed children and bought stale [materials]."[30] The existence of the seminar indicates the establishment of an official Yunnanese organization for public health and an endeavor specifically dedicated to inoculation under Tang Jiyao—but one that still encountered substantial resistance to vaccination, as opposed to variolation. Moreover, this opposition existed among the ranks of medical workers themselves as well as those they sought to vaccinate.

The development of medical services at French consulates complemented these efforts toward governmental public health in warlord-era Yunnan.[31] At first, French physicians did little more than provide services to local Europeans and consular officials. Only a few medical reports survive from the 1910s, probably because the leadership of the French consular hospital at Kunming overturned almost every year. Nonetheless, the report of a Dr. Vadon, a doctor-major in the colonial military and a physician at the French consular hospital there in 1912, gave a vivid picture of its operations. He wrote that the medical post had two primary functions: outpatient consultations for Chinese patients and hospitalization of the gravely ill. Vadon noted that the clinic (see fig. 1) saw a daily

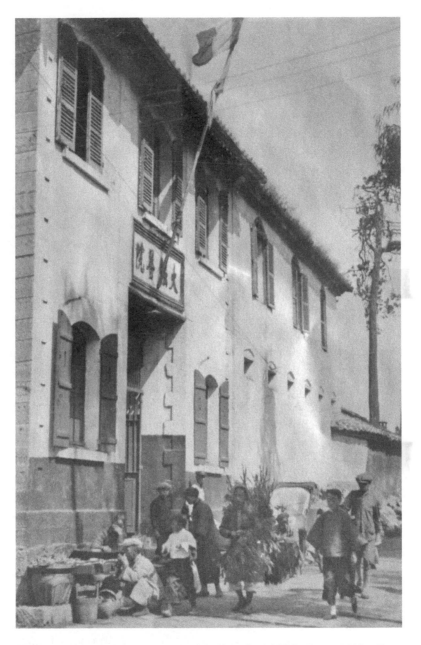

FIGURE 2.1   French consular hospital in Kunming, 1928. Georges Mouillac, "Hôpital consulaire de Yunnanfou: Rapport sur le fonctionnement du poste médical consulaire de Yunnanfou, année 1928" [Consular hospital of Yunnanfou: Report on the function of the Yunnanfou consular medical post, year 1928], box 194, coll. 513PO/A, CADN. Reproduced courtesy of Centre des Archives diplomatiques, Nantes.

average of 231 consultations, adding, "This gives an idea of the crowd that can press itself, on a sunny day, into the hospital courtyard and which sometimes has literally besieged the door of the consultation room." Vadon oversaw a separate service for European and "notable Chinese" patients. This service provided private consultations with a special waiting room that included a library.[32] Such class-based discrimination indicates the diversity of clientele that the consular hospital served as well as its efforts to cater to wealthy Yunnanese.

Vaccination against smallpox was a routine part of French consular medical work. Vadon reported that the hospital adhered to Chinese traditions of seasonal variolation in the late winter or early spring by holding vaccinations every winter. He offered vaccines to Europeans as requested, as well as to Vietnamese and Chinese twice a week. In the north of French Indochina, the Vaccinogen Institute in Tonkin produced these vaccines using cowpox cultivated in its own heifers and sent a shipment to Kunming every week. Vadon believed that the work of the French hospital encouraged Chinese physicians to replace their original variolation procedures with Jennerian methods. The hospital not only offered vaccinations but also sold vaccines to local doctors and taught them how to use the new products. Vadon explained succinctly, "The doctor-variolators are becoming the doctor-vaccinators" and elaborated that "many use old vaccines from Japan or Shanghai but many also come to buy them at the French hospital, where, beforehand, some practical lessons on vaccination are given to them."[33] However, Vadon noted that the popularity of the vaccinations was not assured, saying, "In the first years of the existence of the medical post, these vaccinations did not have great success; but for these past two years, they have followed a constant and very marked progression."[34] His remarks offer no explanation for these trends in receptivity to vaccination, nor do they clarify the means by which vaccines from Japan or Shanghai arrived in Yunnan.

Ultimately, French vaccination work served the ends of empire. The government of French Indochina exercised active control over the work and resources of the consular medical post in Kunming. The post received the joint oversight of the governor-general of French Indochina, its chief financier, and the head of the French legation to China in Beijing. The medical post at Kunming was subject to periodic inspections by "high functionaries" from Indochina, including the governor-general himself, Albert-Pierre Sarraut, in 1913. French military physicians who served in the post usually hailed from the colonial forces in French Indochina, although the First World War briefly disrupted these personnel and financial networks.[35] And many doctors and nurses were themselves individuals of Southeast Asian background who served as cultural and linguistic mediators.

In contrast to the IMCS physicians Chand and Sircar, the Southeast Asian subjects of French colonial rule who did medical work in Yunnan were a larger and longer-lasting group that apparently navigated local and colonial politics with greater ease. The most prominent of these intermediaries, Bui Van Quy, was probably the longest-serving doctor at the French consular medical post in Kunming. A Vietnamese man who had spent several years in France and had graduated from the School of Medicine at Hanoi (École de Médecine de Hanoi), he worked in Kunming for over ten years, from September 1911 to at least June 1922. Bui was often commended not only for his medical knowledge but also for his abilities with the local language and people. One French physician wrote of him, "His perfect knowledge of the Chinese language and local customs and habits, as well as the friendships he has built among civil servants and nobles, make him a very valuable collaborator."[36] In 1920, Bui Van Quy's brother Bui Duc Khang joined him at the consular hospital in Kunming. Many of the nurses who staffed the post had also trained in French Indochina.[37] The work of Vietnamese medical professionals was thus essential to the French medical enterprise in Yunnan.

During the 1910s and 1920s, consular medical outposts became the backbone of a medical infrastructure that reinforced existing links between Yunnan and physicians, bacteriological institutes, and medical schools in French Indochina. By 1921, the staff of the post in Kunming consisted of one French military doctor who liaised with the French consular authorities, two Vietnamese physicians who had studied at the School of Medicine in Hanoi, and five or six Vietnamese nurses who had also received training through the French Indochinese government (see fig. 2.2).[38] Although small, Kunming's medical station offered comprehensive services. Its hospital had about forty beds and provided surgery as well as clinical consultations to European, Chinese, and Vietnamese patients. Regular vaccinations and revaccinations against smallpox were among the most prominent services that the French medical post offered. The table below describes the number of patients that consular medical staff vaccinated from 1921 to 1929. Physicians at the post submitted annual reports on morbidity, mortality, and treatment statistics as well as general observations on epidemiology and general hygiene.

Although consular hospitals relied on resources and personnel from French Indochina, they also actively participated in local medical networks. A key point in the integration of these networks came in January 1922, when Dr. Georges Mouillac arrived from Sichuan to take charge of the consular medical post at Kunming just as an epidemic crisis was gripping the city. The drama of this outbreak and its resolution were decisive for French involvement in Yunnanese public health. A pestilence of unknown provenance, thought to be diphtheria, was raging across the city and had already killed over forty thousand. The provincial government had set up a quarantine hospital in a local brothel under the direction of an English medical missionary, but this was a woefully insufficient step toward resolving the epidemic.[39] The French Antirabic and Bacteriological Institute of Hanoi initially balked at sending antidiphtheria serum to Kunming, in favor of preserving its supplies for French Indochinese hospitals, but even after it relented, the serum proved to be ineffective. The French physicians in command of the consular station had then distributed anticholera injections to no effect.[40]

Upon taking control, Mouillac quickly found a valuable colleague in Bui Van Quy, now the deputy doctor in charge of the consular medical post, and Yunnanese contacts that Mouillac had met in Sichuan, where he had spent fourteen years directing a scientific mission and the provincial government's school of

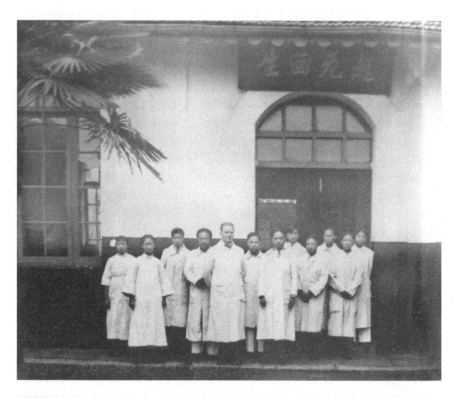

FIGURE 2.2   French consular medical staff with Dr. Georges Mouillac at center, Kunming, 1929. Georges Mouillac, "Rapport sur le fonctionnement du poste médical consulaire de Yunnanfou—année 1929" [Report on the function of the Kunming consular medical post—year 1929], box 194, coll. 513PO/A, CADN. Reproduced courtesy of Centre des Archives diplomatiques, Nantes.

medicine. Mouillac plotted to use these relationships to take command of the isolation hospital that was under English direction, later writing that the English medical missionaries "found their roles reversed and that the French doctor took the place previously given to the English."[41] This initial conflict marked the beginning of a long rivalry between Mouillac and English medical missionaries in Yunnan.

Once Mouillac began treating patients in February 1922, he began to suspect that the epidemic was not diphtheria but scarlet fever. He explained, "I administered anti-diphtheria serum, only to see its ineffectiveness," and the two diseases shared similar symptoms: sore throat, fever, swollen lymph nodes, and gray or white coating of the throat.[42] In a move that demonstrated the integration of French physicians in Yunnan into the medical networks of French Indochina, Mouillac immediately sent word of his theory to the Health Service (Service de Santé) at Hanoi. Subsequently, the service at Hanoi sent a physician named Lafont, the director of the Bacteriological Laboratory at Tonkin, to Kunming. After a microscopic analysis proved inconclusive, Lafont agreed with Mouillac that in many cases the clinical symptoms of scarlet fever were present. Treatment followed according to what Mouillac described a "classic" standard that aimed to alleviate symptoms, and the epidemic subsided by the end of summer in 1922.[43]

Mouillac and Bui won substantial recognition for their work in a theatrical turn of events that underscored the strategic value of epidemic control in Yunnan as well as the increasing prestige of French medicine there. On the morning of Monday, September 4, 1922, Tang Jiyao and Tang Jiyu, his cousin and the mayor of Kunming, arrived at the French Hospital. In thanks for French medical services during the scarlet fever epidemic, they gave Mouillac and Bui Van Quy tablets of honor and commemorative medals to the entire hospital staff. Mouillac later reported, "The tablets were carried with great ceremony upon flowered litters, and, accompanied by musicians of the traditional style, they were carried through a part of the city before arriving at the hospital, where they were immediately fixed in the place where they were intended."[44]

The involvement of the provincial warlord Tang Jiyao in the commemoration suggests that the resolution of the epidemic was as much a political event as a medical one and that it gained French physicians official sanction for their work in the province. Indeed, in the same year, Tang made Mouillac the official physician of his government. Mouillac wrote to his superiors that this action was "a tribute to his [Mouillac's] medical knowledge, and at the same time a sure guarantor of the development of our influence and our scientific methods in this Chinese province, bordering our great Colony of Indochina."[45] Mouillac explicitly sought to establish political influence in Yunnan, and he saw establishing the authority of French medical science and earning the commendation of Tang as key steps in this process.

The 1922 scarlet fever epidemic in Kunming more generally revealed the state of public health under Tang Jiyao. Chinese medical work and administration had persisted under Tang, but he was also open to cooperation with foreign doctors. Although other Western physicians were active in the region, they did not have the training or equipment that Mouillac had. The French consular medical post in Kunming represented not only the efforts of French Indochina to extend its colonial influence north into China but also the increasing integration of Western medicine in Yunnan with French colonial networks vis-à-vis medical research facilities, equipment, and sources of scientific authority. This integration became stronger with the French consular outpost's renewed attempts to vaccinate local Yunnanese against smallpox.

French Medicine and Power in Yunnan

Vaccination was an important part of the expansion of French clinical medicine in Yunnan during the 1920s, although the practice also revealed the limits of French investment in biomedical structures there. Mouillac found that, in contrast to Vadon's experiences a decade earlier, the Jennerian vaccination his predecessors had introduced was increasingly popular. "The vaccinations were strongly appreciated by the Chinese population and the French hospital at Kunming not only practiced there on site a great number [of vaccinations], but also dispatched in the interior many tubes of vaccine with which they had been supplied by the Vaccinogen Institute of Tonkin," he wrote in 1923.[46] Mouillac noted that the Tonkin institute, as well as a vaccine factory at the Pasteur Institute in Chengdu that the French Ministry of Foreign Affairs oversaw, were sufficient to provide for the vaccine needs of the entire region of southwestern China. He reported, "There is not any interest to create in Kunming an establishment of this kind. The proximity of Hanoi permits us to receive in the required time all the vaccines which we may use, and in the best conditions possible."[47] Mouillac's observations demonstrate the utility of Kunming as a frontier city to French administration: the Indochinese government consciously fashioned it as a hinterland outpost meant to expand French influence and perhaps halt epidemics before they reached Indochina but not to become a significant center of medical work (or governance) in its own right.

Vaccination at the French consular hospital in Kunming continued through the 1920s, occurring every Tuesday and Friday afternoon from January to March (see table 2.1). The hospital gave both first-time vaccinations and revaccinations

TABLE 2.1   Vaccinations at the French consular hospital in Kunming, 1921–29

YEAR	FIRST-TIME VACCINATION	REVACCINATION	TOTAL
1921	2,063	375	2,438
1922	1,076	1,047	2,123
1923	2,048	888	2,936
1924	1,844	1,006	2,850
1925	1,389	528	1,917
1927	136	155	291
1928	514	245	799
1929	413	147	560

Sources: Georges Mouillac, "Rapport sur le fonctionnement du poste médical consulaire de Yunnanfou durant l'année 1921" [Report on the function of the Kunming consular medical post during the year 1921], box 559, coll. 513PO/A, CADN; Georges Mouillac, "Rapport sur le fonctionnement du poste médical consulaire de Yunnanfou, année 1922" [Report on the function of the Kunming consular medical post, year 1922], April 2, 1923, box 559, coll. 513PO/A, CADN; Georges Mouillac, "Rapport sur le functionnement du poste médical consulaire de Yunnanfou, année 1923" [Report on the function of the Kunming consular medical post, year 1923], box 559, coll. 513PO/A, CADN; Georges Mouillac, "Rapport sur le fonctionnement du poste médical consulaire de Yunnanfou, année 1924" [Report on the function of the Kunming consular medical post, year 1924], box 559, coll. 513PO/A, CADN; Georges Mouillac, "Rapport sur le fonctionnement du poste médical consulaire de Yunnanfou, année: 1925" [Report on the function of the Kunming consular medical post, year: 1925], box 559, coll. 513PO/A, CADN; "Rapport sur le fonctionnement du poste médical consulaire de Yunnanfou, année 1927" [Report on the function of the Kunming consular medical post, year 1927], box 559, coll. 513PO/A, CADN; Mouillac, "Rapport sur le fonctionnement du poste médical consulaire de Yunnanfou, 1928"; Mouillac, "Rapport sur le fonctionnement du poste médical consulaire de Yunnanfou—1929."

against smallpox that would ensure continued immunity against the disease. In a typical procedure, patients came back several days later so that staff could inspect the site of vaccination to ensure its success. Until 1921, the colonial government at Hanoi provided the vaccines without charge so that the consular hospital could dispense them without charge to Yunnanese. After 1921, Mouillac bemoaned having to pay for the vaccines and pass on the charges to local patients in every subsequent medical report, writing in 1924, "It was an excellent means of propaganda, which now we must make a shortcoming." Yet having to pay for a smallpox vaccine did not seem to deter locals from getting the jab. The year 1923 was the most successful one of the smallpox clinic, with reports of 2,048 people receiving the vaccine for the first time and 888 for the second.[48]

Most of the vaccinations given by the consular hospital were successful, but every year a few cases of smallpox still occurred in the town. Occasionally the outbreak of smallpox epidemics in the southern port cities of Guangzhou and Hong Kong spurred the consular medical post to intensify its vaccination work.[49] Through the early 1920s, the hospital performed about two thousand vaccinations a year for infants of both foreign and local parentage. In accordance with the schedule for traditional variolation that was widespread across China, the consular outpost distributed vaccines in the early spring, and well-off families only brought their children in for vaccination on days deemed auspicious by a local sorcerer. Mouillac wrote of this practice, "The Doctor vaccinator, in order to succeed, must learn well these customs which are widespread in China."[50] In Kunming as in other cities, accommodation of Chinese medical tradition was considered necessary for doctors of Western medicine wishing to inoculate against smallpox.

Local people also feared that vaccination would weaken the body's resistance to other epidemics that threatened Kunming. In May 1922, Mouillac noted that the outbreak of scarlet fever had made many local families unwilling to be vaccinated. "Since the beginning of the epidemics, not a person has presented himself at our vaccination meetings," he wrote. "The Chinese claim that the vaccine attracts the scarlet fever, and moreover—a fair enough thing—the body weakened by the vaccine fights less and allows the germs of scarlet fever to attack easily."[51] Local Yunnanese people thus employed a calculus of risk in deciding whether or not to get vaccinated during the early twentieth century.

While French doctors closely tracked Chinese acceptance of their work in their reports, they eyed competitors with suspicion. The ever-encroaching medical work of English missionaries in Yunnan often appeared in medical reports from the French consular post at Kunming. Spheres of competition included clienteles, staff and their training, and especially hospital spaces. In his yearly reports, Mouillac invariably brought up English missionaries as potential competitors that justified increased expenditures on French medical work. At an unspecified date in 1920–22, the governor-general of Indochina, Albert Sarraut, agreed to fund a new hospital.[52] In 1924, while discussing plans for the new French hospital, Mouillac wrote, "The English have opened with great ceremony, in the presence of the warlord of the Province, a large modern hospital, well constructed and well equipped. . . . We find ourselves at this fact in a state of inferiority."[53]

Although French and British physicians competed for power and patients in Yunnan, the French consular medical service remained committed to the broader project of establishing French influence there. In 1922, Gabrielle Vassal, the wife of a French military physician assigned to Kunming, wrote, "It is much to be desired too that other hospitals should be built like the one at Yunnan Fou which makes French science admired and respected."[54] The explicit, prominent role of science in increasing colonial influence suggests the centrality of modern medical techniques such as vaccination to the French diplomatic project in Yunnan.

Life in the borderlands of Yunnan was difficult, and the hardships that doctors faced indicated the extent of their commitment to state medical endeavors in Yunnan. Occasional uprisings threatened French and French-trained medical staff. By 1910, the colonial government of Indochina had exploited coolie labor for the construction of a railway across the Yunnan-Indochina border where it was charging high customs taxes, leading to widespread resentment of and resistance to French power.[55] This opposition found a target in medical staff. For instance, on the evening of June 28, 1928, a Dr. Jarland was in charge of the French consulate in the southern town of Mengzi. A local man came to the consulate claiming to be an official searching for an escaped prisoner. This proved the pretext for "a band of about fifty soldiers armed with . . . bricks, boards, and daggers, who flung themselves upon our compatriots surprised and unarmed." Jarland survived the attack but suffered heavy bruising and internal bleeding.[56] And in February 1929, an "armed Chinese band" attacked the private residence of one Dr. Dumont, a physician at the Kunming consular hospital, and firebombed his house.[57] Working for the French placed even Chinese medical staff at risk. One physician from Guangxi who had trained at the School of Medicine of Hanoi shut down his medical consultations in the French-controlled mining town of Gejiu for a year in 1921, thanks to a long anti-French campaign in the local press. In May 1922, the French consular authorities, keen to erode the influence of English medical missionaries in Gejiu, came to an agreement with local elites and authorities that permitted him to practice unaccosted every day at the local hospital.[58] These incidents indicate the extent to which French medicine was identified with the power of the French state in Yunnan.

The Rise of Long Yun and the Resurgence of Yunnanese Public Health, 1927–37

While Tang Jiyao ruled over Yunnan, French hospitals and dispensaries remained the basis of medicine and public health in the region. But after his rule ended, a reordering of local public health administration turned Yunnan away from French medical influence and toward the Nationalist government in Nanjing. In 1927, Tang Jiyao's protégé, Long Yun, ousted him and entered a loose alliance with Chiang Kaishek, who was then consolidating control over the newly unified Republic of China as the leader of the Nationalist Party in Nanjing. By 1937, when the Republican state administration arrived in the southwest, Long Yun had been firmly in command of Yunnan for ten years.

Long—a member of Yunnan's non-Han Lolo people, an alleged opium addict, and a deft military strategist—skillfully managed his political relationships with the Nationalist regime. Although he provided military support to Chiang, until 1935 the Republic had little real control over Yunnan, not least because the rural economy, focused on opium cultivation until 1934, was largely independent from the central state.[59] In the medical sphere, this is reflected in the minimal impact that Chiang's 1934 New Life Movement (Xin shenghuo yundong) had in Yunnan. The movement, originating in Jiangxi, sought to reform Chinese culture and create modern citizens by instituting new ideals of hygienic modernity, manners, and Confucian morality. In Beijing, the movement sponsored some free vaccinations for children, and in other major cities, such as Tianjin and Nanchang, hygiene campaigns were a part of its activities. After a few years, the movement dissipated as more a promulgation of moral platitudes than concrete policy changes. In Yunnan, at the fringes of Nationalist control, mention of the New Life Movement rarely appeared in local public health materials during the 1930s, and it did not lead to major health campaigns there.[60]

Despite the limited impact of national policies, Yunnan's public health infrastructure shared a concern for vaccination against smallpox with the Nationalist state. In August 1928, the Republican government in Nanjing issued an order mandating vaccination against smallpox for all citizens (although the ability of the state to implement such an order was severely constrained). In February 1929, it mandated the construction of vaccinator training centers in every province. They were to be established in provincial public health departments or local hospitals and mandated to accept students from twenty to forty-five years of age for training periods of three months, free of charge. Students were to study an extensive list of texts and were to practice smallpox vaccination on no fewer than ten people.[61] The presence of a vaccination training center in Yunnan that predated the national mandate, having been established at the Hongji Hospital in 1914, indicates that Nationalist public health interests and policies were slowly converging with those of provincial institutions.

Other agencies under Long Yun also supported vaccination work in Yunnan—yet this work still did not reach a large percentage of the provincial population. A 1924 gazetteer describes the Kunming City experimental health station (weisheng shiyan suo) as subsidiary to the Municipal Public Affairs Office (Shizheng gongsuo) and responsible for medical experiments, research, production, and distribution. While the experimental and research sections focused on testing of food, drugs, and cosmetics, the production section listed as one of its responsibilities the manufacture of smallpox vaccines and sera (doumiao xueqing). And in 1932, the provincial government established a public health bureau that supported some popular education campaigns. According to its official gazetteer, by 1931 the provincial government counted twenty thousand people among its vaccinated citizens. A 1932 estimate placed Yunnan's population at 11,795,000, so provincial smallpox vaccination rates remained severely limited to less than one percent.[62]

By the early 1930s, smallpox vaccination had become a matter for provincial as well as municipal regulation in Yunnan. In a 1932 report, the Yunnan Provincial Government included a section devoted to smallpox vaccination, which occurred every year from March to May and from September to November. When necessary, the provincial Public Security Office (Gong an ju) was to establish a smallpox inoculation course within municipal hospitals.[63] By this time, Kunming had developed a network of seven hospitals within its city limits, including the Kunhua Hospital (Kunhua yiyuan), the Yunnan Army Hospital (Yunnan lujun yiyuan), the Donglu Hospital (Donglu yiyuan), the Red Cross Hospital (Hongshizi yiyuan), and the Benevolent Yunnan Hospital (Hui dian yiyuan), in addition to the French and Hongji Hospitals. The most important of these was the Kunhua Hospital, which would later become a central base for several wartime biomedical institutions in Kunming.[64]

In a 1936 report, Yao Xunyuan, head of the experimental health station for Yunnan, discussed details of the provincial cowpox inoculation seminar. It built upon programs that had been established at the Hongji Hospital decades earlier (see above), and every winter accepted a class of doctors' assistants, each of whom was recommended by his or her home county. According to Yao, its curriculum "not only emphasized the study of smallpox vaccination skills, but also concurrently conferred knowledge about infectious diseases and public health in order to train general medical personnel." Yao praised the broad impact of this training school, stating that by 1936 it had graduated one thousand students. He claimed that the school had a widespread influence across the province, saying, "Every county has carried out the new method of smallpox vaccination work, and in the hospitals, they also hold vaccinations free of charge."[65] The development of a comprehensive training program suggested that the Yunnanese government under Long Yun was centralizing its medical infrastructure at Kunming. It also underscored efforts to establish Jennerian vaccination across the province.

The networks that supplied vaccines to Yunnan had also changed to reflect growing connections between the provincial government and the Nationalist regime at Nanjing. A 1932 official provincial report on public health specified that according to regulations, when local smallpox vaccine resources were not sufficient to ensure public health, the provincial government imported vaccines from Shanghai. Yet this approach was fatally flawed, because the immunizations often lost their efficacy on the way from Shanghai. The report stated that the provincial government would therefore appropriate excess public funds to establish a vaccine-production facility locally.[66] Such a plan made it clear that supply networks for vaccines had changed. Instead of obtaining the necessary materials from medical practitioners in Burma and Pasteur Institutes in French Indochina as they had in past years, vaccinators in Yunnan now looked to Shanghai as a source of material. Yet the province remained so physically far from the center of Republican medical and economic networks that it was not feasible to mobilize them in order to supply vaccines from Shanghai—suggesting the imperfect integration of Yunnan into the emerging Nationalist social and political order.

In 1937, a city receptive to several different medical traditions awaited the arrival of refugee scientists from China's eastern coast. The colonial ambitions and competitions of Britain and especially France in early twentieth-century Yunnan, as manifested in medical outreach work, had helped establish the hospitals, training schools, and other medical infrastructure that Tang Feifan and other wartime medical researchers would rely on. For instance, when he arrived, Tang would have found a medical school that offered its instruction in French—the Yunnan University (Yunnan daxue)—and French-sponsored hospitals largely staffed by Vietnamese doctors who had trained in Hanoi.[67] Yet much of this infrastructure was also the result of Yunnanese administration under the warlords Tang Jiyao and Long Yun. The relationships that British and French imperial powers formed with Yunnanese warlords rested upon longstanding connections between Yunnan and neighboring states. The efforts of French physicians to use medicine, especially smallpox vaccination, to gain the trust and respect of Yunnanese did not supersede the local autonomy that warlords retained. This dynamic endured and continued to shape public health work throughout the Second Sino-Japanese War, as the warlord Long Yun oversaw the work of visiting scientists and physicians who developed vaccines in wartime Yunnan—in contrast to other parts of the hinterlands, where the central Nationalist state asserted new and more extensive degrees of authority.

PRODUCING IMMUNITY ACROSS THE HINTERLANDS

In December 1939, a French doctor named J. P. Mauclaire submitted a report on a recent journey across southwestern China. He had driven from Kunming to Chengdu to investigate a cholera outbreak that had spread across the region. The latest in a series of incidents, this epidemic had run rampant among refugee populations in Kunming and was reported to have ravaged Guizhou Province. To investigate its extent, Mauclaire, who worked for the League of Nations Health Organization (LNHO), joined a convoy of medical supplies that it was sending to Sichuan. He identified the long-range movement of unvaccinated populations, especially highway truckers and military units, as the probable explanation for why cholera had spread over such a broad area. Mauclaire criticized both the local Southwestern Transportation Company (Xinan yunshu gongsi) for failing to vaccinate its drivers against cholera—the truckers claimed that if they were vaccinated, their arms would be so sore that they could not drive—and the highway health stations that allowed these drivers to cross provincial borders unvaccinated.[1] This negligence, he believed, was at the root of the current epidemic.

In his journey, Mauclaire traced the outlines of a new medical infrastructure that was then developing across the region following the Nationalist state's arrival. From 1937 to 1945, government and philanthropic organizations constructed hospitals, laboratories, and public health units. Vaccination against smallpox, cholera, typhoid, and plague became an important part of their activities.

The cities of Chongqing, Lanzhou, Kunming, and Guiyang hosted wartime organizations that collaborated—and competed—with each other and that perceived immunization as a fast, mobile solution to the problems posed by epidemic crises. Vaccines and sera thus materially and strategically connected global and local medical networks during the war. Facilities established for vaccine production soon took on other responsibilities for local health organizations, such as bacteriological testing and medical education. A swift expansion of services helped integrate medical organizations across Nationalist territory, and these nominally national networks fostered many connections to the world outside China. International aid organizations funded and facilitated Chinese development of vaccines, enfolding the embattled nation into a global community of medical research and a worldwide pharmaceutical supply network that reached as far as Buenos Aires, Bucharest, and Cairo.

In the fields of immunology and bacteriology, the Second Sino-Japanese War reshaped global processes of scientific circulation and translation. The notion of circulation, as James Secord and Fa-ti Fan have interpreted it, describes the geographical movement of ideas and things as part of the production of knowledge—often in messy, incomplete processes that involve multiple layers of translations and transformations. Circulation is a useful concept for understanding transnational and transregional relationships of immunological research in wartime China, although the cities of Kunming, Chongqing, Guiyang, and Lanzhou were also centers of research and knowledge production in their own right. Moreover, historians have shown that conditions of war often facilitated research as medicine became more significant to military operations in the modern era.[2] The case of wartime China generally supports this point, as researchers continued to participate actively in worldwide networks of microbiology and immunology despite financial and logistical limitations.

This chapter surveys the history of vaccine research and development in China's wartime hinterlands during the early years of the war, considering first a major project launched by the LNHO and then, in turn, the major cities of Chongqing, Guiyang, and Lanzhou. (The next chapter will discuss the key role that Kunming and the National Epidemic Prevention Bureau there assumed as the war raged.) Although urban areas were not the only places where medical researchers, students, and administrators worked, they were significant hubs for coordination and exchange. The development of vaccine production in cities coincided with the deployment of new and coercive strategies for immunization, reflecting the ongoing militarization of Chinese society. Yet many urban dwellers welcomed vaccination as a means of defending themselves against disease at a time when the Japanese offensive threatened to cause epidemic catastrophe both directly, through biological warfare, and indirectly, by causing large-scale migrations of refugees and soldiers across the country. Attempts to establish a certification system that connected immunization status to free passage on ships and roads suggested the increasing importance of biology to individual rights and freedoms in wartime China.

At the onset of war, in the wartime capital of Chongqing, the NHA adopted policies of comprehensive vaccination. It also coordinated funding and supply requests from Chinese groups for vaccines and immunological research. To supplement their own funding, educational and medical administrators worked closely with two foreign aid organizations that sent people, money, and equipment to China: the American Bureau for Medical Aid to China (ABMAC) and the Sino-British Science Cooperation Office (SBSCO). The state distributed these funds and supplies locally in Chongqing as well as in subcenters in the cities of Kunming, Lanzhou in northwestern Gansu Province, and Guiyang, the wartime hub of Chinese military medicine and capital of Guizhou Province in the southwest.

Outside these cities, the LNHO contributed significant funds, personnel, and resources to the cause of universal vaccination in China's hinterlands. This early international intervention connected the medical networks that were rising across western China to a global immunological community. In a field crowded with many different interest groups—the Nationalist and Communist Parties, the overseas Chinese, the European members of the League of Nations, even the US military—it was the Nationalist government and the urban populations of western China that benefited most from the wartime influx of financial and material investment.

In examining the emergence of vaccination as a common strategy in medical networks across Nationalist wartime territory, I build upon the work of several scholars. John Watt suggests that the primary wartime achievement of the NHA was its epidemic prevention work via highway health stations, epidemic prevention teams, and support to local administrations. Nicole Barnes argues that the war transformed medicine in China by permitting the increased participation of women in the medical profession as well as by solidifying the significance of both "scientific biomedicine" and Chinese medicine in health administration. Wayne Soon suggests that wartime medical institutions created by overseas Chinese provided important venues for the dissemination of medical knowledge, particularly in military medicine. There exists now a growing consensus that medicine and public health changed dramatically during the war in part because of an influx of new actors from the West and overseas Chinese enclaves and in part because the war forced new configurations of professional identity and traditions.[3] Where Watt, Barnes, and Soon focus on clinical medicine and public health in distinct communities in Chongqing, Yan'an, and Guiyang, I suggest that vaccines provided critical links connecting biomedical networks across unoccupied China, especially through the work of the League of Nations.

Aid from Abroad: The League of Nations in China

In the chaos that followed Japan's 1937 invasion of eastern China, the LNHO sent personnel and supplies to help the Nationalist state control the epidemics that threatened to break out in China's hinterlands. The League of Nations had undertaken a formal program of "technical collaboration" with the Republic of China since the early 1930s. In September 1937, the Chinese delegation to the League of Nations requested medical aid to Nationalist territory, claiming that the influx of refugees that had begun pouring into southwestern China was causing an epidemic crisis. Ludwik Rajchman, a Polish bacteriologist and the director of the LNHO, subsequently planned the creation of three medical units to assist the NHA. In December 1937 and January 1938, the units began operations in Xi'an, Changsha, and Nanning and continued work until February 1939.[4]

Each unit soon focused its efforts on mass vaccination of civilian populations. In undertaking this enterprise, they soon encountered a host of problems in implementing large-scale immunization that required new strategies to ameliorate, if not overcome, these issues. The units worked and sometimes competed with local bacteriological laboratories, eventually coordinating a donation program that supplied the Nationalist government with over eight million anticholera vaccines. The work of the LNHO thus actively enfolded Chinese researchers and health administrators into a global network of immunology.

The staff of the LNHO did not take the decision to intervene in a war zone lightly. When Rajchman informed the Japanese consul-general in Geneva, Usami Uzuhiko, of his intent to provide medical aid to China, the diplomat—whose country had withdrawn from the League of Nations in 1933—responded that "of course he was speaking in a personal way, but he hoped that nothing would be done by the commissioners in any way to impede the military operations." Rajchman understood this comment as a thinly veiled threat and "replied, also in a personal way, that [he] could not imagine any such thing occurring."[5] Military and political considerations did, however, inform the configuration and work of the units. For example, Rajchman asked Borislav Borçic, a Croatian public health expert who had advised the NHA before the war, for his advice on where to place the headquarters of the unit intended for northern China. Rajchman wrote: "In view of the character of the military operations, I anticipate you may advise a place further West—will it be somewhere in Szechwan [Sichuan]?" And the head of the second unit in central China, R. Cecil Robertson, requested to be stationed at Changsha because his former assistant at the Lester Institute in Shanghai—none other than Tang Feifan—was the son-in-law of the provincial governor of Hunan.[6]

Each unit of the League of Nations Epidemic Commission, as it became known, was responsible for a region to the north, east, or south of Chongqing and was staffed by at least six people, including a commissioner who led the operations and a chief medical officer. The units were each equipped with laboratories, delousing baths, automobiles, and a stock of drugs, vaccines, sera, and emergency medical supplies. In addition to military and political constraints, cultural and linguistic considerations shaped the organization of each unit. The units were assigned to integrate with local health administrations and each had liaisons with the central government. All the francophone staffers were assigned to the southernmost unit, which was based in Nanning and Guangzhou, a region that had experienced extensive French colonial influence. It was overseen by Antoine Lasnet, a former French colonial physician and First World War veteran who had previously served in East Africa and Madagascar.[7] The anglophones were similarly grouped together in the second unit. Robertson, an Englishman, was commissioner of this group, which provided support to central China and the Yangzi River basin. Native speakers of German staffed the northern unit, headquartered in Xi'an and led by the Swiss doctor and bacteriologist Hermann Mooser. Mooser also liaised with medical workers at the base camps of the CCP at Yan'an. After an initial misadventure, in which the regional hospital staff there rebuffed the efforts of the LNHO to provide assistance and confiscated photographs and other personal items of its representatives, Mao Zedong sent a representative in July 1938 to apologize and reestablish relations with Mooser's group.[8]

Vaccination quickly became the principal work of each unit, in addition to epidemiological surveillance and quarantines. This was largely because the LNHO staff decided that giving Chinese people vaccinations was easier and more effective than trying to develop hygienic infrastructure across unoccupied China. One early report from Xi'an notes that establishing sanitation work on a large scale was not possible, but that large-scale immunization against smallpox was already under way.[9] The commissioner, Mooser, decided that his unit's "main and first measures" must be the prevention of smallpox and typhoid fever. He commandeered the local Shaanxi Epidemic Prevention Bureau, claiming that the facility's potential for pharmaceutical manufacture made it a necessary acquisition and expense. "We consider our production laboratory as a very essential part of our Unit," explained Mooser, "for the paramount reason that our communications with the sources of [vaccine] supply may be threatened at any time."[10] H. M. Jettmar, a technical expert in the unit, reported after a trip to Pingliang, a city northwest of Xi'an, that "it seems to be one of the most important tasks of our anti-epidemic subunit, to organize here a general vaccination campaign."[11]

The second unit, stationed in Changsha under Robertson, launched a large-scale immunization campaign against smallpox and cholera that immunized 81,973 people against cholera in the summer of 1938 alone. The third unit, under Lasnet in Nanning, commenced vaccination programs against smallpox and cholera immediately upon its establishment (see fig. 3.1). It also began producing smallpox vaccine and preparing typhus vaccine in its laboratory. The unit's chief epidemiologist, Jean Laigret, was a specialist in the manufacture of typhus vaccine with experience in Senegal. He had been assigned to this region specifically because of the prevalence of typhus there.[12] All three units thus organized large-scale vaccination campaigns soon after arrival in China.

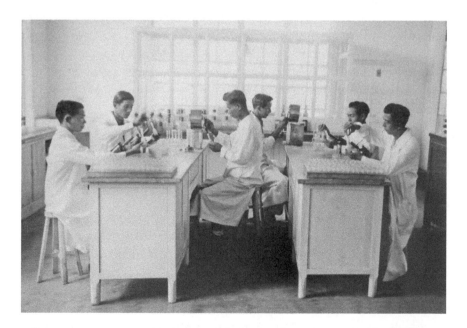

FIGURE 3.1 Packaging cholera vaccine for distribution at a League of Nations unit in Nanning, 1938. "Laboratoire de la Mission Antiepidemique de la S.D.N. en Chine, Unité No. III (Groupe Lasnet), Nanning (Kwangsi), 1938" [Laboratory of the League of Nations Anti-Epidemic Commission, Unit III (the Lasnet group), Nanning, Guangxi, 1938], box 5775, RG 50, ser. 30817, dossier 33627, LON. Copyright United Nations Archives at Geneva.

Local medical communities generally welcomed the vaccination activities of the units, although provincial and municipal governments did not necessarily accommodate their work. For instance, the editors of *Yunnan yikan* (Yunnan medical journal) reported approvingly on the League of Nations aid, noting that financial support for this work amounted to about 1.5 million Swiss francs. They also wrote that the work of the League of Nations intended to prevent epidemics of cholera, malaria, typhoid and smallpox.[13] In some cases, local people eagerly solicited vaccinators. For example, in April 1938, residents of Xi'an "stormed" the unit headquarters demanding vaccines because they had heard rumors that the Japanese army was spreading cholera and typhoid fever from its planes. Mooser dismissed the rumors as specious, although given Japanese initiatives in biological warfare in China, the fears of Xi'an residents appear to have been reasonable. In the same month, although the unit did not carry out a vaccination program of its own, it gave the smallpox immunization to anyone who showed up at the unit's offices requesting one. Approximately twenty-three thousand people were vaccinated.[14]

For every person who crowded into a clinic to ask for a vaccine, the units encountered a number of disobliging officials, malfunctioning vehicles, and recalcitrant targets of immunization. The unit administrators encountered logistical difficulties that demonstrated the hair-raising complexity of obtaining immunological materials and equipment, manufacturing vaccines, and dispensing them on a large scale. In Kunming, Yunnanese officials insisted on the payment of provincial customs duties (*lijin*) on the drugs, medical supplies, instruments, vehicles, fuel, tires, and other supplementary materials that the units imported. The officials often detained shipments in order to collect these taxes. Interprovincial and interport duties also impeded the prompt delivery of parcels, a critical matter when it came to vaccines that might expire after a given date, and so the LNHO arranged for special certificates specifying exemption from taxes to accompany its cartons. "All three Units are working under trying and dangerous conditions, and the regions where they are operating are frequently subjected to bombardment from the air," summarized Rajchman, describing the difficulties inherent in attempting to operate in a war zone.[15] Environmental factors contributed to these problems. The rough terrain of the hinterlands impeded supply lines, while a cold climate and overloaded transportation infrastructure obstructed the administration of vaccines in western China.

Supply and production presented a particularly acute challenge. In Xi'an, Mooser faced broken refrigerators and a scarcity of calves. Without young cattle, Mooser could not produce sufficient cowpox lymph for smallpox vaccinations; without refrigerators, his unit could not store the immunizations they did produce. These were not unique problems. In prewar Sichuan, for instance, the

Pasteur Institute at Chengdu had used local water buffaloes as well as local heifers to cultivate cowpox lymph.[16] In wartime Xi'an, issues of standards as well as supplies mounted. The unit's staff deemed preexisting stocks of vaccine to be of inferior quality and discarded them. Consequently, Mooser focused the short-term work of the laboratory on producing cholera vaccines and simply purchased seven hundred thousand doses of smallpox vaccine in Hong Kong and Bandung for immediate local distribution.[17] Here there were further difficulties. Some imported vaccine was dried and had to be thoroughly ground up and mixed with a glycerin solution for use. Because the mortars that the unit used to grind the vaccine were too large and the dried vaccine was divided into many glass capillary tubes for distribution to vaccination teams, the unit had a much lower yield of vaccine preparations than anticipated. What should have immunized two thousand people against smallpox only inoculated eight hundred. Although the LNHO purchased additional vaccine for Mooser's unit in Hanoi and Canton, it was delayed in transit. "It is well possible that most of the vaccine may have lost its potency on arrival at Sian [Xi'an]," fretted Mooser, "as it has been left for weeks in the offices of the Eurasia Aviation Company at Hong Kong without refrigeration."[18]

The problems did not end at acquiring or preserving a steady, reliable supply of vaccines. Distributing them proved just as fraught with difficulties. Mooser's team attempted to vaccinate year-round but was hindered both by air raids and cold weather. In January 1939, staffer Pan Tai Foh reported that because of frequent air attacks, most people spent their days in the countryside and returned to the city in the late afternoon. "It was very hard to vaccinate them in the country where they were widely scattered," he complained, "nor was it easy to vaccinate them after their return on account of the late hours." The cold weather was an even worse impediment to immunization work. Most people wore heavily padded cotton clothing in the winter, and they could not take off their clothes outside or even physically roll up their sleeves for a shot. In January, then, only 439 individuals were vaccinated against smallpox.[19] Typically the unit vaccinated at least several thousand—sometimes tens of thousands—of people against the disease each month. For example, in March 1938 the unit vaccinated approximately 71,000 people against smallpox; in December 1938, the unit vaccinated approximately 18,800 people.[20]

When cholera broke out in the summer of 1938, the league immediately responded. As discussed above, J. P. Mauclaire attempted to trace the outbreak of the epidemic to its origins while serving with the commission's third unit, stationed in southern China. Each unit helped local health administrations vaccinate travelers who risked spreading the disease, but implementing this practice proved immensely difficult. The first unit, in northern China, focused on aiding the local Shaanxi government in enforcing mandatory inoculation for all passengers arriving in Xi'an by train. "A few brawls were inevitable," wrote Mooser, "but nearly all had to submit to inoculation as the gates were closed against those who had no 'Inoculation certificates,' and to save time all passengers submitted." The certification process thus served to enforce the requirement of vaccines and often entailed forcible immunization. Mooser's explanation of the significance of the certificates exposed the willingness of vaccination teams to use force. He noted that passengers were "all warned to keep [the certificate] as a 'free pass' to enable them to move about the city unmolested by our eager Inoculators."[21]

In Xi'an and other wartime cities, demonstrating one's state of immunity as a vaccinated person became necessary to exert the rights of a citizen and travel freely in one's own country. Yet the efforts of the second unit to implement a similar system in central China revealed that the assumption of such power over urban populations was limited and fragmented. Describing the inoculation certificate system used there, one report explained that it worked well on bus routes but that the "immense volume of traffic" at railway stations made it impossible to fully implement there. As for water transport, the unit could only inoculate and inspect passengers on boats that the local customs officers stopped. "Many small craft escape attention. This is quite unavoidable," explained the report, indicating the limits of LNHO units to address all modes of interregional transportation in their epidemic prevention work.[22]

As the units expanded vaccination programs, they adopted more effective tactics. Mooser's unit employed vaccination teams to go door to door in villages around the city and also stationed inoculators at the city gates. In a subunit at Hanzhong, a city southwest of Xi'an, a vaccination team immunized with both smallpox and cholera-typhoid combined vaccines 601 people who came to a delousing station.[23] The second unit, stationed in Changsha, also adopted the method of combining vaccination work with other hygienic activities. Its commissioner, Robertson, reported, "Refugee populations accept preventive work such as inoculation and vaccination much more readily if it is combined with the general work of a clinic."[24] In a branch office in Jiangxi Province, one senior health officer went so far as to equip a truck as a "vaccination van" for mass cholera inoculation. The truck was decorated with promotional health posters and carried a case full of vaccines and other medical supplies.[25] Strategies such as the combination of immunization with clinical care, door-to-door inoculations, and employing mobile health stations allowed the units to penetrate more deeply into previously unvaccinated populations and regions.

The League of Nations Epidemic Commission also provided assistance to local bacteriological laboratories—although "assistance" sometimes blurred into appropriation. For instance, the northern unit, directed by Mooser, essentially commandeered the Xi'an branch of the Northwest Epidemic Prevention Bureau (Zhongyang xibei fangyi chu, hereafter the Northwest Bureau) for its own work. One report noted that unit personnel were training new staff for the bureau that would remain after the LNHO had concluded its epidemic prevention work. The central unit, led by Robertson, loaned a staff member to the National Epidemic Prevention Bureau in Kunming. The southern unit also provided direct material assistance to the bureau.[26] Tang Feifan had requested aid in procuring standard cultures of pneumococcus, meningococcus, and sera from the Lister Institute of Preventive Medicine in London. When Tang attempted to have them shipped from the United States, the cultures were delayed and "arrived dead or avirulent." Another shipment was addressed to Nanjing by mistake, where the Japanese occupation forces confiscated it.[27] Unit staffer Pierre Dorolle therefore sent the request to Geneva, and staff of the LNHO then contacted the State Serum Institute of Copenhagen to request the cultures on Tang's behalf.[28] The provision of standard cultures was thus another means by which the LNHO supported Chinese involvement in a global immunological network.

In addition to the support of the League of Nations, which supplied two million Swiss francs to the project, the League of Nations Epidemic Commission received many philanthropic donations from European governments, organizations, and companies. Donations of tetanus and diphtheria antitoxin came unprompted from the Danish government and the Danish Red Cross as well as two kilograms of the antimalarial Atabrine from Bayer. The governments of the Netherlands and the Netherlands East Indies also donated funds.[29] In requesting aid from the British Lord Mayor's Fund for the Relief of Distress in China, LNHO administrator Melville Mackenzie noted the importance of supplying food and clothing to the populations that the units served, explaining that they were fundamental to improving resistance to infectious disease. Moreover, they were useful from a psychological standpoint. "Before wholesale vaccination of a refugee camp against smallpox, cholera, typhus, plague or any other disease can be undertaken," he explained, "it is essential to secure the confidence of the population. There is, and can be, little enthusiasm among a destitute semi-starved refugee population in the visit of a doctor armed with an inoculating syringe."[30] Providing food and clothing would make the refugees much more tractable to the real epidemic prevention work of vaccination.

In addition to the immunizations the League of Nations supplied, it organized a massive cholera vaccine donation program for the Chinese government. On July 7, 1938, as cholera spread across Nationalist territory, the NHA sent a telegram to the secretary-general of the League of Nations. It requested assistance in obtaining six million doses of cholera vaccine. The secretariat of the league responded by sending out a request for vaccine donations from governments in the United

States and Europe and from non-Western members of the league. Over the next months, the world responded to China's call. In total, governments across the globe pledged 8,123,000 doses of cholera vaccine—well over the amount requested—to the NHA. The primary donors came from the United States, Romania, and Turkey (see table 3.1), but bacteriological institutes as far away as Cairo and Buenos Aires promised immunizations to China.[31]

The vaccine donors relied on a complex communication and trade network to actually get their materials to China. The example of a gift by the Turkish Ministry of Health is illustrative. On October 26, 1938, twenty cases containing 300,000 cubic centimeters of vaccine left Ankara aboard the steamer *Sivanecya*, bound for Port Said.[32] The Turkish Ministry of Health had already shipped 690,000 cubic centimeters in four lots from August to October 1938.[33] The cases were stored in refrigerators and consigned to the shipping company Jardine Matheson in Hong Kong, free of charge.[34] J. J. Taylor, the representative of Jardine Matheson in Hong Kong, was the primary contact for the vaccines as they made their way toward China. He noted that in addition to the vaccine donations organized through the

TABLE 3.1   Anticholera vaccine donations to China via the League of Nations

INSTITUTE	NUMBER OF VACCINES DONATED
Government of Burma	50,000
Central Committee for Providing Assistance to the Civilian Population of China, Netherlands	60,000
Ministry of Hygiene, Egypt	100,000
Bacteriological Institute of Buenos Aires, Argentina	200,000
Staatenserum Institut, Copenhagen	213,000
Government of Indochina	500,000
Malay States	500,000
Ministry of Hygiene, Australia	500,000
Sanitary Administration, Ceylon	500,000
School of Hygiene, Zagreb (Yugoslavia)	500,000
Institut Cantacuzène, Bucharest	1,000,000
Ministry of Hygiene, Turkey	1,000,000
American Red Cross	3,000,000
Total	8,123,000

Sources: Organisation d'Hygiène, "Rapport au conseil sur les travaux de la vingt-neuvième session du comité d'hygiène (Genève, 12 au 15 Octobre 1938)" [Report on the work of the twenty-ninth session of the hygiene committee (Geneva, October 12 to 15, 1938)], document C.380.M.226.1938.III [C.H. 1381(I)], box 5788, RG 50, ser. 30817, dossier 37258, LON; L. Rajchman, memo to Lester, July 4, 1938, box 5788, RG 50, ser. 30817, dossier 34507, LON; "League of Nations Health Organization: Collaboration of the League of Nations in the Control of Epidemics in China," C.H. 1353, July 26, 1938, LON.

League of Nations, charitable groups in the United States and Philippines had donated vaccines directly to the Chinese Red Cross Society. The Chinese government also bought vaccines from the United States, shipments for all of which had passed through his offices.[35] This gives some indication of the disorganization and logistical complexity that could arise from a global call for vaccines.

After the cholera immunizations arrived in Hong Kong, some were shipped by rail to Changsha (which in 1938 had not yet fallen to the Japanese), to be delivered to the Chinese Red Cross Society.[36] However, the Pasteur Institute at Hanoi sent one million doses to Kunming, and Yugoslavia sent five hundred thousand doses to Canton; Taylor noted in September that Japanese bombings had disrupted the rail line between Canton and Hankou, so that many vaccines had been held up in Hong Kong, although he reassured the league that "the vaccines are being safely stored here, and are not deteriorating."[37] This note provides a reminder of the careful planning that such donations required, since they had to be kept in cold storage and distributed before they expired. The Eastern and Australian Line, the Dutch company Koninklijke Paketvaart-Maatschappij at Singapore, the British India Steam Navigation Company of Burma, and the British Peninsular and Oriental Line all agreed to transport vaccines free of charge.[38] In cases where shipping fees were not waived, such as the shipment of five hundred thousand doses of vaccine from the School of Public Health at Zagreb, the League of Nations picked up the charges.[39] Upon their arrival, both local administrations and units of the LNHO distributed the vaccines.

The elaborate financial and transport networks on which the league relied activated a global immunological community and connected China materially to that community. By sending vaccines to China, bacteriological laboratories around the world signaled their membership within this network, demonstrating their technical skills and production capacities. The vaccines themselves were testament to the ability of these laboratories to produce materials to the specifications of internationally defined standards and to preserve their potency despite traveling large distances. By its conclusion in February 1939, the work of the commission had connected China to a global immunological network, one connected by material goods as well as through theories of bacteriology and virology. The work of the LNHO also illustrated many of the challenges inherent in establishing mass immunization campaigns.

Governing Health in Chongqing

Although the League of Nations Epidemic Commission provided substantial resources and personnel to the Nationalist government, the project was also relatively short-lived. It accomplished the bulk of its work in a single year, 1938, when many Chinese health organizations were busy moving their operations to the southwest. After the NHA transferred its headquarters to Chongqing in late 1937, it built upon the work of the league and oversaw the rise of a medical network across Nationalist territory that would sustain research and development until the end of the war in 1945. The cities of Chongqing, Lanzhou, and Guiyang became important nodes as sites of national health programs that also took on important local functions as medical centers. The collaborative work of developing, making, and distributing vaccines connected these nodes to each other, to Kunming, and to the outside world.

As the wartime capital, from 1937 to 1945 Chongqing was the center of Chinese public health administration. From this craggy, humid city at the confluence of the Jialing and Yangzi Rivers in Sichuan Province, NHA staff attempted to direct medical work across a territory that had been disrupted by invasion and war. Like Yunnan, Sichuan had been under the rule of a warlord, Liu Xiang, until Chiang Kaishek moved the base of Nationalist operations to Chongqing in 1938. During the course of the war, about eight hundred thousand people came to the city from the occupied eastern territories. These wartime refugees included orphans and factory workers as well as government officials and diplomats. A variety of institutions, including banks, the national mint, newspapers, factories, and embassies, moved to Chongqing with the central government. During the war, Chongqing was an infamously grimy city, full of opium, prostitutes, and beggars. But it was also a remarkably cosmopolitan place, home to a large international community that expanded during the war to include many foreign embassies, the Korean government in exile, and the headquarters of a variety of international aid organizations. Among these groups were agencies from the United States and Europe that sought to provide China with scientific and medical aid, notably ABMAC and the SBSCO.[40]

The implementation of coercive vaccination in Chongqing reflects the militarization of society in wartime China. Before and during the Second Sino-Japanese War, the political activities, economic and social policies, and environmental management of the Nationalist state sought to mobilize resources for war.[41] In the sphere of public health, universal, mandatory vaccination in the service of controlling wartime epidemics became a major aim of national health policy— especially in the wartime capital. In late 1937, the NHA made its headquarters in the village of Geleshan, just outside Chongqing. It fell under the directorship of Yan Fuqing from 1938 to 1940, then Jin Baoshan after 1940. In Geleshan, the NHA attempted to continue prewar efforts to build a modern public health infrastructure. Throughout the war, it fostered the growth of county health centers in the provinces of Gansu, Guizhou, Yunnan, and Sichuan; set up regional training institutes for midlevel health personnel in Guiyang and Lanzhou; and designated centers of medical education in Kunming, Guiyang, Chengdu, and Chongqing.[42] In 1941, Jin Baoshan declared that the primary wartime goal of the NHA was to preserve civilian lives through epidemic prevention and medical relief. From Geleshan, he oversaw the construction of highway health stations, malaria surveying work, and an epidemiological intelligence service. The NHA also established thirty-five antiepidemic units to carry out "preventive inoculations on a large scale" as well as disinfect drinking water, build delousing stations, and set up mobile isolation units. In addition, it directed funding from the central government to subsidiary organizations such as the National and Northwest Epidemic Prevention Bureaus.[43] This funding was tied to oversight and control, given that the NHA reserved powers to appoint the organization's head and had exerted them in the transfer to Kunming.[44]

The NHA paid special attention to establishing and enforcing mass vaccination in its would-be model city, Chongqing. As Nicole Barnes has shown, the Nationalist leadership sought to remake the wartime capital along the lines of Nanjing and the other eastern coastal cities it had abandoned. In service of this project, it invested heavily in local health infrastructure. In November 1938, the NHA established the Chongqing Bureau of Public Health, a municipal health administration that imposed hygienic reforms on such everyday activities as waste disposal and food and drink sales. Shortly after beginning operations, the bureau mounted extensive public vaccination campaigns. In December 1938, it requested six hundred vials of smallpox vaccine from the NHA and then arranged for local health organizations to provide these vaccinations free of charge. Thereafter, it distributed smallpox and cholera-typhoid vaccines every spring and fall. In May 1939, cholera broke out in the city. Working with local police, the bureau implemented forcible vaccination, sending teams door-to-door to deliver immunizations, and donated vaccines to hospitals and clinics. Forty teams operated vaccination stations in densely populated areas such as transit stations, teahouses, and refugee camps. In 1940 and 1941, the bureau vaccinated over 150,000 people against cholera a year and reported no subsequent cholera cases, demonstrating the success of the NHA in its own backyard.[45]

By war's end, the NHA had mandated immunization against smallpox as well as the explicit use of force to implement this order. A national government announcement on March 13, 1944, proclaimed ten rules for smallpox vaccination. The plan was for local organizations to target children of one, five, and eleven years of age in campaigns during the spring and autumn. Kindergartens and schools were to inspect their students, and any unvaccinated individuals would be reported and immunized. Vaccination teams were to hand out certificates that could serve as proof of inoculation, and the regulations stipulated that "in cases where there is a smallpox epidemic, county and city hygiene departments must hold forcible vaccination." Moreover, in cases where people had not been immunized according to this schedule, they were to be forcibly vaccinated and charged a fee of about thirty yuan, or about one-third the cost of a bag of rice.[46]

In Chongqing, the NHA coordinated with two organizations that sought to provide financial and material medical aid to the Nationalist government throughout the war: ABMAC and the SBSCO. While ABMAC funded public health programs across Nationalist territory that vaccinated local populations, the SBSCO provided aid to scientific researchers who found themselves in the hinterlands, arranging for publications, research equipment, and personnel to be sent back and forth between China and Allied territory as needed.

The Sino-British Science Cooperation Office

While the work of the League of Nations, as well as ABMAC, fell to a number of secretaries, liaisons, and staffers, that of the SBSCO relied primarily upon one man. A tall, bespectacled Englishman, Joseph Needham was a biochemist at the University of Cambridge, a radical Marxist, and a devoted Christian with fast-growing interests in the history of Chinese science. In 1943, the British Council, an organization of the United Kingdom established in 1934 to promote intercultural exchange, sent Needham to Chongqing at the head of an outfit meant to provide China with material support to scientists and help them continue their research. Needham wrote that the unpredictable and oft-censored nature of China's wartime postal service made it impossible to send scientific manuscripts out of the country and posed "a menace to the morale of our Chinese colleagues." The SBSCO, he argued, could help fulfill this demand for more reliable, extensive communications.[47]

The two primary contributions of the SBSCO to wartime medical work were to survey research efforts in southwestern China and to facilitate communication among units in the hinterlands and with the outside world. As part of their work, from 1943 to 1946, Needham, his wife Dorothy, and his assistant, Huang Tsing-tung (H. T. Huang), surveyed scientific work in universities, laboratories, and factories across unoccupied China, from Gansu to Yunnan. In the course of their travels, Needham and Huang visited scientific research units, gave lectures at local universities, and met with researchers. Needham meticulously documented his travels through correspondence, diaries, and photographs. His immediate impression was that scientists in China were beset by supply interruptions and communications breakdowns. For example, he wrote of an apparently wide-spread practice in which smaller scientific organizations packed all their equipment up whenever the leadership changed. The purpose of this "extraordinary bureaucratic caper" was to prevent new officials from knowing the extent to which the current inventory might have differed from its state under past leadership, presumably to facilitate graft.[48]

The practical value of Needham's surveying work lay in the communication it permitted for researchers in China. When Needham visited scientific organizations in China, he or his wife, Dorothy, made lists of supplies that the institutes required and sent orders for these supplies via Chongqing to London.[49] In conversations with individuals, the Needhams also gathered practical questions from Chinese researchers. For example, when they met Li Guanhua, a biochemist at the Emergency Medical Service Training School (EMSTS), a military training school for the health professions in Guiyang, Dorothy wrote that Li wanted to know the best way of maintaining cultures that tended to become pleomorphic (displaying no spores, just white mycelium). She also made a note to get "Tang P.S."—probably Tang Peisong at the General Physiological Institute of Tsinghua University in Kunming—to send penicillin cultures to Liu Bing Yang, a bacteriologist at the school.[50] SBSCO thus facilitated communication of Chinese microbiology researchers with each other as well as with foreign colleagues.

Such exchange did not merely consist of getting materials and knowledge into and across China. Needham's organization also arranged for the submission by airmail of 139 scientific manuscripts from China to leading English-language journals such as *Nature, Annals of Applied Biology*, and *Proceedings of the Royal Society of Tropical Medicine and Hygiene*. These articles ranged from general descriptions of scientific work in wartime China and investigations of the southwestern environment to the results of highly technical experiments in physics, chemistry, and biology.[51] Their publication through SBSCO provided a means for Chinese researchers to continue professional work amid the hazards of war and revealed conditions and research interests in wartime China to Anglo-American scientific communities in a broad spectrum of disciplines.

The American Bureau for Medical Aid to China

The American Bureau for Medical Aid to China provided a means for conveying money and medical equipment from benevolent parties in the United States to the Nationalist government during the war. Founded in October

1937 by overseas Chinese in New York, ABMAC provided a common source of funding and professional connections for the many medical projects that arose across wartime Nationalist territory. The organization also projected Chinese-American wealth and political power. It called upon alumni of the PUMC, Chinese-American students, and the famous novelist Pearl S. Buck to raise funds in the United States for medical support to China. Over the course of the war, the organization sent a total of $9.5 million to China.

In Chongqing, NHA staff reviewed applications for ABMAC funds that subsidiary organizations submitted. ABMAC also relied upon the Chinese Red Cross to distribute the funds that it sent for the purchase of medical supplies and equipment such as vaccines, microscopes, and ambulances. Outside China, ABMAC sponsored projects to obtain textbooks, journals, and anatomical and pathological microscope slides in the United States and send them to medical schools that had transferred to the wartime southwest. They also supported postgraduate fellowship training for Chinese candidates at American medical schools, thus furthering medical education in the wartime hinterlands. The organization also supported the first blood bank in China, established at Kunming in 1943.[52] The principal involvement of ABMAC in vaccination work was its support in establishing a vaccine plant at the EMSTS. In this respect, ABMAC played a vital role in making the city of Guiyang a major medical center in wartime China and connecting this provincial capital to the new national capital at Chongqing.

Chinese Military Medicine at Guiyang

Although Chongqing and Lanzhou became wartime medical centers largely because they had long been established administrative hubs, Guiyang rose to prominence largely because of one man, Lin Kesheng, and the military medical community he established there. Guiyang was the capital of Guizhou, a province much like its neighbor to the west, Yunnan. Subtropical climates and rich biodiversity characterized both provinces. Also like Yunnan, Guizhou was home to non-Han peoples, primarily the Miao, and had generally eluded the reach of Chinese government until the Qing.[53] When Lin came to Guiyang in 1939, then, he found himself in a remote area, even by the standards of the hinterlands.

Born in Singapore to a prominent overseas Chinese family and trained in medicine in Scotland, Lin had been a professor of physiology at PUMC before the war. In 1937, Minister of Health J. Heng Liu (Liu Ruiheng) recruited Lin to be the head of the Chinese Red Cross Medical Relief Corps (CRCMRC). Lin then traveled to Hankou to establish a headquarters and supply depots for treatment of soldiers wounded in action. In May 1938, Liu asked Lin to build a medical school to serve the NHA, the CRCMRC, and the Army Medical Services. Lin opened the EMSTS shortly thereafter in Changsha, but in February 1939, the advance of the Japanese occupation forced the school to withdraw to Tuyunguan, a forested village outside the remote city of Guiyang, where they built new facilities out of bamboo, mud, and rice straw.[54]

After 1939, these makeshift structures became the military medical center of Nationalist China. At Tuyunguan, the EMSTS offered a few basic courses from two to six months long as well as a full medical school curriculum.[55] A variety of other military medical endeavors soon joined the EMSTS and CRCMRC there, among them a military hospital, a medical supply warehouse, several clinics, and an artificial limb factory. Outside Tuyunguan, the Chinese military established the Army Medical College in an old Qing-era barracks on the marshes surrounding Anshun along the route between Guiyang and Kunming. Like the EMSTS, the Army Medical College was a transplant, in this case from Nanjing. Although military medical work in Guizhou was extensive and supported by ABMAC and the NHA, life was hard for the doctors and support staff who came to Tuyunguan and Anshun. Most physicians wore simple blue cloth Red Cross uniforms with cotton-padded coats and received a paltry monthly salary of about 120 yuan. By 1942, this sum would have bought about one and a half kilograms of rice in Chongqing.[56]

Vaccine production was a fundamental component of military medical operations in Guiyang, although the process was marked by technical difficulties and reliance on external funding. An Institute of Bacteriology and Immunology at the Army Medical College operated under the leadership of Maj. Gen. Li Chenpin, who had studied with the American virologist T. M. Rivers at the Rockefeller Institute (now Rockefeller University) in New York City. Rivers and Li had been first to cultivate *Vaccinia* (the virus closely related to cowpox that was used to make the bulk of twentieth-century smallpox vaccines) and yellow fever viruses in explanted fibroblasts, a type of cell typically found in the connective tissue of animals that had been transplanted to a nutrient medium. Such processes of cultivation were crucial to the development of virology and of vaccines against viruses. In Anshun, though, Li's institute was not capable of such work. When Joseph Needham visited the Army Medical College, he found that Li was "overburdened with administrative duties." Furthermore, a severe lack of equipment limited the potential for original research in Guiyang. For example, instead of using beef broth in cultures, Li used soybean sprout juice. However, the institute at Anshun continued to produce smallpox, cholera, and typhus vaccines.[57]

By 1939, after the Battle of Changsha in September marked the launch of a major Chinese offensive, the need for vaccines for the armed forces grew more pressing. More money and equipment to support vaccine manufacture began to trickle into Guiyang. At the end of the year, Lin Kesheng requested funding from ABMAC to establish a vaccine plant there to supply the Chinese military. In his application for $15,000 to purchase equipment to set up the plant, he cited "the large amounts of vaccine and sera required by the Red Cross alone, and the inability of government laboratories to furnish the demands made upon them."[58] He estimated that such a laboratory could produce five hundred thousand doses of (unspecified) vaccines a day.

In February, Lin's application was successful. ABMAC purchased the necessary equipment and shipped it from the United States on February 27 and also sent funds to construct the laboratory building itself. In September, the materials arrived in Guiyang. Chen Wengui, a researcher who had worked with cholera and plague expert Robert Pollitzer, assumed leadership of the vaccine plant after its establishment. It produced an average of twelve million doses of smallpox, cholera/typhoid, tetanus, typhoid, and plague vaccines a year. From March 1941 to June 1942, the plant produced 6,043,920 doses of smallpox vaccine, 6,200,000 doses of four varieties of bacterial vaccines, and 500,000 cubic centimeters of tetanus-typhoid combined vaccine.[59]

These vaccines found their way to an army of several million Chinese soldiers through several routes. The plant donated five hundred thousand cubic centimeters of combined tetanus-typhoid vaccine directly to the Army Medical Administration, and the rest were sold "at nominal cost" to the Army Medical Administration, the CRCMRC, and other medical organizations. Mass vaccination was one of the main practical field programs that the EMSTS undertook in its work to educate military medical staff, as part of the control of waterborne diseases such as cholera and typhoid. By 1940, the CRCMRC had given soldiers nine hundred thousand (unspecified) vaccines over the course of a year. Records clearly varied, then, and were not necessarily centralized, but in at least some cases administrators made efforts to specify the number of times they gave soldiers a particular vaccine. For instance, in August 1944, Army Medical Administration and EMSTS units operating in Yunnan reported that over the previous six months they had given soldiers 19,483 vaccines against smallpox; 43,020 inoculations against cholera, of which 10,854 were second injections; 77,094 cholera-typhoid combined immunizations, of which 21,017 were second injections; and 49,647 antityphus shots, of which 23,957 were second injections.[60]

In their efforts to supply the military, vaccine manufacturers in Guiyang corresponded and collaborated with researchers across China, especially those at the National Epidemic Prevention Bureau in Kunming. For example, bureau chief Tang Feifan sent his deputy, Wei Xi, from Yunnan to Guiyang to study typhus. In a 1943 application for ABMAC funding, Wei wrote, "With good luck and good success we wish we can carry the work further on toward the goal of mass production of anti-typhus vaccine in this laboratory, as it is not only a wartime emergency but also a demand that may persist until the postwar days."[61]

Once at Guiyang, Wei worked with Liu Pingyang, a classmate from the Xiangya Medical College and former student of Hans Zinsser. Together, they sought to cultivate typhus *Rickettsia* bodies within the bodies of silkworm larvae and pupae rather than chicken embryos, as was more typical. Needham explained the stakes of this research, saying that if successful "it would greatly simplify the preparation of the Cox vaccine under Chinese conditions, where incubators are not available but silkworms are." (The Cox vaccine was the first successful antityphus vaccine, which made use of *Rickettsia* strains grown in chicken egg yolk membranes, a technique that American researcher Herald Cox had pioneered in 1938.)[62] The focus of research in Guiyang, as with so many other immunological research projects during the war, was not necessarily on developing totally new vaccines but rather on coming up with new methods and components for manufacturing them on a large scale.

The national project of military medical work made Guiyang an important local medical center. In 1944, the NHA established the Central Antimalaria Office (Zhongyang kangnüe suo) and a provincial hygiene experimental station to research local diseases and manufacture smallpox inoculations and other vaccines.[63] Joseph and Dorothy Needham noted that Guizhou benefited from the presence of medical workers who had evacuated their original institutions. "Before the war, the province had no University," wrote the Needhams in 1944, "but the University of Kweichow [Guizhou] was founded 3 years ago and is gradually being built up at Huachi. Similarly the Kweiyang [Guiyang] Medical College has been newly founded to provide for future medical education in the province." However, since the staff of these institutions was primarily composed of wartime refugees who were "only awaiting the chance to go back to the east," their futures remained uncertain. The Needhams added, "At the Kweiyang Medical College we were told that only one student enrolling this year is a Kweichow native. There is now a hospital in every hsien [county] of the province, but only 10 Kweichow doctors."[64] Although the scope of military medical work at Guiyang was similar to research in Yunnan, then, it seems that interactions between national medical workers and local people were more limited there than in Kunming or another frontier city in Nationalist territory, Lanzhou.

Immunization on the Outskirts of the Hinterlands: Lanzhou

Outside Chongqing, other urban centers arose as administrative hubs for vaccine projects that covered large regions of Nationalist territory. As discussed above,

Guiyang became a center of military medicine with Lin Kesheng at the head of its landmark EMSTS. Kunming was another such center for southwestern China and the most prominent producer of vaccines, as the next chapter will explore. The city of Lanzhou became the primary Nationalist focus for hospitals and civilian medical training programs in northwestern China. As in Guiyang, Lanzhou took on important roles as a center for local public health during the war because it hosted national biomedical institutes.

Capital of Gansu Province and the largest city in northwestern China, Lanzhou was a major secondary administrative site for the NHA after 1937. This dusty city on the upper reaches of the Yellow River had been a trade and administrative hub on the Silk Road between China and the West. In the early twentieth century, it became a center of commercial enterprise and industrial activity in the northwest. The advent of war and the Japanese occupation of eastern China made Lanzhou a strategic supply and manufacturing site.[65] The capital of Gansu also took on new political importance because of the proximity of the CCP. In 1935, the party had established its base of operations in the mountains outside Yan'an, in Shaanxi Province near the border with Gansu. In 1937, as part of the Second United Front alliance that the Nationalist and Communist governments formed against Japan, Chiang Kaishek had granted the CCP formal administrative authority over the region around Yan'an. Yet Nationalists and Communists were uneasy allies. Given its proximity, Lanzhou became an important wartime base for the Nationalists because it provided a potential bulwark against Communist influence in the northwest.

The capital of Gansu also became a regional center of medical administration. After a 1943 visit, Joseph Needham wrote that Lanzhou was "as important a medical as an industrial centre." In addition to a pharmaceutical factory and a training institute for paraprofessional health workers such as vaccinators and sanitary inspectors, the NHA sponsored the development of the National Northwest Medical School (Guoli xibei yixueyuan) and the National Northwest Hospital (Guoli xibei yiyuan) in Lanzhou. The capital of Gansu was also home to the Northwest Bureau.[66] The NHA had established it in 1934 to address widespread problems of epizootic disease, scarlet fever, diphtheria, and other epidemics in the region. Although largely autonomous in its financing and daily work, the Northwest Bureau was a subsidiary of the National Epidemic Prevention Bureau and corresponded closely with the Kunming headquarters. Although originally focused on epizootic disease prevention at its establishment in 1934, when the war began the Northwest Bureau expanded its remit to include more work on human diseases. To this end, it added more technical staff, constructed a private glass factory and livestock facilities, and imported supplies from Hong Kong and French Indochina.[67]

During the war, the Northwest Bureau became the primary distribution center for vaccines in northwestern China. It fell under the directorship of Yang Yongnian, a graduate of the Mukden (Shenyang) Medical College and Tokyo's Keio Medical College. Like Tang Feifan, Yang had also studied with Sir Henry Dale in London.[68] During the war, Yang oversaw the construction of a new factory at Pingliang to produce smallpox vaccine. He also established Northwest Bureau sales and distribution offices in Chengdu and Xi'an. From 1939 to 1942, the Northwest Bureau manufactured over 10.5 million cubic centimeters of cholera vaccines, 25 million cubic centimeters of cholera-typhoid vaccines, 1.7 million cubic centimeters of plague vaccine, and 4.5 million smallpox vaccines. The Northwest Bureau sent approximately 80 percent of the vaccines it produced to the Chinese army and continued to produce vaccines against livestock diseases such as cattle and sheep anthrax and rinderpest. The bureau in Lanzhou benefited from its proximity to the front lines of Japanese occupation. It had a large herd of ponies and horses, some of which had been captured from the Japanese army, and obtained large supplies of agar smuggled from Japan for use in bacterial cultures. However, unlike in Kunming, where a mild climate reigned year-round, the dusty countryside of Gansu impeded work during the summer because it made sterile conditions practically impossible to maintain.[69]

As it became a powerful regional vaccine manufacturer, the Northwest Bureau also took on new local importance. A major responsibility of the bureau in Lanzhou was the surveying of infectious diseases in northwestern China. For part of this work, Northwest Bureau staff communicated with local public health departments to gather epidemiological data, sent staff out to distribute vaccines as needed around the northwest, and operated two mobile clinical units equipped with materials to set up temporary fifteen-bed hospitals. The Northwest Bureau also developed new programs that connected it more extensively to surrounding populations, such as the construction of a chemical research laboratory to study local herbs and traditional medicines. In 1940, it established a Department of Pathology that performed autopsies, taught pathology to students at the nearby Gansu Medical College, and evaluated tissue specimens that local hospitals sent in for diagnosis. The Northwest Bureau also provided serological, chemical, and bacteriological testing for Lanzhou-area hospitals.[70] The expanding scope of the Northwest Bureau, combined with the presence of many NHA-sponsored clinical and training programs, thus made Lanzhou a prominent medical center in the wartime northwest.

From 1937 to 1945, a variety of organizations rushed to meet a dire need for epidemic control in China's hinterlands. Many of these groups and regional adminitrations focused on vaccinating local populations against cholera, typhoid fever, and other diseases. It is surprising that, given the constraints of environment, air raids, and economic inflation, medical researchers and public health administrators in China were able to continue work, communicate with each other, and send supplies to each other. Vaccines in particular provided a common cause to disparate groups of medical personnel and the basis of a material circulation of scientific knowledge in wartime China. In some places, they also took on significance as administrative tools through certification systems that made proof of vaccination against cholera conditional for travel.

The war also marked a turning point in which Chinese microbiologists worked more extensively with American colleagues. Although Chinese scientists had long been making journeys abroad to study, the arrival of American and European medical experts in southwestern China provided new avenues for exchange. Meetings with League of Nations commissioners, Joseph Needham and his associates, and ABMAC representatives permitted Chinese researchers to gain access to new publications, develop extensive exchanges with foreign colleagues, and transmit their works to Western journals. Over the course of the war, Chinese researchers made new international connections, and the staff of Nationalist medical institutions found some measure of stability in their wartime shelters.

THE EMERGENCE OF MASS IMMUNIZATION IN WARTIME KUNMING

Public health initiatives facilitated the growth of medical networks across unoccupied China. They also emphasized vaccine research and development in the southwest. The city of Kunming presented particular challenges to medical professionals and biological researchers who made it their temporary home. Poverty, air raids, and epidemics threatened the lives of those who found themselves in wartime Yunnan Province. Although refugee researchers such as Tang Feifan and Wei Xi had reestablished laboratories and teaching centers by 1937, they were not necessarily prepared to respond to the specific epidemiological risks Yunnan posed. Local outbreaks of plague, cholera, malaria, and typhus in the late 1930s and early 1940s presented severe threats to the Nationalist wartime effort in southwestern China. Responses to these epidemics could have taken a variety of forms, from sewer construction and quarantines to investment in clinical care, but the biomedical community at Kunming made the manufacture of vaccines its top priority. Why did this city emerge as an important center of Chinese immunological research and production during the war?

Mass immunization was a strange response to disease outbreaks in Yunnan. Distributing vaccines to almost twelve million people over 152,000 square miles of mountains, subtropical forests, and rivers presented a host of logistical, financial, and epidemiological challenges.[1] The material requirements for vaccines and sera seemed insurmountable at a time of economic crisis, especially when compared to cheaper strategies such as quarantines. And, in fact, province-wide vaccination rates in Yunnan are difficult to estimate but do not seem to have risen above a small fraction—about 5 percent—of the population during the war. However, mass immunization remained a major wartime administrative goal. To national health officials facing epidemic crises, vaccines were not just medical technologies that could prevent illness or produce bodily immunity in individuals. They were also strategic defenses against an enemy that was actively using biological weapons to spread infectious diseases. Researchers and administrators in wartime Kunming therefore devised systems to produce and distribute large quantities of immunizations across the province not just as a hygienic measure but also as part of the Chinese war effort.

Amid the many epidemics that beset wartime Yunnan, one acute outbreak of cholera in 1942 provoked an unprecedented response from local health administrators and the National Epidemic Prevention Bureau. To control the crisis, a state-sponsored immunization project sought to reach an entire provincial population in both urban and rural areas. The state employed a strategic combination of persuasion and coercion to achieve its goals. Researchers in Kunming collaborated with local public health administrators to develop a system to produce large quantities of anticholera vaccines and distribute them widely. This coordinated effort reflected changing relationships between medical science and public health in southwestern China. Researchers and physicians not only introduced new public health strategies and concepts to many parts of Yunnan for the first time, they also began to see themselves as participants in the developing field of modern immunology and found ways to develop research agendas within the relative constraints of vaccine development. From its focus on diseases endemic to Yunnan to addressing the particular health needs of the city of Kunming, the system of mass immunization that medical researchers developed during the war was thoroughly a product of southwestern China.

In examining the immunological community that formed at Kunming, this chapter reconstructs a world that pulled its members from local health administrations, research laboratories, medical school clinics, and local factories. This diversity of perspectives and actors accords with recent trends toward understanding immunology in the context of medical practice and production as well as within the laboratory.[2] It also helps articulate the involvement of researchers and medical workers in health initiatives that supported state-building processes. The sera and solutions they produced required distribution to populations often unfamiliar with the techniques of vaccination, and orders to immunize encompassed both coercive and persuasive methods. The increasing use of force to compel vaccination reflected the growing power of the Nationalist state—especially at provincial and national borders, where the examination and enforcement of immunization requirements contributed to the increasing control of political authorities. It also suggested the significance of biological characteristics such as one's immunization status in shaping individual rights and freedoms to travel.

Biomedical Research amid Bombings and Bankruptcy

The first chapter discussed the difficulties that hindered biomedical institutes' reestablishment of their prewar work in Kunming. The challenges of aerial bombardment, economic inflation, and epidemic outbreaks continued to shape and curtail biomedical work in the city throughout the war. While Japanese air raids soon became predictable, albeit greatly disruptive, events that primarily endangered facilities and equipment, the economic and epidemiological dangers of Yunnan posed more serious problems for the researchers who found refuge there.

Although most organizations found temporary facilities on the outskirts of town, those that remained in the city of Kunming became the targets of Japanese bombs. Feng Youlan, a philosophy professor at Lianda, remembered that in the early years of the war, Japanese planes typically arrived from Wuhan after ten o'clock in the morning—so regularly that Lianda and other schools in downtown Kunming rearranged their schedules to plan daily breaks for lunch and evacuation from ten o'clock to three o'clock in the afternoon. One of his colleagues remarked upon the ineffectiveness of the raids, saying, "Hah! I used to hear that five bombs were all it would take to flatten Kunming. They must have dropped over five thousand bombs by now, but Kunming is still the same as ever."[3] Although reliable statistics do not exist for the total number of air raid casualties in Kunming during the war, they were typically low thanks to a well-developed shelter system. In 1941, the arrival of the American Volunteer Group—the aviation unit led by US Army major Claire Chennault known as the "Flying Tigers"—also mounted a defense of the region's airspace. Japanese air raids therefore disrupted but did not prevent or totally destroy the work of educational and research institutes.

Despite their routine nature, air raids did pose a special danger to organizations conducting medical research with dangerous microorganisms. After the war, Tang Feifan reflected on the challenges of his time with the National Epidemic Prevention Bureau in Kunming, writing, "During this time we underwent some of the most terrible experiences of our lives, when we had to prepare plague vaccine or to perform animal experiments with plague bacilli, without any protection from the enemy raiders." The rats that infested the Western Hills outside the city, where the bureau built its laboratory, combined with Japanese air raids to make Tang's work with the plague bacillus especially dangerous since the rats could transmit plague and would spread it quickly if an explosion compromised the integrity of the laboratory. "We were fully aware of the great responsibility resting on our shoulders, if this dreaded infection should ever be disseminated as a result of an air raid," explained Tang.[4] But the work carried on, reflecting an assumption that the potential risks of an accidental plague outbreak did not outweigh the consequences of failure to produce antiplague vaccines and sera.

Although air raids rarely caused heavy fatalities, they occasionally wreaked physical havoc, forcing institutions to reconsider their settlement in Kunming. Although the Japanese invasion of mainland China had stalled by 1939, in September 1940, the Japanese army occupied northern French Indochina. This development disrupted Allied supply lines into Yunnan that used the railway between Haiphong and Kunming. It also permitted the Japanese to launch air raids on Kunming from the much closer city of Hanoi. A particularly severe attack on October 13, 1940, employed twenty-seven airplanes that used bombs and machine guns. "Flying daringly low the aircraft systematically raked the city north and south," claimed one report. "An immense pall of smoke hung over the city after the bombardment, which seemed to destroy the entire city."[5] A report by an anonymous student on the bombing of Lianda noted the extent of the destruction. Where once a biology laboratory had stood, there were only "wrecks of library book-shelves with splinter-ridden volumes of much-used reference books." The extent of the ruins suggested the fragility of educational endeavors in Kunming as well as the physical danger that they sometimes posed. Books and glassware could swiftly become shrapnel in an air raid. After the raid ended, a student in the biology department was spotted picking up specimens from the debris; the student did not panic but rather "was scrutinizing those slides one by one, almost as calm as during his regular laboratory hours."[6] These pieces of apparatus would have been precious objects in the hinterland of Yunnan, to be carefully preserved and organized in the face of destructive air raids. The 1940 attack forced several medical schools to leave Kunming for ostensibly safer ground in the provinces of Sichuan and Guizhou.[7]

Refugees in Kunming watched not only the skies with trepidation but also their own dwindling pocketbooks. Wartime monetary inflation posed special economic challenges to scientific and medical research endeavors and made it impossible to maintain prewar standards of production. Jin Baoshan, head of the NHA in Chongqing, noted that the National Epidemic Prevention Bureau and its subsidiary branches struggled because it could not raise the prices of vaccines and other biological products to a level commensurate with manufacturing and transport costs. "This makes it especially difficult to produce enough to meet the wartime needs and to distribute to distant areas," he wrote. The bureau faced a constant challenge to keep vaccine prices artificially low. In 1945, Tang Feifan had to request $7 million in emergency funds from ABMAC to help cover a budget shortfall.[8]

Wartime inflation not only decreased incentives to work in wartime scientific endeavors but also considerably reduced the standard of living for those who did so. "The scale of pay has risen only seven times while the cost of living in Yunnan has risen 103 times," wrote Joseph Needham after a 1943 visit to survey scientific infrastructure in wartime China. "It is often hard for men whose names are well known in Europe and America to get enough to eat."[9] Academics often packed their families into tiny two-room apartments and subsisted on a diet of rice and vegetables. "Salaries paid to university professors are worth perhaps one tenth of their pre-war value," explained the Needhams.[10] Zhu Hengbi, president of the National Shanghai Medical College, observed that medical professors with inadequate monthly salaries sought extra income, sometimes by taking on additional teaching. "They could not concentrate on their work, teaching efficiency deteriorated and as a result the standard of their work was seriously affected," he noted.[11] Such a frank acknowledgment underscored the detrimental impact of inflation and economic hardship upon medical education and practice in wartime China.

For researchers in the life sciences who had come to Kunming, wartime deprivation was more than a matter of limited diet and cramped quarters. It also made them susceptible to the very diseases that they studied. "Malnutrition due to economic stringency affected the health of the teachers and quite a number fell victims to tuberculosis," wrote Zhu, explaining the link between poverty and illness for professors in medical schools across the wartime southwest. "Once they fell ill, there was no one to care for them at home, and the expensive fees of hospitalization were well beyond the reach of their puny incomes." Zhu claimed that the incidence of tuberculosis among medical students crept up to 10 percent, due in no small part to cramped housing situations that encouraged the spread of infection. "Their living quarters were so crowded that when one person became ill, the rest were exposed to danger of infection," he wrote, noting, "Students not infrequently succumbed to disease and death before they could finish their course."[12]

Yunnan more than lived up to its fearsome reputation as a pestilence-ridden province. A variety of contagious illnesses spread across the province from 1938 to 1940, the most severe of these being an outbreak of plague in western Yunnan in 1939. Approximately one-third of the workers building the Burma Road contracted malaria, and outbreaks of bubonic and pneumonic plague occurred among this population. Whereas bubonic plague primarily affected the lymph nodes, causing characteristic lumps, or buboes, that preceded more severe symptoms such as gangrene, seizures, and high fever, pneumonic plague attacked the lungs and often soon led to respiratory failure. Pneumonic plague also passed directly from person to person, increasing its deadliness. In 1940, NHA authorities in Chongqing sent Robert Pollitzer, an Austrian disease prevention expert with the League of Nations, to Yunnan to investigate the epidemic. They also ordered Tang Feifan and Miao Ancheng, the head of the Yunnan Provincial Department of Public Health (Yunnan sheng weisheng chu), to send medical workers to the affected area. Their orders were specifically to "coordinate with local public health organs to carry out large-scale preventive injections" and to enact quarantines. Despite the combined efforts of experts from the League of Nations, the National Epidemic Prevention Bureau, the NHA, and the Yunnan Provincial Department of Public Health, epidemics continued to break out in Yunnan throughout the war. From 1938 to 1950, 6,899 people contracted plague and 2,448 died of it.[13]

Other diseases endemic to the southwest soon reared their heads in Yunnan. Beginning in the autumn of 1939, cholera spread to Kunming and twenty-six surrounding counties from Guiyang, thanks to wartime refugees. From July to November, 4,700 people caught the disease, and 3,487 died, yielding a mortality rate of almost 75 percent. In August 1940, the provincial experimental health station planned to form disease prevention teams in order to prevent the spread of cholera and distribute them along public roads and in the city of Kunming, where they were to give free "anti-cholera injections," or vaccinations. Malaria was also widespread in Yunnan from 1933 to 1940, killing approximately thirty thousand people. Schistosomiasis was also prevalent in the region during the early 1940s.[14] The diseases endemic to Yunnan continued to cause epidemic crises throughout the war, as refugees, soldiers, and workers moved across the province.

Local Trade, National Health, and Vaccine Production in Yunnan

The severity of early wartime epidemics brought researchers and physicians in southwestern China into contact with local health administrators, who requested their help in controlling outbreaks. These responses typically included a variety of measures, such as disinfection of wells, toilets, and houses of families with sick people; quarantines; and careful investigation of potential cases of the disease.[15] Vaccination featured prominently among epidemic control strategies. In Yunnan, a place that had heretofore remained on the fringes of national public health measures, the work of the National Epidemic Prevention Bureau and other wartime medical institutes in Kunming signaled a significant step toward the integration of the province into central health administration. Because many hospitals in Kunming did not have sufficient laboratory facilities to carry out their own clinical tests, they relied on the bureau for many services. Private clinics in the city sent samples of blood, urine, and other materials to the sales office of the bureau in downtown Kunming. At the bureau laboratories, they were tested for everything from Kahn reactions (to diagnose syphilis) and gonorrhea to signs of pregnancy. The bureau sent back its reports via a pharmacy down the street from its Jinbi Road store, near the Kunhua Hospital.[16]

Although a national outfit, the bureau advertised its work and wares locally. At Jinbi Road, the bureau sold vaccines for smallpox, cholera, rabies, typhoid (combined), meningitis, pertussis, and other diseases.[17] It also published advertisements in *Yunnan yikan* (Yunnan medical journal), a publication intended for local physicians. This journal reported steadily on the work of the bureau and other medical organizations in Kunming. "Since the National Epidemic Prevention Bureau moved to Yunnan, it has worked hard to carry out all work," read one article in 1939. "And as every place needs large quantities of every kind of vaccine and smallpox inoculation, they have really worked overtime to hasten production. Now they have already produced smallpox vaccine, and distributed it to every medical service site." The unnamed author continued his or her praise, adding that "furthermore, their prices are relatively inexpensive. Before long, [their products] can be spread among the people in every place."[18]

The development, manufacture, and dissemination of vaccines became a national priority from 1938 to 1943 because they directly aided the war effort. Public health administrators in the southwest considered vaccines an essential tool to prevent disease outbreaks among both military and civilian populations. In 1940, American scholar Dorothy Borg noted that epidemic control was "the primary wartime function" of the NHA at Chongqing.[19] Jin Baoshan, director of the NHA, wrote that one of the primary tenets of wartime public health was "preventive vaccination: to hold large-scale dissemination of smallpox inoculation and to inject vaccines for cholera, typhoid, etc." Vaccination was a major strategy of epidemic prevention alongside environmental health measures such as street sweeping and garbage collection—and it was the responsibility of the National Epidemic Prevention Bureau to ensure this tactic succeeded, as the national organization tasked with production of vaccines and sera.[20] In Kunming, Tang Feifan described the bureau's priorities as "first to supply the needs of our own fighting forces, then the allied armed personnel and finally to our civilians." Tang personally visited army camps across the southwest, reflecting the bureau's attention to military medical work.[21] Vaccine production in Kunming was therefore a key component of national antiepidemic work. It also manifested the ongoing militarization of society during a time of war.

In addition to the need to control outbreaks of endemic diseases, concerns over Japanese biological warfare also contributed to health officials' focus on vaccines in epidemic control. Fearing that the Japanese were employing biowarfare tactics to disseminate infectious diseases in Nationalist territory, Nationalist health authorities used vaccination to try to strengthen the resistance of the Chinese people to the illnesses the Japanese might spread.[22] A 1941 radio broadcast given in Chengdu and published in the magazine *Zhanshi yizheng* (Wartime medical administration) discussed the nature of biological warfare, suspicions of its past and future use by Japanese forces, and methods by which China could resist such weapons. Potential Japanese transgressions included sending traitorous Chinese agents to poison wells and rivers with deadly bacteria, contaminating cigarette rolling papers and food, and using planes to disseminate plague via aerosol in Zhejiang Province.[23]

Vaccines provided an important means of Chinese resistance to such nefarious measures. "The officers and soldiers at the front, and fellow citizens at the rear, should all receive preventive injections, or vaccinations, against cholera, dysentery, and typhoid," said the broadcast. "After receiving preventive injections, the body has immunity, so that even though disease may be transmitted it may not have lethal danger."[24] As a safeguard against biowarfare, then, vaccination was not only a basic hygienic activity but also a military tactic that the Nationalist government employed against the Japanese.

The strategic importance of vaccines meant that their development became the primary wartime work of the National Epidemic Prevention Bureau and other institutes during the early 1940s. This contrasted strongly with the variety of research projects that had characterized the prewar activities of these bureaus, from nationwide epidemiological surveys to morphological research on the *Vaccinia* virus and etiological studies of trachoma.[25] In Kunming they focused almost all their resources on developing vaccines, sera, and other Western medicines necessary for emergency medical relief. A letter to Tang from a colleague overseas suggests the frustration that this might have evoked. On June 10, 1938, P. P. Laillau at the Medical Research Council in London wrote, "I hope you are flourishing, and that it will not be long before you are back again on research work which I am sure you will find much more interesting than making vaccines, although in the circumstances that is clearly a very useful bit of work." Whether researchers themselves liked it or not, vaccines remained the mainstay of the bureau's work, reflecting broader governmental priorities during the war.[26]

As microbiologists and physicians focused their efforts in Kunming on developing and manufacturing vaccines, they made the city a center for medical research. For instance, Tang explored novel ways to accelerate vaccine production. In 1939, he discovered that applying ether to cowpox lymph was an effective antibacterial measure, and this became the bureau's standard procedure for mass production of smallpox vaccinations. However, during the course of the war Tang and his second-in-command, Wei Xi, encountered a demand for dried vaccine, for which this procedure was useless. The dried immunization required "crude lymph," or organic material harvested from the scabs of a mammal infected with the *Vaccinia* virus, to age for several months in a refrigerated glycerin suspension. This reduced the bacterial content of the lymph to safe levels while preserving the live virus for use in the vaccination process. Wei explained the unsuitability of this preservation method to wartime conditions, saying, "There was such a constant, urgent and heavy demand by both the military and civilian medical services for this vaccine, that [the prior preparatory] method was considered too slow to cope with the requirements." Wei undertook a project to determine whether gum acacia, more easily available locally, might be a legitimate alternative. He first inoculated a calf with a strain of *Vaccinia* from Beijing and obtained lymph from it seven days later. Then Wei ground the lymph into a fine powder and added a solution of gum acacia that he had prepared using materials from a laboratory in Calcutta. After dessicating the mixture, he tested it on rabbits and found that compared to their glycerin-treated counterparts, vaccines that used gum acacia were equally potent in preventing smallpox.[27] Although American virologists had published research on the ability of gum acacia to preserve live viruses in 1936, Wei and Tang appear to have been the first to demonstrate its usefulness in the mass production of dried smallpox vaccines.

A medical research conference held in Kunming in 1940 demonstrated the new focus on epidemic control and vaccination that medical experts there had adopted. From April 2 to April 5, 1940, the Chinese Medical Association held its Fifth General Conference in Kunming. Over three hundred delegates, students, and guests attended the conference, including consular officials from England, France, and the United States, as well as representatives from the Yunnan provincial civil administration, the NHA, and the Departments of Education and Military Medicine. They presented papers on wartime medical relief, education, public health, clinical medicine, pathology, and pharmacology. Staff members of the National Epidemic Prevention Bureau reported on their research endeavors in Yunnan, demonstrating the significant scope of wartime biomedical research in the southwest. Tang gave a paper on the acceleration of smallpox vaccine development, and Wei Xi spoke about his recent research on typhus. Senior Bureau researchers Huang Youwei and Shen Dinghong gave a paper on the viability of reusing agar for cultures as a consequence of wartime supply shortages.[28]

The meeting was also an exposition of medical research, education, and practice in Yunnan. Local medical colleges, health administrations, research institutes, and hospitals hosted delegates and arranged day trips to sites of local interest, one of which was the laboratory of the National Epidemic Prevention Bureau at its Western Hills complex.[29] The Kunming conference in 1940 was one of few wartime opportunities for China's national medical community to convene and exchange news and findings on a large scale. In its meetings and exhibitions, it demonstrated that Kunming had become a critical hub in China's wartime medical networks. As the previous chapter has shown, important work was also happening in Guiyang, Lanzhou, Chongqing, and other cities, but Kunming was a critical center for the integration of work from these sites.

A Cholera Crisis

Two years after the Fifth General Conference showcased the growing potential of regional institutions for epidemic control and prevention, an outbreak of cholera put those capabilities to the test. In early May 1942, the disease struck rural parts of western Yunnan. On the twelfth of the month, it reached Kunming when two hospitals there received twelve patients, all refugees from Burma, who displayed symptoms of the disease. Thereafter, cholera ravaged the city, causing 886 cases and killing approximately one-third of those afflicted in Kunming by July 28. The clinical stages of this epidemic, as in most outbreaks, began with diarrhea—the most severe cases had more than thirty bowel movements in the first twenty-four hours—and was followed by exhaustion and dehydration. Then the diarrhea became less frequent, but stools became atypical, generally appearing pale and milky. If patients recovered, they did so within three to seven days. But most victims did not get better. By September, *Yunnan weisheng* (Yunnan journal of public health) reported that twenty-six counties in Yunnan had been affected and 3,487 people had died. The resultant provincial mortality rate of 74 percent stood in stark contrast to that of the capital city, where epidemic control was comparatively well supplied and organized.[30]

Although this was not the first time that cholera had struck the province in recent memory, the 1942 outbreak was different. The presence of leading medical researchers, their growing capacity to produce vaccines and sera, and the urgent need to control epidemics in a time of war and migration all contributed to the local establishment of a comprehensive immunization system centered in Kunming. As soon as the first signs of the disease had begun to manifest in places such as Zhongdian, a rural township near Yunnan's northwestern border with Tibet, local public health authorities turned to the National Epidemic Prevention Bureau for help. Tang and his staff used stool samples to confirm that the epidemic spreading across Yunnan was cholera and began preparing vaccines to send to affected towns. The cholera immunization then popular in China was Kolle's vaccine. German bacteriologist Wilhelm Kolle had developed this vaccine in 1896 while working as an assistant to Robert Koch, and it had quickly become the global model for cholera prevention in the early twentieth century.[31]

Tang and his collaborators at the bureau saw the cholera outbreak as a great danger but also a research opportunity. Japanese investigators had recently suggested that the cholera bacillus took several serologically distinct forms: the microorganism Koch had originally observed, or the Inaba type, and a variant known as the Ogawa type.[32] Tang decided to examine the serological types of cholera patients in Kunming to learn more about their frequency and incidence. This information could yield insights about the geographic origins of the epidemic. Staff from the bureau used cotton swabs to take samples from the patients' rectums and prepared agar cultures from these samples. They acquired 129 rectal specimens from 110 patients who presented with cholera symptoms and successfully obtained 83 strains of vibrio. To ascertain the serological types of these samples, Tang and his collaborators prepared Inaba and Ogawa type-specific sera using samples of each type that he had obtained from the Central Research Institute at Kasauli, in northern India. They mixed bacterial suspensions of the samples with each of these sera and recorded which mixtures agglutinated, or exhibited clumping of particles. Such a reaction identified the sample in question as belonging to the same type as the sera with which it had been combined.

Upon completion of all experiments, Tang and his collaborators found that sixty-four strains, or 93 percent of the cases in question, agglutinated when combined with the Inaba type–specific serum. The remaining five—all of which were drawn from patients toward the end of the epidemic, in August 1942—were similarly identified as Ogawa-type cases. Moreover, the team used the same agglutination tests to evaluate stock strains that the National Epidemic Prevention Bureau had collected from eight epidemics across the nation from 1912 to 1939. They found that all but two of these were the Inaba type. Tang and his colleagues concluded that although the Inaba type was definitely the primary strain of cholera responsible for the epidemic and had originated in Burma, the Ogawa type suggested that another source of cholera was contributing to the epidemic, perhaps from India or Guizhou Province. They recommended the inclusion of both serological types in the future preparation of cholera vaccines as a practical measure that could help curb future epidemics.[33]

Although Tang and his collaborators drew conclusions of interest for public health in the wartime southwest, their work had one shortcoming: they did not carry out control tests to ensure that stock Inaba- and Ogawa-type vibrios agglutinated with the Inaba and Ogawa type-specific sera they had created.[34] Perhaps for this reason, Tang's work appears to have been a scientific dead end, with no significant subsequent citations. The study's assertion of the multiple origins of the epidemic does provide some insight into where the 1942 cholera epidemic may have begun, contrasting with more recent allegations that Japanese biological warfare in China was entirely to blame for the outbreak.[35] Although the actions of Unit 731 and other Japanese biological warfare units in spreading infectious diseases in eastern China have been thoroughly documented, the invasion of Burma in March 1942 meant that many refugees may have spread the disease without any further efforts on the part of the Japanese.[36]

The article also demonstrates that although the wartime bureau faced straitened circumstances in Kunming, it had retained a significant number of stock strains from past epidemics in China and that Tang was able to draw on a transnational network of contacts to acquire stock samples from laboratories in India. International connections were an important aspect of research at the bureau, and Tang sent staff abroad on several occasions to gain more knowledge and research experience on how to make vaccines. International agencies often facilitated such foreign exchanges. For instance, the Rockefeller Foundation sponsored Wei Xi's travel to the United States Typhus Commission in Myitkyina, Burma, to study scrub typhus with American military medical researchers, as well as Huang Youwei's journey to Mumbai's Haffkine Institute to study plague vaccine manufacture. Tang also sent senior staff member Shen Dinghong to India to study methods of developing vaccines against plague.[37] These international exchanges sought to rectify specific problems that the bureau faced in its vaccine research and development but also allowed bureau staff to form new connections in global networks of immunology and bacteriology.

Despite the opportunities that the 1942 cholera epidemic afforded for microbiological research, the chief function of the bureau in this crisis remained the production of cholera vaccines in large quantities. Over the course of the year, it manufactured over four million cubic centimeters of the vaccine. It also synthesized 3.8 million combined typhoid-cholera vaccines. In creating a heat-inactivated, whole-bacterial-cell vaccine, Kolle's method of making anticholera vaccines required growing cholera vibrios in agar and heating them in solution. Because agar supplies were severely limited in the wartime southwest, senior technician Huang Youwei developed a method that took advantage of reused agar. Joseph Needham praised the efforts of the bureau to continue producing materials and to maintain a sterile atmosphere in conditions of scarcity, claiming that its staff had preserved "high standards of cleanliness in the stables and animal houses in spite of the lack of any running water supply." He also noted that Tang had organized the construction of a private glass factory at the Kunming site to prevent impurities in the packaging process.[38]

The bureau proved the most enduring source of cholera vaccine for Yunnan's beleaguered health authorities. In September, the Kunming Temporary Medical Treatment and Disease Prevention Committee (Kunming linshi yiliao fangyi wei-yuanhui) formed and met with local medical groups. One of the main decisions they made was to hold free immunizations provided by the local experimental health station.[39] It drew on its existing stock of vaccines, along with some provided by the NHA, to mail a total of 78,000 one-cubic-centimeter doses to every county in the province for use starting May 12. But within a week, these supplies were exhausted, and the administration began to purchase cholera vaccine from the National Epidemic Prevention Bureau instead. By June, it had bought 298,000 cubic centimeters of vaccine.[40]

In Kunming, a variety of local and refugee groups coordinated efforts to disseminate these vaccines. The Yunnan Provincial Health Administration sent materials to fifty-four public and private hospitals so that they could offer free immunizations. Medical schools and other organizations directly under the administration of the city public health bureau directed students or workers to organize thirty-three vaccination teams to vaccinate local residents. The National Tongji University Medical College and other local schools of medicine and nursing contributed personnel to these teams. Some Lianda students set up clinics to promote hygiene in the town of Lijiang and Mojiang County; their activities would have likely included vaccination work. The Zhongzheng Medical School and the National Shanghai Medical University joined together to open a local clinic in Kunming as well as an experimental public health station outside the provincial capital, in the town of Qujing in eastern Yunnan.[41]

Vaccination against cholera and other diseases proceeded across the province via these initiatives. Yet they met with substantial local resistance from rural villagers, and public health authorities employed a mixture of persuasion and coercion to disseminate the anticholera vaccine. They dispensed free vaccines through hospitals and schools but also occasionally employed forcible inoculation at city gates and major roads. For example, in planning its anticholera efforts, the town of Yuxi, to the south of Kunming, drew up a list of mandates for immunization. After specifying that six small teams of vaccinators should set up stations at transport hubs, these regulations stated that health administrators should "make full use of text and word of mouth, in order to make people understand clearly the importance and therefore volunteer to be immunized, and when it is necessary they must implement it by force [*qiangpo shixing*] at the city gates and on the streets."[42]

While coercive tactics were generally implemented at the discretion of vaccinators in local towns, they tended to target travelers. On May 15, the provincial government sent an announcement to local media saying that "for all people entering or leaving [the province], those without vaccination certificates are not allowed to buy train tickets and airplane tickets."[43] When people tried to enter and exit Yunnan, they had to supply a certificate showing proof of inoculation: "Those who resist must be forcibly vaccinated with the aid of the local police." These vaccine certificates became necessary to buy train and airplane tickets for travel into and out of the province. A detailed order stating these restrictions on travel was reprinted in the *Yunnan Journal of Public Health*, underscoring its significance.[44] The requirement was an issue of particular concern for laborers who came to work at factories in Kunming, and these plants assumed the responsibility of helping new workers get vaccine certificates along with other necessary paperwork.[45] One's vaccination status thus determined his or her ability to cross provincial borders freely.

These measures were not unusual for the time and place. A few years earlier, in 1939, similar regulations had applied in the case of a cholera outbreak in the city of Chongqing. But in Yunnan, local administrators tended to avoid coercive immunization when possible. One 1942 article discussing anticholera work in the *Yunnan Journal of Public Health* explained, "As for this year's epidemic prevention work, despite encountering all kinds of financial difficulties, it nonetheless proceeded smoothly thanks to colleagues from every health organization providing kind assistance. This city [Kunming] still has not implemented mandatory vaccination, and all departments independently and enthusiastically requested immunization."[46] The article's presentation of this outcome as very positive indicated that voluntary inoculation was preferable to the use of forcible methods—and, perhaps, that the former was rare enough to merit mention and praise. Available records do not permit a full reconstruction of what local people in Yunnan actually thought about mass vaccination or the precise extent to which they avoided it. Yet the evolution of a dialogue about forcible vaccination against cholera and its desirability within the medical community suggests that coercive techniques remained a feature of public health throughout the war and so did unwillingness to receive vaccines.

Despite the variety of measures and institutions that contributed to vaccination efforts, immunization against cholera during the 1942 Yunnan epidemic only reached a fraction of the affected population. It was not enough to prevent high mortality rates. From April to November 1942, a partial survey of forty-four counties in Yunnan reported that 5,953 people had contracted cholera. Of these, 3,041 had died, yielding a death rate of about 50 percent.[47] Popular reports suggest that the final province-wide death toll may have reached two hundred thousand. By June 1942, the *Yunnan Journal of Public Health* reported that provincial authorities had overseen 282,736 vaccinations against cholera. Since a 1932 census had estimated the population of Yunnan as standing at 11,795,000, this meant that after one month, anticholera vaccinations had only reached about 3 percent of the total population of the province at most.[48] Furthermore, because Kolle's vaccine required two or three injections over the course of about a week, it is unclear whether these statistics represented three hundred thousand individuals receiving the cholera vaccine.[49] However, this figure does indicate the novel, essentially unprecedented scale of vaccination work in Yunnan. Given that no clear records of anticholera vaccination exist for the province before 1938—only smallpox vaccination was well known there—and that even smallpox vaccination had only reached twenty thousand Yunnanese by 1931, the bureau basically introduced anticholera vaccination to the province during the war.[50]

Although more people were being vaccinated than ever before, the protection against cholera that they gained was also likely limited to a year or two. In 1902, the developer of the most widely used anticholera vaccine, Wilhelm Kolle, had claimed that large-scale use of his vaccine in Japan was 80 percent effective—but his study lacked a control. It was only after the war, in the 1960s, that controlled studies in Pakistan and Manila successfully tested the effectiveness of this vaccine. In East Pakistan, where cholera was endemic, researchers found that the vaccine provided over 70 percent protection against the disease in adults for the first year and declining efficacy over the next two years. In the Philippines, where cholera is usually not present, it provided protection to about 26 percent of those immunized during an outbreak there, suggesting the highly variable efficacy of the vaccine.[51]

In wartime Yunnan, the efficacy of the combined cholera-typhoid vaccine that the National Epidemic Prevention Bureau manufactured was also unclear. The bureau used three different strains of typhoid obtained from the United States Army Medical School in Washington, DC, in combination with heat-killed *Vibrio cholera* bacteria: the Rawlings strain of *Bacillus typhosus*, the Kessel strain of *B. paratyphosus A*, and the Rowland strain of *B. paratyphosus B*.[52] Given the contemporary consensus that killed whole-bacterial-cell vaccines such as TABC provide immunity for a relatively limited period, it likely had an efficacy similar to Kolle's cholera vaccine—highly variable and possibly good for one year or less.[53]

Given their limited scope and effectiveness, what lasting impacts did anticholera vaccination in wartime Yunnan have? The establishment of this practice represented novel efforts and ambitions on the part of the Nationalist state to use vaccines to enact collective biological protections against disease. Immunization initiatives in the wartime southwest against smallpox and typhoid fever, as well as cholera, demonstrated the growing power of the central state. This power manifested itself both in contributing to the health administration of a province that had long functioned independently and in the new establishment of immunization mandates that encompassed coercive and persuasive methods—which in turn shaped individuals' abilities to travel freely. The case of anticholera work in one village in rural western Yunnan, as seen through the eyes of a hapless but observant anthropologist, illustrates some of these dynamics.

Implementing Vaccination in Rural Areas: The Case of West Town

The 1942 cholera epidemic emphasized the dangers—and research opportunities—that wartime Yunnan presented to the wider scholarly community that had gathered there. One of the professors who came to Kunming with the Yunnan-Yenching Institute of Sociological Research was a young anthropologist named Francis Lang-Kuang Hsu (Xu Langguang). Hsu had completed his doctorate under Bronislaw Malinowski at the London School of Economics in 1940 and shortly thereafter took up his first teaching post in Kunming. After the war, Hsu immigrated to the United States, where he became the president of the American Anthropological Association, defined the field of psychological anthropology, and taught at Columbia, Cornell, and Northwestern Universities.[54]

Hsu's ethnographic scholarship provided a rare observation of local Yunnanese reactions—and resistance—to the 1942 anticholera vaccination campaign. In May 1942, Hsu was conducting fieldwork on kinship dynamics and social mobility in western Yunnan when cholera erupted in the village of West Town, near the city of Dali. West Town was home to about eight thousand people, most identifying as part of the Bai ethnic group. Before the outbreak, Hsu found the place unremarkably unhygienic. "Personal habits of the people are like those in most other villages in China," he wrote, singling out their "drinking of unboiled water, eating exposed and uncooked food and raw vegetables, considering flies on food as a matter of course, and taking no bath."[55]

The cholera epidemic began in May and lasted for a month. It came to West Town from the Burma Road a few miles away. At its peak, there were six or seven deaths per day. Given the comparatively small population of West Town, this represented an alarmingly high mortality rate. The primary popular response was to hold prayer meetings celebrating the cult of Marshal Wen, a widely popular deity who could "release and arrest all evil spirits causing any form of epidemics." In late imperial China, local festivals such as these prayer meetings had constituted a critical intermediary space in which agents of both state and local society participated. The appearance of a prayer meeting that appealed to the Wen god confirmed the lasting impact of this popular cult into the twentieth century. It also suggests that these prayer meetings may have shaped local receptivity to immunization drives, since Hsu noted that the directors of the meetings were often seniors whose advice was highly influential in the community.[56]

In addition to the prayer meetings, posters also appeared in the streets suggesting measures to combat the epidemic. This advice ranged from providing written prescriptions of traditional medicines to recommending that townspeople do good deeds in order to avert disaster to advising that healthy locals receive vaccines against cholera. The "anti-cholera injection" of which Hsu wrote was probably Kolle's vaccine. West Town's local hospital, missionary college, and local middle school provided these injections to the public. The hospital gave out free shots, sent out nurses into the streets to inoculate residents, and disseminated public health posters advertising the treatment.[57]

But many villagers refused vaccination. Although Hsu did not collect detailed statistics for vaccination or mortality in West Town, only surveying thirty-one recipients of the vaccine, he observed that most children received immunizations through schools. Young boys were more likely than girls or older people to receive a vaccine. This tallies with observations of gender-based disparities in immunization elsewhere. In wartime Chongqing, cholera vaccination rates were generally lower among women. This difference may have been due to population imbalances, the public nature of some immunization stations, a perceived need to focus medical care on male populations, a preference among women to visit medical centers with which they were familiar regardless of whether they offered shots, or other factors.[58]

Although adults avoided immunization in West Town, they could not always escape it. "Not everyone who took the injection did it willingly," wrote Hsu, although he did not specify whether local authorities actually employed forcible vaccination. Many adults only accepted inoculation because of pressure from peers. For instance, one worker at a local missionary college mess hall only agreed to the immunization because the faculty who ate there threatened to have her fired if she did not.[59]

Women like the cafeteria worker often avoided getting cholera inoculations in West Town because, they claimed, "It is too painful."[60] This was a legitimate concern. American physician and researcher Richard Strong wrote of both Haffkine's and Kolle's vaccines, "Such methods will probably never come into general use, owing to the great discomfort and sometimes even serious results to which they give rise in the inoculated." Strong described a typical reaction to the vaccine as including a fever of 102 to 103 degrees Fahrenheit, severe body aches, and faintness. If the limb that had received the injection felt pressure or even moved slightly, intense pain could result. Strong summarized, "The reaction is so great that the method is not likely to be generally submitted to voluntarily."[61] Resistance to vaccination in the 1942 Yunnan epidemic supported this conclusion.

Despite the pain, most villagers in West Town accepted the practice of vaccination, but not exclusively. They saw the anticholera injection as "*another* device against the epidemic, not the only device or even the most important one," to be used alongside other measures such as prayers. For Hsu, such ambivalence meant that in the case of West Town, scientific knowledge coexisted with, rather than replaced, traditional beliefs in the causes and proper treatments for cholera.[62] Because Hsu was concerned with refuting the anthropological distinctions among magic, religion, and science that his mentor Malinowski had developed, he focused on the connections between scientific and religious responses to cholera in West Town. Hsu argued that these connections showed that science and religion were inextricably bound together for villagers and that to achieve widespread acceptance, "science has to be cloaked by magic."[63]

Hsu was captivated by the relationship between religion and science in West Town not only in terms of what villagers believed about the cholera epidemic but also in terms of how these beliefs shaped outside observers' perception of West Town's residents. Western-trained doctors who came to the village expressed disdain and intolerance for traditions such as prayer meetings. Hsu believed that this phenomenon posed an obstacle in establishing modern hygienic practices in China more generally because the scorn of these doctors aroused local ire and noncompliance with their public health measures. He expressed his frustrations in observing physicians who "never look at the social environment of their less fortunate sisters or brothers," derisively concluding, "In the end they settle in one of the big cities making their pot of money, while occasionally wondering why the country as a whole makes no progress in public health and scientific medicine. They will never understand."[64]

This analysis is provocative in the context of Kunming. It was precisely this sort of person—trained in Western medicine, who had settled in a major city with a prestigious position—who staffed the wartime research institutes in Yunnan's capital. Hsu emphasized the potential for cultural clashes between these professionals and Yunnanese. But the exigencies of war meant that cooperation, as well as conflict, characterized many of the relationships between the researchers who developed vaccines in Kunming and the local residents they sought to immunize.

Lessons of 1942: The Cholera Epidemic in Professional and Popular Imaginations

By the autumn, cholera had subsided in Kunming. Yet the programs that had developed there to encourage vaccination against the disease remained and grew. The National Epidemic Prevention Bureau expanded its vaccine production and research. Its staff began to see—and market—themselves as immunological specialists. Moreover, their work had a substantial impact on public health in southwestern China. It not only distributed many vaccines to Yunnanese for the first time but also encouraged popular education about and understanding of immunology and public health in the southwestern borderlands.

The year 1942 marked a significant shift in vaccine production for the National Epidemic Prevention Bureau as it moved its focus from smallpox vaccines to accelerate the manufacture of cholera and cholera-typhoid combined immunizations. From July 1937 to December 1941, the bureau produced approximately 12.6 million cubic centimeters of cholera vaccine, 21.7 million cubic centimeters of cholera-typhoid combined vaccine, over 1.6 million cubic centimeters of plague vaccine, and almost 64 million doses of smallpox vaccine.[65] For the years 1942 and the first half of 1943, the bureau reported new production figures to ABMAC that included 6.5 million cubic centimeters of cholera vaccine, 4.2 million cubic centimeters of cholera-typhoid combined vaccine, 5 million cubic centimeters of plague vaccine, and 1.4 million doses of smallpox vaccine. For comparison, in 1931, the provincial government of Yunnan had reported that just twenty thousand citizens had received the smallpox vaccine. In 1942, the bureau in Kunming produced almost fifty times that many, or 960,622 doses.[66] These numbers also compare favorably to major Chinese cities before the war. For example, at the height of vaccination campaigns in Shanghai in 1933 and 1934, 246,063 people received smallpox vaccines, and 577,200 received anticholera inoculations. Manufacturing figures for the bureau in Kunming also exceeded its own prewar production levels. For instance, when cholera struck Beijing in 1932, the bureau had produced 5,513,000 milliliters of cholera and cholera-typhoid combined vaccines for distribution across the region, only about half as much as it manufactured in wartime Kunming.[67]

In addition to ensuring continued mass production, bureau staff continued developing new methods of making vaccines, although wartime exigencies continued to shape and limit their work. Most notable among these was the work of Wei Xi, who collaborated with the United States Typhus Commission in Burma and military medical researchers in Guiyang on projects to develop a vaccine against typhus (see previous chapter). After returning to Kunming, Wei also worked on a project to use silkworm pupae, rather than the more typical rats or guinea pigs, to produce rickettsial suspensions for use in producing vaccines. When he published this research in 1947, Wei specifically cited "the shortage of laboratory animals and other essentials resulting from the war" as a motivating factor for the project. Supported by a grant from the Rockefeller Foundation's

International Health Division, Wei cultivated three different silkworm variet-ies using local eggs and tested each variety for susceptibility to typhus using a murine strain of typhus rickettsia that he had obtained from his contacts in the United States Typhus Commission. He found that rickettsial bodies usually began to grow in the intestines and ovarian tubules of silkworm pupae a few days after injecting them with the strain. This propensity made the pupae a suitable medium for producing rickettsial suspensions that could aid in the preparation of typhus vaccines and further experiments.[68] Although this method did not become a popular or widespread means of cultivating rickettsia, Wei's research on local silkworms demonstrated the use of fauna native to southwestern China as experimental objects.

The importance of local conditions to biomedical research was apparent to foreign observers. Joseph Needham noted the effectiveness of the bureau's vaccines over those of non-Chinese provenance. "The vaccines prepared by the National Epidemics Prevention Bureau," he wrote, "were used in prefer-ence to western-made sera since there are local differences in strains of patho-genic bacteria, and the local vaccine confers more protection."[69] This comment emphasizes the importance of the natural environment of southwestern China to the Nationalist development of vaccination programs during the war. The frequent presence of cholera, plague, and typhoid fever strains endemic to Yun-nan and its surroundings prompted researchers to develop vaccines suited to local conditions.

Wartime vaccine development in Kunming also changed the way that researchers saw their work and presented it to others. At this time, vaccines were considered to be "biological products" alongside drugs, cultures, and other organic materials used for research. A 1940 ad for the National Epi-demic Prevention Bureau in one local medical journal advertised the bureau as a developer of biological products that was also active in bacteriological and immunological research. The author went on to claim that the bureau "takes the utmost care to do research, and has expertly produced every kind of bio-logical product, and consults and follows the newest international methods."[70] Comparison with a 1935 advertisement for the bureau, which merely describes itself as a maker of sera, vaccines, and medical equipment, demonstrates that it was in Kunming that bureau staff first presented themselves to potential purchasers of vaccines as an institute specializing in immunology and bacte-riology.[71] This self-identification on the part of a national institute marked a new phase of self-awareness in the development of an immunological com-munity in China.

In Yunnan, wartime medicine and public health popularized the practices and concepts of this emergent field of study. The terms for "immunity," *mianyixing* and *mianyili*, began to appear more often in local medical journals during the war. Discussions of the etiology, treatment, and prevention of specific diseases often dedicated entire sections to immunity, discussing whether vaccines were available for a particular illness and other means by which immunity might be attained. For instance, one article on smallpox notes, "After one instance of inoculation . . . immunity against smallpox will be supported for about five years."[72] These trends suggested a growing local engagement with biomedical science as well as integration of the southwest into the scientific and medical networks of the Republic of China.

The popularization of immunological knowledge may have been a consequence of local involvement in research and development as well as the newfound prevalence of vaccination in Yunnan. The National Epidemic Prevention Bureau employed locals to help out with vaccine manufacture, exposing them to new concepts and procedures. When Joseph Needham visited the bureau's laboratory facilities in 1943, he took a photograph partially

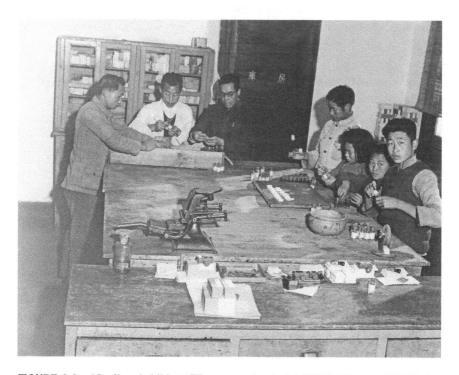

FIGURE 4.1   "Staff and children filling ampoules in the NEPB / National Epidemics Prevention Bureau (Zhong yang fang yi chu), Hsishan (Xishan) near Kunming." August 1944. Wartime Photographs Archive, NRI. Reproduced courtesy of the Needham Research Institute.

titled "Staff and children filling ampoules" (see fig. 1). The black-and-white image showed three men gathered around a table in the background, while four figures—one woman, two young children, and a juvenile male—stood around another side of the table, each working with individual ampoules of an unidentified vaccine. That children could fill the ampoules speaks to the compartmentalized production that characterized vaccine manufacture at the bureau by the wartime era.

That bureau staff would have employed young children in this way is particularly noteworthy given that a number of local Yunnanese people sent letters to the bureau requesting employment there. For example, one Kunming native named Peng Shuchang wrote (in English, because the bureau required that its clerks have training in that language), "I am very anxious to be employed in our national organizations or other institutions instead of other foreign firms, for it seems to me a man [who] cannot do his duty for his own country is a great shame indeed!"[73] A surface reading of the application suggests the patriotic ideal that characterized many workers' approach to the work of the bureau as well as the symbolic prominence it held as a national biomedical organization. However, given that the likely alternative for many men like Peng was conscription into the Nationalist army, the letter also suggests that working at a government office such as the bureau might have been a way to avoid military service. Tang took a strong interest in the development of the local staff and workers that the bureau did hire in Yunnan, holding weekly meetings to discuss research developments in China and abroad as well as the technicians' progress on their work.[74]

The 1942 cholera crisis in Yunnan did not reach pandemic status, and it only lasted a few months. However, it mandated the development of a vaccination program that sought to reach all members of the population, urban and local. The 1942 epidemic also led to the enactment of regular immunization against multiple diseases in Yunnan. This chapter and the preceding one have suggested that despite logistical and financial challenges to its establishment, mass immunization emerged as a response to crises of the wartime southwest, born of its unique epidemiological environment and specific fears on the part of Nationalist administrators about biological warfare. Yet despite its contingent origins, this strategy would become a key feature in public health programs that would expand to a national scale after the war with Japan ended in 1945.

The biopolitical dynamics that mass immunization policies created in the southwest also endured and spread. These initiatives provided room for both persuasive and coercive methods, underscoring that the act of immunization was rarely straightforward, and potentially fraught with violence and pain. Vaccinators themselves faced a complex set of concerns in complying with orders, correctly administering a new medical technology, and accounting for their actions by taking records and issuing immunization certificates, often interacting with people who had very different backgrounds, educations, and worldviews in the process. Their actions represented the beginning of several trends—toward accounting, toward the targeting of populations, toward the use of biological definitions to shape the rights of citizens—that would continue and even accelerate in the postwar years.

NATIONALIZING MASS IMMUNIZATION AMID CIVIL WAR AND REVOLUTION

On September 9, 1945, Japanese forces in China formally surrendered to Chiang Kaishek. Shortly thereafter, Tang Feifan and two colleagues set out from Kunming for Beijing, where they planned to recover the old facilities of the National Epidemic Prevention Bureau at the Temple of Heaven. Those researchers lucky enough to get a seat on an airplane or space in a truck to return east in 1945 embarked on an uncertain journey. Nationalist military forces were not the only soldiers left in China: in the northeast, the Soviet Union had invaded Manchuria, and the Communist People's Liberation Army (PLA) was gathering strength in the northwest. When Tang arrived in Beijing, he and his colleagues discovered that the Japanese occupation, and then the Nationalist military, had left their former offices in a state of thorough disrepair. "When we reached here, we found all our buildings in a most dilapidated condition," said Tang in a January 1947 lecture delivered at the reopening of the bureau, "and it was estimated that it would be more economical to rebuild the premises than to attempt to make adequate repairs to the ruins."[1] After eight years of conflict and exile, plans for reconstruction offered a fresh start for institutions, buildings, and people long battered by war. And at the Temple of Heaven, a site that held particular cultural and national significance, the prospect of renewal carried special meaning.

The conclusion of the Second Sino-Japanese War in 1945 did not put a stop to armed conflict in China. But it did mark the end of exile for many medical experts—even if only for a few years. After the end of Japanese occupation, these scientists returned with the Nationalist government from the hinterlands to China's eastern coast, eager to reclaim their old spaces and positions. The supplies and facilities that the Nationalists left in the western borderlands—and which they appropriated from the Japanese occupation—provided the basis for a novel national infrastructure of biomedical production. Meanwhile, the CCP strengthened its power base in rural northern China and prepared its own bid for power. The military forces of the Nationalist and Communist Parties almost immediately launched a series of skirmishes that quickly escalated into full-blown civil war, culminating in the withdrawal of the Nationalists to Taiwan and the establishment of the PRC in 1949.

This chapter examines the expansion of mass immunization in China during the calamitous period from 1945 to 1949. The reestablishment of biological research and production bases in the newly repossessed eastern cities solidified the authority of Chinese immunologists such as Tang Feifan, Wei Xi, Xie Shaowen, and others as prominent contributors to Chinese public health. At the same time, as the capacities of state administrations were stretched and strained, new dialogues emerged over the role of coercive immunization, its relationship to legitimate governance, and the ability of microbiology to contribute to national reconstruction.

Medical researchers and clinicians especially championed one vaccine at this time: the BCG immunization against tuberculosis. The immunization itself proved difficult to produce and implement, but its promotion reflected the changes that the war with Japan had wrought in China's public health system and its adoption of mass immunization programs. Nationalists and Communists alike embraced the vaccines that these researchers developed and manufactured—although from 1945 to 1949, the ability of both to manufacture and distribute large quantities of vaccines fell far short of their ambitions.

The history of medicine during the Chinese Civil War challenges prevailing views in which cities broke down under corrupt Nationalists, Communists converted peasants to their views, and the hinterlands quickly fell back into obscurity and isolation.[2] An examination of vaccination policies and practices in this period suggests that after Japanese withdrawal, China's major coastal cities actually became more, not less, socially and economically integrated with the nation's borderlands—at least in terms of health administration. Wartime medical networks in southwestern China continued to function after 1945, and the Nationalist state maintained the relationships it had developed with provincial authorities. These officials co-opted materials and structures that the national government had built during the war, often to deal with local outbreaks of infectious disease—especially tuberculosis.

Although scholars have begun to understand the modern history of tuberculosis in global terms, China's place in those narratives has remained unclear. Historians have discussed the significance of this disease as a leading cause of mortality in early twentieth-century China and the key role it played in prompting Chinese translations and appropriations of the germ theory of disease.[3] Moving this work into the mid-twentieth century, a survey of medical research and writing reveals that Chinese researchers and physicians participated actively in global efforts to promote the BCG vaccine in the immediate postwar era. Contemporary accounts suggest that antituberculosis immunization did not begin in China until after the PRC was founded in 1949.[4] Yet scientists working for the Nationalist administration actually laid the groundwork for that campaign years earlier. Unlike Western models of tuberculosis management, in which vaccination coexisted alongside social reform movements that encouraged the development of structural sanitation and personal hygiene, before 1949 the Republic of China lacked the money and human resources to develop comprehensive sanitary infrastructures. Instead, medical researchers promoted BCG as an effective, cost-efficient means of preventing tuberculosis that would save China from economic and demographic ruin—even though actually distributing the vaccine on a national scale remained impossible.

Postwar Reconstruction

In the months immediately following the Japanese surrender, Chinese biomedical researchers who had gone to western China returned to the metropolitan centers they had left in 1937. They rejoined colleagues who had stayed behind in occupied territory and reclaimed facilities and materials that the Japanese army had left in its wake. In Beijing, Shanghai, Nanjing, and other cities, they reestablished institutions, administrations, and research projects, maintaining connections with international research communities even as political and economic crises led China to slip further and further into outright civil war.

On January 1, 1947, the National Epidemic Prevention Bureau reopened as the National Vaccine and Serum Institute (Beijing shengwu zhipin yanjiusuo). Substantial manpower, financial investment, and logistical planning had enabled the institution's postwar reconstruction. Along with the British Red Cross, both the China National Relief and Rehabilitation Administration and the United Nations Relief and Rehabilitation Administration, organizations set up after the war's end to facilitate the reestablishment of social order and welfare, had supported the erection of new facilities in Beijing. In February 1946, work began on a new complex at the Temple of Heaven site. This included fourteen new buildings and laboratories, among them a stable for experimental animals built on the grounds of the old Altar of Agriculture.[5]

Even after the expansion was complete, Tang worried about adequately outfitting the new buildings. "The vaccine, serum, plague, standardization and other laboratories are only temporarily equipped with whatever material we have on hand," he fretted, awaiting the arrival of a shipment from the United Nations.[6] Tang's concern with the physical apparatus of the laboratories, like the new name of the organization itself, reflected a transformation in mission: the Institute no longer sought generally to control or prevent epidemics but instead focused specifically on the manufacture and distribution of vaccines, sera, and other "biologicals" that could provide immunity against disease.

A focus on vaccine production clearly did not preclude the institute or its leaders from wide-ranging ambitions. A formal reopening ceremony included speeches from Minister of Health Jin Baoshan and Peking University president Hu Shih, as well as an academic conference in which Chinese immunologists at the institute and other research organizations presented over fifty papers on recent research. "With the arrival of new equipment and increased personnel, we hope that we shall be able to make increasing contributions in the field of biological production in China," declared Tang at the opening session. "It is our aim to develop our Temple of Heaven headquarters into a strong base for scientific endeavor." He envisioned the National Vaccine and Serum Institute as the new flagship of a nationwide network of institutes that would foster research on drugs, vaccines, and communicable diseases to "work for the protection of the health of our masses," drawing explicit comparisons to the Pasteur Institute in Paris and the Lister Institute in London.[7] This mission represented a new, more expansive set of goals for the organization. Before the Japanese invasion, it had focused its work on urban immunization campaigns and epidemiological data collection. Tang articulated an ambition for the institute to play a central role in research, as well as health administration, from this point forward.

The National Vaccine and Serum Institute was not the only Nationalist health institution seeking a triumphant return, in the face of uncertainty and at great expense, to the formerly occupied cities on China's eastern coast. The central NHA had to reshuffle many of its personnel to accommodate its return to formerly occupied territory—especially in the capital, Nanjing, where Minister of Health Jin Baoshan had found most of the NHA's original headquarters in a shambles when he and his staff returned from Chongqing.[8] Yet although war had destroyed much of the prewar medical infrastructure that existed in China's eastern and southern urban centers, the Japanese occupation had not left a tabula rasa in these cities. Many biomedical researchers and clinicians became involved in projects to take control of medical facilities established by the Japanese occupation.

During its occupation of China, the Japanese had established medical research and educational programs that shaped the development of immunology in the regions under its administration, especially Manchuria in the northeast. The occupying army had a large bacteriological laboratory and vaccine factory in Dalian as well as a series of quarantine stations along major transportation routes in the region. Three medical schools in Shenyang, Harbin, and Tianjin provided clinical instruction. The most infamous Japanese medical research facility, however, was that of Unit 731 in the city of Harbin. This organization oversaw the central laboratory for Japanese development of biological and chemical weapons. From 1932 to 1945, its staff, led by Gen. Ishii Shirō, conducted brutal experiments on local Chinese subjects that contributed to Japanese germ-warfare initiatives in central and southern China.[9] Less well known were Unit 100, established in 1936 at Changchun to develop weapons for veterinary and agricultural sabotage operations, and Unit Ei 1644, established in 1939 in Nanjing for the development of chemical and bacterial weapons.[10]

In addition to its experiments on human subjects, Unit 731—formally titled the Kwantung Army Epidemic Prevention and Water Purification Department (Guandong fangyi jishui bu benbu)—had managed a major vaccine production site. Its headquarters at Harbin had produced at least twenty million doses of immunizations every year against eighteen different diseases, and Ishii conducted clinical trials to test the merits of plague and cholera inoculations produced via ultrasonic and conventional means. The Japanese occupation forces distributed these vaccines as part of a broad-ranging and intensive investment in public health programs that emphasized immunization. For instance, in 1939, about two hundred thousand anticholera immunizations and vaccinations against smallpox were given to the residents of occupied Tianjin.[11]

Although the Soviet army removed large amounts of industrial machinery from northeastern China after 1945, the fate of medical laboratories and equipment has not been so thoroughly examined. Upon Japanese capitulation in 1945, the staff of Unit 731 and many military research facilities destroyed their work and their equipment—although Chinese diplomats have claimed that after 1945, Japanese biowarfare programs left approximately one hundred tons of toxic chemical agents and shells across Manchuria and the occupied territories to its south.[12] The Nationalist administration rushed to take control of the structures that remained, assigning National Epidemic Prevention Bureau staff to help take over epidemic and epizootic disease research stations in northern China (including the site in Changchun that had been the former home of Unit 100).[13] Although the Nationalist government sought to possess Japanese structures in northeastern China, it was the CCP that eventually assumed administration of these sites, as it seized control of more and more territory.

Along with the reclamation of physical spaces and structures came the recovery of professional roles. While the first skirmishes of the civil war were breaking out in northeastern and northwestern China, the cities of Beijing, Nanjing, and Shanghai were once again becoming centers of biomedical research and development for the Nationalist government. Upon their return from the hinterlands, many microbiologists enthusiastically resumed research and teaching, with immunology the subject of many scientific publications from 1945 to 1949. In the pages of the *Chinese Medical Journal*, researchers published on serological and immunological studies of cholera vibrios, production of the BCG vaccine against tuberculosis in China, and methods of producing vaccines against smallpox and other diseases.[14]

Immunological specialists assumed prominent roles in postwar research and education. In many cases, they reunited with colleagues who, like Xie Shaowen, had stayed behind during the war. These researchers were generally not vilified as collaborators with the Japanese occupation but typically resumed prewar positions. After Tang left for Beijing, Wei Xi, his deputy, stayed behind in Yunnan and assumed leadership of the National Epidemic Prevention Bureau headquarters in Kunming, which became a branch institute of the National Vaccine and Serum Institute. However, Wei soon moved to Shanghai and became head of the institute's branch office there as well as a professor of microbiology at the Shanghai Medical School. In 1946, Xie Shaowen temporarily joined the National Vaccine and Serum Institute while it was rebuilding and his home institute, the PUMC, remained closed. After the college reopened in 1947, Xie resumed his professorship there in the Department of Microbiology and began accepting students again. In 1946, Liu Sizhi assumed a professorship at the Peking University School of Medicine as chair of the Biochemistry Department. In the same year, Lin Feiqing and her husband, Rong Dushan, also a noted microbiologist, traveled to the United States for advanced training at the Ellis Fischel Cancer Hospital in Missouri, where Rong worked with leading radiotherapy specialist Juan del Regato. Upon their return in 1947, the pair took positions at the newly established National Defense Medical College in Shanghai.[15] The researchers who had been instrumental in developing Chinese immunology since the 1930s seemed well on their way, then, to resuming leading national roles in public health.

Chinese scientists also continued cooperative work with American research scientists and funding agencies that had begun during the war with Japan. For example, after the National Vaccine and Serum Institute was reestablished in Beijing, the ABMAC continued to subsidize its work on penicillin. In a letter to ABMAC requesting financial support to continue the domestic production of penicillin, Tang Feifan wrote, "Now since we are established in Peiping [Beijing] we consider it necessary to request for supplements so to ensure continuous production of penicillin for at least one year and to figure on expansion as soon as working conditions allow."[16] This indicated the institute's enthusiasm for, and continued dependence on, foreign funding. Given the severe lack of cash that the Nationalist government faced by 1946, international aid provided a critical supplement to vaccine research and development in China.[17] These programs also demonstrated Chinese researchers' continued engagement with global research communities.

Vaccination in Civil War China

In the spring of 1946, a doctor named Fang Gang made a mistake that almost cost him his life. Fang, a technician in the Bacterial Testing Group of the Nationalist Central Health Laboratory in Nanjing, had been working with plague bacilli to prepare cultures for antiplague vaccines when he suddenly fell ill with fever, chills, and tell-tale swollen lymph nodes. Fang had accidentally infected himself with bubonic plague. Once the diagnosis was confirmed, the laboratory immediately—and secretly—isolated Fang and gave preventive medicines to the people with whom he had been in contact. They injected him with antibacterial sulfonamides, and he "completely recovered in wondrous fashion. Others did not know he had even been sick."[18]

This incident demonstrated severe security flaws in Chinese health administration and research—and the power of antibiotic drugs, which had recently been introduced to China—but it also revealed that that system was more sophisticated than one would have expected in a nation devastated by war. The episode also threatened the reputation and integrity of the NHA at a fragile moment in its postwar reconstitution. At a time when the Nationalist government was reasserting control over eastern China, no one needed to know that the country's primary hygienic laboratory had been so easily compromised. But this incident also demonstrated strategies of swift response to potential epidemic outbreaks, using strict quarantine and new drugs, which the NHA had developed during the war—as well as a continued emphasis on developing and manufacturing vaccines as a means of epidemic control.

Although many researchers and physicians returned to the urban centers of Beijing, Shanghai, Nanjing, and Guangzhou immediately after war's end, the connections forged between the central Nationalist government and its hinterlands persisted in medical administration through the late 1940s. Likewise, mass vaccination in these regions had demonstrated strategic value as a means of epidemic control during the war with Japan and remained a major part of Nationalist—and Communist—health policies.

After 1945, Nationalist health policy mandated mass immunization for the newly reunited nation, although total immunization rates for this period remained low, only reaching a fraction of any given population. In an August 1946 national directive to hold summer health campaigns (*xialing weisheng yundong*), the Nationalist Ministry of Health ordered that preventive health teams carry out "preventive injections and vaccinations against cholera, typhoid fever, smallpox, diphtheria, and other contagious diseases." The directive also stipulated that workers should observe local conditions and carry out health work as they saw fit. Other actions to be taken alongside the vaccinations included using propaganda to publicize the campaign from May to August, holding sanitary competitions, assembling health personnel from schools, factories, and public places to hold health lectures, and holding campaigns to eliminate vectors such as mosquitoes, flies, and rats that could transmit contagious diseases.[19]

The command to immunize reached many urban populations. For example, from May to August 1946, the city of Shanghai vaccinated 2,050,884 people against cholera. In the cities of Chongqing, Qingdao, and Guangzhou, smallpox and cholera vaccines were the mainstays of intensive immunization work; in 1946 the Qingdao Municipal Health Department (Qingdao weisheng ju) inoculated as much as 64 percent of the population of the city (484,959 people) against cholera.[20] The Philanthropic Hospital of Kunming, in its report of activities from 1948 to 1949, noted that giving smallpox inoculations and other vaccines was part of its work in children's health. It also recorded giving vaccines and prophylactic sera against smallpox, cholera and typhoid (combined), diphtheria, and bubonic plague. However, only 1,524 people—less than 1 percent of the city's population—were vaccinated in these initiatives, suggesting their continued limitation.[21]

The certification of vaccination also continued in cities. After 1945, Nationalist health administration united the certification systems established in the cities of the wartime hinterlands with similar programs that hygienic authorities had employed in zones of Japanese occupation.[22] Such a convergence suggested the growing coverage of systems that could facilitate state surveillance of vaccination status on a national scale. For instance, in Kunming in 1946, the Red Cross Hospital prepared stock immunization certificates that read in English as well as Chinese, "This is to certify that Mr./Ms. [name] has been vaccinated against smallpox, cholera, typhoid, and paratyphoid in our hospital." The certificates were to be signed by physicians at the hospital.[23] Circular notices in the same year from the Shanghai Quarantine Service, under the NHA, informed other municipal governments and shipping companies of epidemic outbreaks at Chinese ports and any corresponding requirements that the service placed upon passengers. For instance, a notice issued on September 10, 1947, announced that all incoming and outgoing passengers in Shanghai must possess certificates showing that they had received a cholera vaccine. "Those who are not in possession of such certificates will be inoculated by the quarantine officers before being permitted to land," warned the notice in English as well as Chinese. A follow-up bulletin informed readers that the port of Hong Kong had defined a valid certificate as showing immunization had occurred from six months to six days prior to departure, including a photograph of the holder stamped with an official seal, and bearing the signature of an official health administrator occupying a government position in public health.[24] This list of requirements suggested the extent to which documentation of individuals' inoculation statuses—and commensuration of these credentials across time and space—had become a part of epidemic control.

Outside cities, provincial programs sponsored inoculation against multiple diseases. For instance, in 1946 teams in Fujian Province distributed 126,614 vaccines against smallpox, 469,304 antiplague vaccinations, 49,524 combined immunizations for cholera and typhoid fever, and 12,745 antimeningitis shots. However, provincial vaccination drives were far from comprehensive. Fujian's population was officially reported to be 11,100,680 in 1947.[25] And in 1946, Guangdong Province reported that although it had purchased enough smallpox vaccine to immunize 658,585 people, this figure represented only about 2 percent of the provincial population. Similarly, during the Summer Hygiene Campaign of 1946, Guangdong only distributed enough cholera vaccines to inoculate 1,018,600 people, or about 3 percent of the population.[26] Although vaccination programs were becoming a widespread feature of postwar public health, their reach remained limited.

As the fighting between Nationalists and Communists slowly advanced toward China's major cities in 1947 and 1948, the production of vaccines expanded. In southwestern China, health administrators in the interior continued to make use of formerly national scientific facilities and processes. The southwest remained connected to the immunological centers forming on China's eastern coast. Municipal educational authorities claimed the physical remnants of the institutions that had left—even today Yunnan Normal University still occupies the former buildings of Lianda—and vaccination remained an important part of public health work, especially in Yunnan.[27] For example, when plague struck the province in 1947, the Western Yunnan Plague Prevention and Treatment Committee (Dian xi shuyi fangzhi weiyuanhui) quickly formed. It drew members from a wide variety of national and international organizations still stationed in Kunming, from the medical and supply divisions of the American military base there to the administrative command of the Eastern Burma Road. Other participants included the Chinese Red Cross, the American Red Cross, the Chinese

Army Office of Public Health (Zhongguo lujun zong siling bu weisheng chu), the National Epidemic Prevention Bureau, the Tengchong County Government, and the Yunnan Department of Public Health. Mass immunization was a major part of antiepidemic work in 1947. Local officials were advised to distribute antiplague vaccines within twenty-four hours of discovering the plague in any given location and reminded of the necessity to sterilize the instruments used for immunization. Infection with contaminated needles, it was thought, would cause workers to lose faith in vaccination, indicating an ongoing concern with public acceptance of this practice.[28] In Baoshan, a small town in western Yunnan where the 1947 plague epidemic hit hardest, local public health authorities purchased over 300,000 cubic centimeters of immunizations. Disease Prevention Brigades, county public health clinics, and private physicians distributed these vaccines for free from June to August.[29]

One report noted a remarkable local receptivity to antiplague vaccination. A local administrator wrote, "The effectiveness of these preventive injections is clear not only in terms of the clinical statistics, but also in that afterwards, the populace also had a much better understanding of it. When I went to inspect the area, the people most urgently wished that they could receive injections of the new vaccine."[30] In contrast to the wartime resistance against cholera vaccination that Francis Hsu had described (see previous chapter), local Yunnanese were reported to seek out immunizations against plague rather than fear or avoid them. This change in attitude may have been due to the fact that although coercive techniques had been commonly used during the war, by 1945 most authorities agreed that less aggressive tactics were more effective. For example, a 1947 article published in the *Yunnan Journal of Public Health* asserted, "In immunizing, those who use forcible methods do not vaccinate as many as those who use persuasive techniques, at the end of the day."[31] The article did not explain what "persuasive" (*qifa*) methods might entail, and some ambiguity remains in the use of that term, given that the force of the state to compel immunization would have underlain any rhetoric that vaccinators used.

The southwest was not the only borderland that focused its postwar health administration on vaccination. People and organizations in northwestern China also integrated the remnants of Nationalist organizations into regional medical administration and continued to play an important role in national public health structures. Although the staff of the NHA's hospital and medical school and the Northwest National Epidemic Prevention Bureau in Lanzhou returned to Nanjing, Shanghai, and other cities after 1945, these facilities themselves remained and continued to provide the basis for a major regional medical center. For instance, in August 1945, the director of the Northwest Bureau, Yang Yongnian, returned to Shanghai, where he established the Central Biological, Chemical, and Pharmaceutical Production Laboratory (Zhongyang shengwu huaxue zhi-yao shiyan chu). In January 1946, the Lanzhou laboratory became a subsidiary production center for Yang's laboratory. In September 1948, after a number of financial troubles, it was reabsorbed into the National Vaccine and Serum Insti-tute network as a branch office.[32] In 1946, the former NHA Central Hospital, renamed the Lanzhou Central Hospital (Lanzhou zhongyang yiyuan), continued working with a Northwestern Advanced Nursing School (Xibei gaoji hushi xuex-iao) to meet local needs. The medical school in Lanzhou, which the Nationalists had appropriated during the war, also returned to local jurisdiction and eventu-ally merged with Lanzhou University to become the Lanzhou University Medical School (Lanzhou daxue yixueyuan) in 1946.[33] Facilities established during the war thus integrated into local and regional networks during the civil war period, even as they maintained institutional and personal connections to the national administrations then reforming.

In developing a national system of health administration that employed mass vaccination as a key feature, Chinese immunologists worried about the geographic expansion of their work and its associated logistical demands. In 1947, the researcher Cai Hongdao discussed cholera inoculation in the journal *Yichao yuekan* (Monthly medical currents). He gave a detailed explanation of what the vaccine was, how it was made, and the kinds of physical reactions people might experience after receiving the immunizations. His discussion also suggested the kinds of technical problems that inoculators of the period com-monly encountered. "Often people will ask whether or not they may use an expired vaccine. In fact, the expiration date printed on the vial containing the vaccine is a fairly abstract date. The important thing is still that one looks to see whether its daily maintenance is appropriate," wrote Cai, referring to the need to preserve the vaccine in a refrigerated environment. "Furthermore, the so-called expiration refers to the fact that immunity may slowly diminish; it is really not saying that after a certain date it suddenly loses efficacy and is totally useless." Cai justified the use of technically expired vaccines by saying that it was better than nothing. "Suppose that one needs to immunize and only has one vial of vaccine on hand that expired not too long ago," he conjectured, "then in that case it can still be injected, because it is harmless, and moreover this injection is generally better than no injection at all."[34] This discussion sug-gested that vaccine shortages and faulty supply lines—as well as the question of whether and how much to bend the rules of immunization—were common issues in anticholera work.

The Nationalist Party's administration was not the only one to enact epi-demic prevention measures in China during the civil war period. The CCP also invested in immunization, especially as a means of disease control in the plague-prone border regions where the party had gained footholds in the early years of the civil war. For instance, in June 1947, bubonic plague struck Harbin, the primary base of CCP operations in Manchuria. The CCP attributed the outbreak to the release of flea-infested rats from the site of Unit 731. (During the war, Tang Feifan had worried about just such a calamity happening in Yunnan if a Japanese air raid destroyed his laboratory.) Thirty thousand died, and the epidemic only subsided after the imposition of strict controls on travel, combined with other public health measures such as quarantine and propaganda distribution. Physicians in Harbin founded a public health group that organized many preventive health activities, which included killing rodents and antiplague vaccination.[35]

In 1949, as the PLA consolidated power across central China, it continued to incorporate health administration into its work. The CCP newspaper and propaganda outlet *People's Daily* published a number of articles promoting vaccination. One such article encouraged immunization as a means of increasing resistance to disease. It read, "From the development of medical science, we know that through methods of manpower, we may produce vaccines, and after injecting these vaccines into people, their bodies produce a kind of resistance. . . . This resistance may not only counter the vaccine, but also may resist the contagious disease with which the vaccine identifies."[36] The article referred simply to "medical science" as evidence of the method's legitimacy and stressed a narrative describing internal struggle within the body that was suited to Maoist rhetoric of contradiction and conflict. Another 1949 article on public health in Beijing said, "Before the Liberation, immunization mostly used forcible methods, but this year we have used methods of persuasion and education, so the people of the city all spontaneously go to the Disease Prevention Stations to get immunizations." The piece did not describe what these methods of persuasion and education involved, merely stating that the regime had vaccinated more than 377,000 people against cholera by August 5, 1949.[37]

It is possible that presenting immunization as a voluntary action was a convenient means for the Communist administration to obscure its logistical inability to vaccinate all the people under its control, using coercive *or* persuasive methods. Regardless, such a statement shows that even before the establishment of the PRC, CCP authors were using the question of forcible immunization to draw explicit comparisons between the Nationalist and Communist regimes. This aligned with a broader strategy to evince positive public impressions of the CCP and its soldiers in contrast to Nationalist troops and officials.[38] CCP rhetoric took advantage of a widespread postwar lack of confidence in the Nationalist state to promote a Communist alternative in which, propaganda suggested, problems of economic mismanagement, military corruption, and intellectual suppression would be absent—and the state would provide comprehensive, competent public health services in the face of epidemics.

The Threat of Tuberculosis and Promotion of BCG in China

One epidemic especially threatened China in the civil war period: tuberculosis. In the early twentieth century, while smallpox, cholera, and other diseases caused temporary but urgent crises, pulmonary tuberculosis remained a leading cause of mortality in China.[39] BCG vaccination offered China the first practical opportunity to prevent tuberculosis on a mass scale using immunological methods. However, although Chinese researchers and physicians promoted the vaccine in medical journals and in popular media, actual immunization rates remained very low from 1945 to 1949. This outcome was likely the result of both the complexity of producing the vaccine and the fact that it could only be administered to people who did not already test positive for exposure to tuberculin, a protein extract of the tubercle bacillus; sensitivity to tuberculin generally indicates that an individual has already been infected with tuberculosis. This condition excluded much of the Chinese population, except newborns and young children, from eligibility for the immunization. However, the postwar campaign for BCG suggests the lasting impact of wartime vaccination work upon Chinese public health. A variety of actors—from clinicians to researchers and administrators—mobilized in support of one vaccine; they cited the United States, rather than Japan, as a model of immunization practice; and they participated in transnational antituberculosis health programs. While any of these developments might have happened before 1937, they converged to shape the wartime experiences of many biomedical researchers.

Tuberculosis is a chronic disease that in twentieth-century China typically spread when one inhaled an infected droplet that a tubercular person had exhaled. The disease is caused by the tubercle bacillus (*Mycobacterium tuberculosis*), which Robert Koch discovered in 1882. Resistant to heat, the bacillus can survive in dark spaces for six to eight months, so tuberculosis infection rates tend to correlate with dark, damp, stuffy, and crowded spaces. Because the bacillus reproduces slowly, it is possible for infected persons to become disease vectors without realizing the extent of their illness.[40] Those who catch the disease may therefore live for many years before developing the telltale symptoms of the disease, such as a cough expelling sputum or blood, night sweats, fatigue, fever, and weight loss. In late nineteenth-century and twentieth-century China, urbanization and the rise of factory production in cities created crowded, unsanitary conditions that permitted infectious diseases such as tuberculosis—then associated with a traditional pathology called "wasting disease" (*laobing*)—to spread rapidly. By 1935, tuberculosis caused approximately 1.2 million deaths per year and accounted for four hundred of every hundred thousand deaths in the nation.[41] The disease particularly threatened Chinese industry because it spread so easily through the urban workforce.

Western nations had employed a variety of public health measures in response to tuberculosis since the nineteenth century, but China lacked the resources to do the same. For example, in the nineteenth-century United States, Americans responded to infection by entering sanatoriums or migrating to what they considered more favorable environments. After the identification of the tubercle bacillus in 1882, preventive tactics that altered individual and collective behavior became intertwined with Progressive Era social reforms. Everything from the establishment of sewers, water purification, garbage collection, and food inspection to the regular use of white porcelain toilets, vacuum cleaners, and refrigerators became a part of American infrastructure and daily life by the early 1900s as a result.[42]

In China, growing awareness of tuberculosis precipitated the selective assimilation of Western germ theory into Chinese medical, political, and social spheres. This development coincided with the rise of practices associated with *weisheng*, or hygiene, which sought to bring many of the reforms mentioned above to China. In the 1930s, the most extensive specific antituberculosis efforts in China—those enacted in the city of Shanghai—consisted primarily of education through media campaigns and the establishment of a few sanatoriums outside the city. But these efforts had not been very effective. In Shanghai, a 1948 survey suggested that as many as seven out of ten Shanghai cotton-mill workers who served on night shifts had contracted tuberculosis.[43]

After the war with Japan, China could not afford to construct more sanatoriums or build more hygienic infrastructure. In 1945, state revenues only amounted to about one third as much as expenditures. After the war, the government of Chiang Kaishek failed to implement effective price controls, continuing instead to print money steadily. Labor soon responded by demanding higher pay. Emergency reform measures in 1947 and 1948 to freeze wages, fix commodity prices, and prohibit private hoarding and export of capital failed.[44] In the face of this economic crisis and the absence of investment in antituberculosis work by the bankrupt Nationalist state, scientists and physicians adopted the belief that BCG vaccination could save the health of the Chinese labor force and, by extension, the economy.

The BCG vaccine is the oldest vaccine still in widespread use today and the only extant immunization that offers protection against tuberculosis. On December

28, 1908, Albert Calmette and Camille Guerín announced their development of "biliated tuberculosis bacilli" in the French city of Lille. In July 1921, Benjamin Weill-Hallé first gave the live, attenuated vaccine to a Parisian infant orally and successfully saved the child from the disease that had killed its mother. In 1924, the Pasteur Institute began to distribute the BCG strain around the world.[45] After Norwegian physician Johannes Heimbeck conducted successful clinical trials with the vaccine in 1926, the League of Nations declared that the oral BCG vaccine was safe in 1928.

The announcement was ill timed. A year later, in 1929, 250 babies in Lübeck, Germany, received an oral vaccine that had been contaminated in the laboratory with virulent bacilli, with seventy-two dying. The Lübeck incident, as it became known, made the BCG vaccine notorious, and health departments in many nations consequently hesitated to employ it. English, Scottish, Irish, and American cities generally avoided the vaccine, while France, Norway, and the Health Section of the League of Nations maintained their support of the immunization.[46]

Although BCG vaccination in China is usually dated to the early Communist period, it actually began in 1933, when Wang Liang—a student of Calmette—carried the original BCG strain to China from France, produced the vaccine in his laboratory at the Shanghai Pasteur Institute, and used it to immunize 248 children without incident. He continued to produce BCG after moving to the Pasteur Institute at Chongqing at an unspecified date, vaccinating about eight hundred children there in total.[47] In retrospect, Wang presented his research in France as a fundamentally patriotic endeavor. "Thinking of the needs of our nation to fight tuberculosis," he wrote in 1948, "I traveled across the oceans, and went to Calmette's laboratory."[48] By 1936, the Shanghai Pasteur Institute had a special department for antituberculosis work. By 1937, the institute was preparing BCG once a week and supplying private doctors and local hospitals with the vaccine. Procedures for manufacturing the vaccine generally conformed to international norms—using potato cultures to preserve the BCG strains and a solution called Sauton's medium to prepare them—but institute staff made some changes to accommodate their environment. For example, in 1942, they replaced asparagine, an ingredient in Sauton's medium, with sodium glutamate, a common ingredient in Chinese cuisine. By 1948, the institute had distributed seventy-five hundred vaccines in Shanghai.[49]

After the Second World War, tuberculosis infection rates quickly rose across Europe. The international health organizations that emerged in the wake of the war promoted BCG as a solution to this transnational crisis. The typical means of controlling the disease were sorely absent in the wreckage of war-torn Europe. Clinicians lacked both the equipment and electricity to conduct diagnostic chest

radiography, and a total collapse of administration precluded any serious public health efforts to identify and isolate people suffering from tuberculosis. Mass
vaccination with BCG provided a means of controlling the spread of the disease in the absence of such infrastructure. In May 1947, the Danish Red Cross
commenced a pilot program in Poland to test children for tuberculin, immunize
those who tested negative with the BCG vaccine, and train local doctors, nurses,
and medical students in the testing and vaccination processes.

In 1948—the year the First International BCG Congress was held, in Paris—
the success of the Danish program led the nascent United Nations International
Children Emergency Fund (UNICEF) and the WHO to fund a pan-European
antituberculosis enterprise. The International Tuberculosis Campaign, in which
twenty-two nations participated, established an International Tuberculosis College to train epidemiologists, physicians, and laboratory staff; a research unit to
evaluate data collected by field workers; and field units that distributed BCG
vaccines from laboratories in Denmark, Sweden, France, India, and Mexico. The
campaign lasted from 1948 until 1951 and eventually reached beyond Europe
to South Asia, the Middle East, North Africa, and Central America. In total, its
agents tested nearly thirty million people for tuberculin and vaccinated almost
fourteen million with BCG.[50]

One of the subsidiary projects that the International Tuberculosis Campaign
funded was a scholarship for three Chinese researchers to visit Denmark in
November 1947. For six months, Chen Zhengren, Wei Xihua, and Zhu Zongyao
studied BCG vaccine production, standardization, and distribution at Copenhagen's State Serum Institute and Anti-Tuberculosis Dispensary. After completing
their studies in Denmark, the trio toured BCG immunization and antituberculosis projects in Norway, Switzerland, Italy, France, England, and the United States.
In October 1948, they returned to China with freeze-dried samples of the Danish
strain of BCG. Chen set up a laboratory within the National Vaccine and Serum
Institute in Beijing to produce the vaccine, and Wei followed his example at the
Shanghai branch of the institute.[51]

Chen and Wei's efforts were accompanied by a new focus in the medical
press on tuberculosis, the dangers it posed to the Chinese population, and the
potential for BCG to provide an economical means of controlling the disease.
A series of articles in the *Chinese Medical Journal* and other publications presented economic imperatives for adoption of the vaccine, exploiting popular
(and legitimate) concerns about China's economic collapse in the face of hyper-
inflation and civil war. In September 1947, Wu Shaoqing wrote that BCG vaccines represented a chance to break pernicious cycles of tubercular infection that
weakened China's labor force: "More ignorance and poverty, more tuberculosis!
More tuberculosis, more poverty!" Wu stressed the potential of the vaccine, in

combination with socioeconomic measures, to control the disease.[52] A year later, Qiao Shumin, at National Lanzhou University, also advocated for widespread BCG use. Qiao pointed out that mass immunization would cost "but an infinitesimal fraction of the millions of dollars it costs to run sanatoria."[53] Another 1948 article suggested that the implementation of BCG immunizations would be as transformative and beneficial as the introduction of Jennerian vaccination.[54] All the authors stressed the economic benefits of BCG, asserting that vaccination provided a feasible practical means of saving China's labor force from consumptive collapse.

These authors outlined plans for the implementation of BCG in China that stressed the use of immunization alongside other, social measures of improving public health. Wu claimed that since the vaccine had only proven partially effective, it should be combined with preventive means such as teaching proper nutrition and quarantining active cases. Qiao laid out a stepwise plan to roll out BCG immunization across the country. He proposed the use of the National Vaccine and Serum Institute as the first site for vaccine production and the establishment of mobile laboratory units that could help establish vaccination in China's interior. He presented an ambitious vision in which all infants were vaccinated with BCG at birth "because the risk of exposure to open cases of tuberculosis in China is so ubiquitous."[55]

The distribution of the vaccine on a national level posed many logistical issues, which Wang Liang, still at the Chongqing Pasteur Institute, discussed in a 1948 article in the journal *Xin Chongqing* (The new Chongqing). After a long period of cultivation, the live vaccine could only be used during a fleeting window of fifteen days. "One cannot transport it to far places for use," worried Wang, "and if it stays local, one must abandon lots of expired vaccines, so it is really not economical." Furthermore, vaccinated infants had to be tested for tuberculin sensitivity before receiving BCG, complicating and lengthening the immunization procedure. After receiving the immunization, babies still required quarantine from the outside world to avoid coming into contact with infected persons. Wang recommended that they remain isolated in a nursery for six to eight weeks before returning home—an arduous requirement for new parents.[56]

Because the BCG vaccine required such extensive interventions in the care of infants and children, pediatricians became important figures in its implementation alongside bacteriologists and public health administrators. In May 1949, pediatrician Song Jie wrote, "In the fight against tuberculosis, the pediatrician stands at the first line of defense." He warned that any pediatrician should carefully explain the risks and limits of immunization "so as not only to protect himself, but also to protect the reputation of BCG." Song suggested several points for physicians to stress before they vaccinated to ensure the success of the procedure: the limited immunity that the vaccine conferred, the importance of doing a tuberculin test to make sure that the child was not already infected with tuberculosis, and the need for prolonged isolation periods before and after immunization. "To enlighten the public in a BCG vaccination campaign, such points, minute as they seem to be," cautioned Song, "may prove essential."[57] This advice suggested some obstacles to introducing mass BCG vaccination as well as the critical intermediary role that doctors played in recommending the practice to parents.

The complex technical requirements of the BCG demanded special consideration in planning for its production on a large scale. Qiao discussed means of manufacturing the vaccine, noting that the "inherent character" of BCG as a living vaccine meant that it could not be imported from overseas and required domestic production. Moreover, the vaccine had to be preserved in heat for fifteen to twenty days as it developed, while most other bacteria used for vaccine production only required twenty-four hours for the same process. Qiao suggested the potential for Soviet manufacturing methods, which used a dry glucose vaccine easily stored at room temperature, to work in China's less accessible borderlands. The dry vaccine was not as fresh, or as effective, as those prepared in suspension, but to Qiao its capacity for long-term storage was worth the trade-off.[58] This attention to means of employing vaccines in China's distant borderlands indicates that immunologists were thinking about vaccination on a national scale—and turning to new models for medical research and development. This point was underscored by the 1948 publication of an article in the *Chinese Medical Journal* on BCG vaccination in the Soviet Union. The success of trials in the Ukraine and Russia during the 1920s had resulted in a nationwide movement there in 1937.[59]

The Soviet Union was not the only potential model to follow in implementation of the BCG vaccine. Authors discussed the precedents that a variety of nations had set in producing and distributing it. Wu Shaoqing cited the Soviet Union, Denmark, Norway, Sweden, Canada, the United States, and even the former enemy, Japan, as models that had already begun instituting regular BCG immunizations. Wang Liang presented an overview of the efficacy of BCG vaccination programs in Europe, Canada, Brazil, and Uruguay as well as the United States. "If BCG was not effective at all, it would have been abandoned a long time ago," he claimed, "and would not have reached a point today where American scholars plan to establish manufacturing offices to produce the vaccine for American children."[60] This statement is odd, given that BCG vaccination was never widely implemented in the American population. It is possible that Wu and Wang drew on scientific evaluations of BCG in medical journals in making this claim.[61] Nevertheless, the possibility that they misinterpreted or overstated the commitment of the United States to the BCG vaccine is indicative of how Chinese physicians built consensus around public health measures. Wu and Wang relied on global standards of assessment and especially on the authority of American biology to reassure their audiences that the BCG vaccine worked. This reinforces the point that the United States had become a model, if not the only one, to which biological researchers in China looked for guidance.

Despite the ambitious plans of Wu, Song, Wang, and others, BCG vaccination rates remained low in China during the civil war. The Shanghai Pasteur Institute claimed that from March 1937 to May 1948, it immunized 7,511 babies with BCG orally and 1,089 children parenterally (via injection).[62] Since about 3.7 million people lived in Shanghai under occupation, the vaccine had only reached a fraction of the population. Such an outcome suggests that researchers who sought to apply BCG on a large scale faced significant logistical obstacles that included widespread preexisting infection with tuberculosis that precluded application of the vaccine, difficulties in preparing it, and further problems with transporting it to appropriate distribution sites. Actually implementing mass BCG immunization did not happen on a large scale until after 1949. Yet its promotion in China during the period from 1945 to 1949 reflected researchers' attention to antituberculosis work on a global stage, perceived connections between the prevalence of tuberculosis in China and its state of economic crisis, and a genuinely national vision for public health and immunization work.

The Advent of Liberation: Decisions, 1949

As the CCP assumed control over more and more territory, many scientists and physicians fled China for Taiwan, Hong Kong, or the West to protect their money, families, and lives. An ABMAC report on the National Vaccine and Serum Institute gives a sense of the sudden exodus, saying that in April 1948, a chemist named Y. C. Ma had been appointed as head of its penicillin laboratory. However, soon thereafter, Ma received a fellowship from the newly founded WHO for advanced training in antibiotic development. By September 1, he was in Toronto. "With the rapid political development in the country at large and in North China in particular we are most keenly concerned with the future of this laboratory," the report read. "Plans were made and instructions asked for, but as there is safety and peace nowhere even had we the finances for any major removal, we have decided finally to let this laboratory—together with the other NEPB laboratories— remain at the Temple of Heaven, and Heaven only knows what is in store there for the future."[63] Despite this ominous prediction, Tang Feifan, Wei Xi, and other immunological experts chose to remain on the mainland during the final months of the war and after the CCP founded the PRC. Why?

No one answer can explain such contingent and difficult decisions. Many researchers in a variety of fields had attained—and perhaps believed that they could retain—good professional placements as the leaders of prominent institutions under the Nationalist regime. After all, Chinese immunologists had generally found themselves well employed after the war with Japan ended. Tang became the chief of the National Vaccine and Serum Institute. Xie Shaowen held a prestigious professorship at the reopened PUMC as chair of the Department of Bacteriology and Immunology.[64] Wei Xi was both a professor at the Shanghai Medical School and branch chief of the National Vaccine and Serum Institute there. It is also possible that immunologists were merely following orders predicated on the belief that the Nationalist government would either not fall or would quickly regain power. For example, in December 1948, the NHA ordered Tang Feifan to keep his institute in Beijing, and Tang had resolved to keep it operating for as long as possible.[65]

Alternatively, some immunologists may have been dissatisfied with Nationalist administration during the civil war and subsequently decided not to follow Chiang's government to Taiwan. For example, in 1947, Xie Shaowen decried in the pages of the *Chinese Medical Journal* the nation's lack of graduate training opportunities for medical scientists.[66] Unlike Tang Feifan or Wei Xi, Xie had stayed in Beijing and Tianjin throughout the Japanese occupation rather than follow the Nationalist government to China's southwest. A retrospective account claims that when the subject of the war came up in discussions with colleagues, Xie criticized Nationalist corruption and that his sympathies lay with the CCP.[67] Although one may be skeptical about the extent of Xie's dedication to the Communist cause before 1949, reports of his dissatisfaction with Nationalist governance correlate with his 1947 article and his decision not to go to the southwest during the war.

Some scientists may have even explicitly endorsed the Communist cause. In 1949, Wei Xi was the head of the Shanghai branch of the National Vaccine and Serum Institute and a professor at the Shanghai Medical School. Liu Juanxiang, a hematologist who assisted Tang, claims that in 1948, Wei Xi, allegedly a Communist sympathizer since medical school, was contacted by the underground CCP in Shanghai. The movement asked Wei to go to Dalian—then still under the control of the Soviet army, which was cooperating with the CCP— to establish a biological production facility there; with Tang's approval, Wei agreed to go to Dalian, and the Communist underground helped transport him there secretly.[68] Other biographies of Wei report a similar version of events, noting that he took his family to Dalian via Hong Kong and became a deputy chief of the Dalian Biological Products Research Institute (Dalian shengwu zhipin yanjiu suo) as well as a professor at the Dalian Medical School (Dalian yixueyuan).[69] Given the large number of historical accounts about the Chinese Civil War that claim that various historical figures were underground members of the CCP, and the obvious reasons one would have for claiming this political heritage, one would do well to treat these claims with skepticism. That said, they cannot be definitively disproved, since Wei Xi seems to have disappeared for a period in 1949 and was established, by 1950, as a professor of microbiology at the Dalian Medical School. The case of Wei suggests that immunologists, like other professionals, may have considered it advantageous to strike early alliances with the CCP.

It is also possible that some immunologists—Tang Feifan among them—genuinely retained the idealistic belief that they could help rebuild China and thought the CCP could foster their work. Liu suggests such a motivation at the beginning of his hagiographic biography of Tang. Liu begins the book by describing the deserted family home in Shanghai's French concession in early 1949, explaining that Tang, his wife He Lian, and their infant son Duoduo were emigrating to the United States. They had already shipped their luggage and bought plane tickets for the journey. But, Liu claimed, Tang was disquieted by the decision. On April 5, the day that the family was scheduled to fly out of Shanghai, he and his wife were taking a last look at their home when Tang exclaimed, "My spirit is not happy to leave its own country and live under another's roof." After this episode, Liu claims that Tang and his wife "calmly awaited Liberation" and that "it was as though the entire family put down their burdens and exhaled in relief."[70]

Liu's histrionic account is best interpreted as a dramatized version of events as Tang may have related them. The descriptions of Tang's emotions employ a wealth of hyperbole that makes it impossible to take the narrative at face value. Similarly, Liu attributed Tang's desire to stay on the mainland to a patriotic dedication to China, claiming that he "deeply loved our country and the people."[71] Although this statement comes across as politically motivated and pro-CCP, it is reasonable that immunologists such as Tang may have believed they would be valued in the PRC, especially since the Communists prioritized vaccines early on in their management of epidemics. And during the last eight years of war with Japan, scientists had seen their journeys to the southwest and manufacturing of vaccines as patriotic endeavors. Certainly Tang Feifan had expressed a dedication to the cause of public health in China in the National Vaccine and Serum Institute's opening ceremony in 1947, when he had claimed that the institute would soon constitute "an important and integral contribution to the public health programme of the Republic of China."[72] The republic, however, was destined for more years of war, turmoil, and eventual exile.

The civil war was a strange, strained moment for medical researchers in China. As institutions transplanted back to the eastern coast, the ordinary rules of laboratory life warped. One technician accidentally infected himself with plague, others disappeared almost overnight, and as the clock ticked down to October 1, 1949, many of those with the means wondered whether to stay in China or, finally, flee. The decisions that biomedical experts faced were not unique. During the war, professionals across the spectrum of society had served a common cause—the survival of China—but now they had to choose sides: Communist or Nationalist? Mainland or Taiwan? Or Hong Kong or the West? Stay or go?

Participation in vaccination campaigns demonstrated a form of community and national belonging, even when the very existence of the nation was in question. Immunological research during the Second Sino-Japanese War formed the basis of vaccination strategies during the civil war as immunization against smallpox, cholera, and typhoid fever became a key public health strategy that was implemented across China to varying degrees. Hygiene also connected the interior to formerly occupied and newly regained urban centers since provincial governments absorbed wartime health structures into their own administrations and maintained connections to national research organizations. Even when immunization campaigns were not very successful—as in the case of BCG—they demonstrated the growing prominence of vaccination in public health. With the rise of the CCP also came the suggestion that coercive immunization policies might have demonstrated the inadequacy of the Nationalist state, placing vaccination squarely within public debates over the legitimacy of the CCP. These debates would only grow more pressing after the withdrawal of the Nationalist Party to Taiwan and the establishment of the People's Republic.

VACCINATION IN THE EARLY PRC, 1949–58

The 1949 establishment of the PRC formally ended the conflicts that had engulfed China for almost twenty years. But the new nation was still in crisis. The PLA continued to wage military campaigns in Tibet and Xinjiang, war loomed in Korea, and infectious diseases still threatened the country's population. In 1949, bubonic plague struck Tianjin and Beijing, and in the following year smallpox broke out in Shanghai. The establishment of national vaccination campaigns, first against smallpox in 1950 and then against tuberculosis, diphtheria, and other diseases in 1952, signaled a national commitment of the new regime to epidemic prevention.[1] Such an achievement was possible, this chapter argues, because new systems of recordkeeping, surveillance, and accountability accompanied the implementation of public health policies. These programs built power over life by self-consciously protecting it from epidemic catastrophe.

As the previous chapters have demonstrated, the CCP's promotion and implementation of mass immunization campaigns was not novel or sui generis. These activities drew upon existing infrastructure, technologies, and knowledge to continue and expand systems of vaccination that had taken shape during preceding decades. The context for this expansion was another war—the conflict in Korea—and reflected the ongoing military and political mobilization of Chinese society. Immunization against smallpox, typhoid fever, and tuberculosis featured prominently in health policy from the establishment of the PRC, especially after the state accused the United States of using bacteriological weapons in the Korean War in the early 1950s. Chinese immunologists assumed prominent positions as scientific authorities who confirmed the allegations. Because these claims stressed a danger to public health, the CCP launched a nationwide movement, the Patriotic Hygiene Campaign (Aiguo weisheng yundong), which began in 1952 and promoted vaccines alongside other public health activities as scientific, modern means of combating germ warfare. The intensification of mass immunization established party authority over health administration and bolstered the legitimacy of the central government, even as the party's growing power was necessary to implement these programs and make people accept vaccination.

Sources from the Kunming Municipal Archives allow a detailed case study of immunization during the early 1950s. Examining one urban and provincial context in detail sheds new light on a central demographic question about the early years of the PRC: how did China lower its mortality rate so quickly? In 1950, the crude death rate of China was probably close to thirty deaths per thousand people per year. By 1957, this figure is estimated to have dropped below twenty per thousand. Demographers credit a broad range of preventive health measures, including immunization, with causing this dramatic if imprecise reduction.[2] What specific role did mass vaccination in the early 1950s play in lowering Chinese mortality rates?

Although Yunnan's epidemiological profile and medical history hardly make it representative of other places in China, by the early 1950s the province was integrated into regional and national frameworks that made it less exceptional in terms of medical administration than it had been. Kunming therefore provides a case study that both indicates the extensive character of immunization campaigns during the early 1950s and suggests that these campaigns employed new ways of monitoring and recording the biologies of individual citizens. Arunabh Ghosh and Thomas Mullaney have suggested that in the 1950s, the CCP rapidly expanded its information-gathering activities via statistics and census taking.[3] Records from Kunming reinforce that observation and suggest a major increase in the capacity of Chinese authorities to administrate health, as vaccination records began to employ classifying markers such as gender and age and to track the immunization statuses of individuals. These practices indicated a growing capacity for surveillance and identification of those who escaped the reach of state mandates.

The implementation of orders for mass immunization against smallpox, typhoid fever, and tuberculosis in Kunming was far from smooth. Analysis of the propaganda that promoted public health campaigns reveals the ideals against which the state measured the work of vaccination teams and shows how the state portrayed and used immunization to build authority. Radio broadcasts, articles, posters, and other promotional materials are, of course, not records of what actually happened. Yet they show that during the early 1950s, the CCP promoted immunization as a critical means by which the central state took care of the people's health, delineating a newly benevolent relationship between the state and its citizens and encouraging an association between effective vaccination policies and legitimate, functional government.

Patriotic Hygiene: Immunization in the New China and the Korean War

Mass vaccination was a part of Communist health policy from the establishment of the new nation. In 1950, at the First National Health Work Conference in Beijing, the CCP established four guiding principles for medical administration: focus on serving workers, prioritize preventive health, use mass movements, and unite Western and traditional Chinese medicine. The Soviet Union also became an overt model for Chinese health policymakers at this time. China's ally sent a number of advisers to the new Ministry of Health (now titled Zhonghua renmin gonghe guo weisheng bu), and the PRC developed a five-year plan along Soviet lines to rapidly improve and modernize hygiene work in China.[4] Because immunizations were often classified as a form of preventive medicine, the Ministry of Health prioritized their distribution after 1950, especially in areas where infectious diseases were endemic.

One of the first health laws that the new government announced, on February 10, 1950, focused on seasonal disease prevention. The regulation stipulated that vaccination was to be a key line of defense against epidemic outbreaks and gave details on the proper use of vaccines against smallpox, diphtheria, and measles. It emphasized the need for regular immunization against smallpox and other diseases and ordered that doctors of Chinese medicine be trained in Jennerian vaccination. In this respect, the order reflected broader trends in which the mandate to unite different medical cultures made use of the manpower of traditional practitioners to serve novel ends. However, health administrators in Kunming regularly complained about the quality of these practitioners' work as vaccinators, reinforcing the argument of Kim Taylor that such an encounter was far more complex than it might seem.[5]

Further legislation in 1950 mandated and regulated annual smallpox vaccination campaigns. Early immunization policies anticipated issues of inadequate personnel and unfriendly reception, especially in rural populations that had not been exposed to as many immunization campaigns as their urban counterparts. The new regulations noted that limiting the period of immunization by season, as was consonant with traditional beliefs about the proper time for variolation, was not "scientific" (*kexue*). A commentary signed by Zhou Enlai, premier of the Government Administrative Council (Zhengwu yuan), specified that vaccination was to be free of charge and that, since many people might still be unaccustomed to the practice, local governments must emphasize propaganda, education, and patient "persuasion" (*shuofu*).[6] Yet further legislation mandated that "all residents within the borders of the People's Republic of China, no matter their nationality, must receive the vaccine" and noted that "if persuasive education had no effect, each health organization must implement forcible methods" to vaccinate those who refused inoculation without a valid reason.[7] The official language thus acknowledged that some people might still find vaccination a strange practice in 1949—but it still mandated this intervention throughout the year, even if it broke with traditions of seasonal immunization and even if local administrations encountered resistance.

To streamline the distribution of biological products, the ministry consolidated vaccine- and serum-manufacturing institutes across the country and placed them under the aegis of the National Vaccine and Serum Institute in Beijing, led by Tang Feifan at the Temple of Heaven until his death in 1957. Subsidiary research stations were located in Shanghai, Wuhan, Lanzhou, Changchun, and Chengdu. One biography of Tang claims that by 1951, this network had increased its production of vaccines and sera sevenfold from 1949 and that in 1952 the bureaus were generating thirteen times as many vaccines as in the previous year.[8] This process completed and consolidated the nationalization of biomedical institutes that had begun during the civil war.

By 1952, vaccines were enshrined in the health legislation of the PRC. In that year, they also reassumed familiar roles as weapons of war. The outbreak of the Korean War placed immunizations, and the medical workers who made them, at the forefront of Chinese discussions about health. In October 1950, the PLA entered the "war to aid Korea and resist America" on the side of the Communist Workers' Party of Korea, which later formed the Democratic People's Republic of Korea north of the thirty-eighth parallel. Likewise, the United States sent troops to support South Korea, then an American protectorate. China and North Korea soon accused the United States of using bacteriological weapons in the conflict. Allegations of germ warfare publicized Chinese microbiologists as figures whose scientific credentials lent authority to the accusations. They also made vaccines prominent armaments in the state's public struggle against biological weapons.

As early as 1951, articles began to appear in China's domestic press claiming that the United States was dropping strange bombs filled with dead flies, spiders, and other unusual objects. Chinese and North Korean media outlets asserted that Chinese bacteriologists had proven that these items were infected with smallpox and other infectious diseases.[9] In 1952, the PLA captured two American airmen who signed confessions that they had participated in acts of bacteriological warfare. The PRC then set up an International Scientific Commission (ISC) that brought in European experts, most of whom had leftist political leanings, to support the findings of the Chinese researchers. Its propaganda organs also released films asserting the allegations in Chinese and also in English for global dissemination.[10]

Controversy over whether the accusations were true continues today, and bacteriologists and immunologists were involved in the debate over their veracity from the beginning.[11] One of the military doctors involved in the accusations, Wu Zhili, wrote, "The matter of bacteriological warfare was settled by being left unsettled." His autobiography states that the bacteriologist Wei Xi provided an early testimony suggesting that the allegations were false. Then the head of bacteriology at Dalian Medical College, Wei was one of the first researchers called in to verify the accusations, but he and colleague He Qi initially said that the samples they inspected were not bacteriological weapons and that the concern was merely a "false alarm" (*xujing*). After Wu reported this finding to Peng Dehuai, the general in charge of Chinese military operations, Peng denounced Wu, claimed that he was parroting the speech of American imperialism, and immediately convened a meeting in which colleagues accused Wu of rightist sympathies.[12]

It is unclear what exactly transpired next, but Wei subsequently changed his story. In a special 1952 edition of the *Chinese Medical Journal*, Wei coauthored an article in English titled "Peace and Pestilence at War" that supported the accusations of biological warfare, saying that "like an octopus, [the United States] was stretching its tentacles far to the rear of the battle front."[13] Wei's recanting suggested that if the accusations were false, then other microbiologists were faced with the same choice: deny the allegations because the evidence was unconvincing, or support them for the sake of political survival. Because Wei had worked with American scientists during the Second Sino-Japanese War, his public support of the allegations provided a politically useful example of Chinese rejection of American power.

True or not, the charges increased the public prominence of Chinese microbiologists. Fears about germ warfare in China shaped the discourses, strategies, and personnel involved in setting national health policy during the early 1950s. Immunologists gained new prominence because they confirmed the veracity of the allegations. From 1950 to 1952, the Ministry of Health sent Tang Feifan, Wei Xi, Xie Shaowen, and other immunologists to laboratories at the Korean front. Films, newspaper articles, and scientific journals cited these researchers as scientific authorities who had definitively isolated pathogenic bacteria from sources near suspicious bombs in northeastern Chinese villages. Tang and Xie published articles in the *People's Daily* confirming and condemning American germ warfare. Tang, now president of the Chinese Society for Microbiology, also published an article in the *Chinese Medical Journal* supporting the claims.[14] Collectively, Tang, Xie, and twenty-six other microbiologists signed a June 1952 editorial in the *People's Daily* rebutting American assertions that the United States was innocent of using bacteriological weapons. The authors hailed from a select group of prestigious institutes including PUMC and the Peking University School of Medicine as well as the National Vaccine and Serum Institute. "We have," they wrote, "already totally proven that the American army has dropped bombs on North Korea and Northeast China that contained many worms and other poisonous organisms. Bacteriologists in every place, using all different kinds of experiments, have already extracted every kind of illness-inducing bacterium from the organisms."[15] In this way, reports of the allegations made microbiology part of a political discourse in which Chinese researchers took leading roles.

In verifying the charges, microbiologists made claims for the authority and proficiency of Chinese scientific expertise on a global stage. The ISC investigated the allegations in coordination with the World Peace Council, a European group of left-wing intellectuals who opposed atomic, chemical, and biological weapons. The commission presented its deliberations as that of an impartial panel of foreign experts, although its members—especially Joseph Needham—had leftist political leanings. It framed its report as the inevitable, logical result of a "mass of facts" and noted close cooperation with Chinese and Korean scientists in affirming that the United States had used bacteriological weapons.[16] A 1952 propaganda film titled *Oppose Bacteriological Warfare*, a Chinese-Korean production that was made in English apparently for consumption in the West, prominently featured "eminent specialists" analyzing specimens, signing reports confirming their discovery of pathogenic bacteria, and discussing these findings with each other. Xie Shaowen was one of the researchers on camera. The film showed him looking through a microscope and displayed his signature on a report confirming plague bacilli in a spider found in a northeastern Chinese village.[17] Propaganda pieces like this film did not merely present microbiologists as knowledgeable people who confirmed political allegations. It made their laboratory work the centerpiece of the show, emphasizing their scientific expertise, authority, and objectivity.

Even as these accusations prominently featured microbiologists, they took place during a perilous time for Chinese scientists, especially those trained in the West. To consolidate its power, the CCP conducted a series of nationwide campaigns to purge bourgeois elements throughout the 1950s. These included the Campaign to Suppress Counter-Revolutionaries in 1951, the Three-Antis and Five-Antis Campaigns from 1951 to 1953, and thought reform of intellectuals in 1953. The second of these identified government, political, and industry officials who had retained positions of power since the Nationalist era and accused them of the three offenses of corruption, waste, and bureaucratism.[18]

Against the backdrop of anti-American sentiment in the Korean War, intellectuals with American training were targeted, and immunologists were no exception. An article in the journal *Xinan weisheng* (Southwestern hygiene) denounced researchers who had gone to the southwest to serve the Nationalist government during the Second Sino-Japanese War. "Some people will say, 'I was driven to the hinterland during the War of Resistance. I am from another province, but now that Liberation has come, there is no need to return to my hometown,'" wrote Lu Zhijun, then director of the Health Bureau of the Southwestern Administrative Council.[19] Lu cautioned that these people were untrustworthy, writing that during the tumult of the 1949 revolution "property that should have been turned over to the People's Republic was instead divided up by these so-called 'scholars,' 'scientists,' and 'technicians!'" He cited the case of Shen Dinghong, who had worked under Tang and Wei at the National Epidemic Prevention Bureau and become head of the Kunming branch in their absence. Lu claimed that Shen, who now owned a pharmacy in Kunming, had embezzled over two billion yuan. Although Lu did not specify Shen's fate, intellectuals targeted in the Three-Antis Campaign were often publicly denounced and stripped of their positions and property.[20]

In this uncertain environment, endorsing allegations of bacteriological warfare provided a means for Chinese immunologists to both maintain political legitimacy and build intellectual authority. Just as scientists such as Shen and professors at renowned research institutes such as the former PUMC were losing their jobs and undergoing criticism in the *People's Daily*, the same newspaper was presenting Tang Feifan, Wei Xi, Xie Shaowen, and other immunological workers as experts serving their country faithfully.[21] To support accusations of germ warfare was therefore a fundamentally political act—not just an opportunity to declare one's support for the CCP but also a means of temporarily avoiding its persecution.

In addition to supporting the party's anti-American policies, allegations of germ warfare in the Korean conflict justified broader state investments in preventive health for both military and civilian populations. For instance, in a March 1952 memo to Zhou Enlai, Mao Zedong wrote, "Please prepare to vaccinate all soldiers east and west of the Liao River. Central and East Hebei, as well as Beijing and Tianjin, should also make preparations."[22] (Mao did not specify which immunizations, however, to prepare.) A medical history of the PLA notes that one of the army's primary responses to the allegations was "to supply large quantities of plague, typhus, and other vaccines and carry out urgent immunization among the troops—and to simultaneously give vaccinations to residents near military encampments."[23] The imperative to inoculate united soldiers and civilians, reflecting the militarization of society over decades of mobilization and transformation.

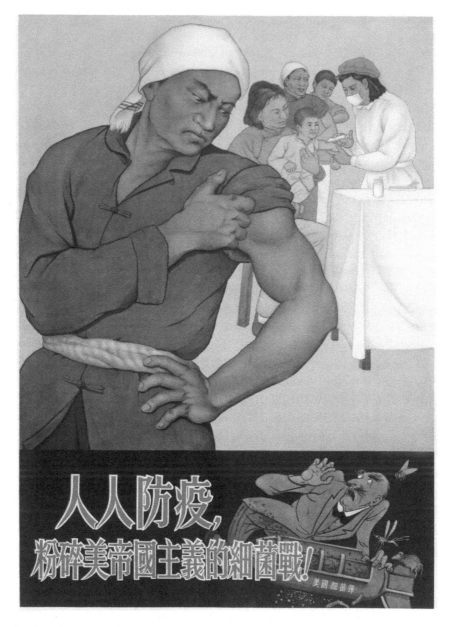

FIGURE 6.1   "Everybody must take precautions against epidemics to smash the germ warfare of American imperialism!," 1952. Ye, "Renren fangyi." Reproduced courtesy of IISH/Landsberger Collections.

These processes of militarization quickly expanded in scope to assume a national character. In 1952, the Chinese Ministry of Health launched the Patriotic Hygiene Campaign, a mass movement that provided a means for immunization against multiple illnesses to become a nationwide health practice. The campaign mandated a variety of hygienic activities, from street sweeping and latrine building to eliminating vectors of disease by killing flies and rats. These policies emphasized direct links between fighting bacteriological warfare and strengthening health work through mass movements. Their goal was the total eradication of infectious diseases, an aim that was also a symbolic response to China's recent history of warfare and environmental disaster.[24]

Vaccines came to the forefront of the Patriotic Hygiene Campaign as an efficient tool of disease prevention—and a means of protecting the Chinese population from alleged American bacteriological weapons. The latter function took on more significance than the former. For example, toward the end of the propaganda film *Oppose Bacteriological Warfare*, a series of clips of Chinese soldiers, civilians, and children receiving shots flashes across the screen as the narrator says, "We must protect the lives of our children. We must protect the lives of all peoples. They must not fall victim to US bacteria."[25] The video drew explicit attention not just to soldiers but also to civilians and especially children as the targets of immunization campaigns, emphasizing the symbolic role that inoculation played in concepts of protecting the health of the nation. Similarly, a 1952 poster (see fig. 6.1) proclaimed, "Everybody must take precautions against epidemics to smash the germ warfare of American imperialism!"[26] It displayed a Chinese worker with his sleeve rolled up in preparation to receive an immunization. This striking iconography articulated a direct means—immunization—by which civilian citizens could contribute to the ongoing military conflict. Such an emphasis suggested that it was not enough for state agents to simply invoke potential benefits to public health in persuading people to get vaccinated. The poster's creators instead stressed the patriotic, not the medical, value of immunization as a reason for their audience to accept this intervention into their lives.

Campaigns on the Ground: The Case of Kunming

How successful were inoculation campaigns in the 1950s—and how might one measure such success? The records of district health stations in Kunming suggest that from 1949 to 1953, a noticeable rise in immunization rates occurred there. Reported smallpox vaccination rates did increase to at least 90 percent in most areas of the city by 1953. This represented a significant change, given that province-wide rates never rose above 5 percent before the late 1940s. Typhoid fever vaccination rates also approached 90 percent in populations under individual health stations in 1953, although typhoid fever continued to occur at a rate of around fifty per ten thousand people until the 1980s. BCG immunization against tuberculosis took longer to implement in Kunming because it was only useful for people who had not already been infected with the disease. By 1953, health stations were supervising the vaccination of hundreds of newborns with BCG.

In rural Yunnan, immunization drives in the uplands, where large groups of non-Han ethnic minorities lived, were initially not entirely successful. Smallpox continued to appear there until 1960.[27] In 1959, 672 people exhibited symptoms of the disease in Cangyuan County, a region in Yunnan's far southwest that borders contemporary Myanmar. It was primarily inhabited by members of the Wa ethnic minority, a highland people who speak a Mon-Khmer language. Since Cangyuan was so mountainous, Yunnan health officials traveled there on horseback, carrying vaccines in ice cream coolers. Health workers staged Chinese opera performances to explain immunization and its importance. Whether or not these methods worked, the incidence of smallpox was sharply reduced. The number of sick people rapidly dwindled until March 1960, when a twenty-three-year-old man named Hu Xiaofa, a member of the Lahu people who lived in the district of Lancang, was identified as the last person to contract the disease in Yunnan and in China. He recovered after three months in an isolation ward.[28]

Establishing a comprehensive system of immunization before and during the Patriotic Hygiene Campaign was easier said than done. Local governments had to rely on a variety of organizations to distribute vaccines and keep records of vaccination in the early 1950s. In Kunming, this state apparatus comprised the municipal bureau of hygiene (*shi renmin zhengfu weisheng ju*), hospitals and clinics, work units, and local subdistrict offices (*renmin zhengfu jiedao banshichu,* literally "people's government street office") that complemented and superseded work units. Because Yunnan was one of the last provinces to be "liberated," in the vocabulary of the CCP, the PRC was slow to establish health administration there. The party began to assume control in late 1949, but Kunming only came under full Communist governance on February 20, 1950.[29] The CCP incorporated personnel from preexisting health systems, as well as local medical workers and cadres, into its new health institutions.[30]

The particular administrative configurations that supported immunization teams reflected the rise of new institutions to supervise public health work throughout the 1950s. In most cities, disease prevention teams or health stations performed immunizations as well as street sweeping, quarantining, and epidemiological surveillance. These teams typically associated themselves with local public security bureaus or police stations and sent smaller, subsidiary groups to neighborhoods under the jurisdiction of the security bureau or local subdistrict office.[31] The latter organization usually demarcated populations within urban areas and were themselves divided into residential communities or neighborhoods. They took responsibility for neighborhood tasks of street sweeping, fire safety, public security, mediating petty disputes, political surveillance, and public health.[32] In Kunming, the municipal bureau of hygiene divided the city into sectors and established health stations in each one that would oversee these teams. The stations also took responsibility for suburban and rural areas in the vicinity of the capital, and their reports stressed the difficulties of inoculating in outlying townships or villages.

A major part of epidemic prevention campaigns involved the organization and training of vaccination teams. In Kunming, people recruited as vaccinators were drawn from local work units (*danwei*) or neighborhood committees. Many were untrained in medicine, so these vaccinators attended short courses to learn the techniques and principles of immunization before beginning work. For example, one training class for BCG vaccination in Kunming was planned to last for two weeks and cover the basics of immunology, the pathology of tuberculosis, and how the BCG vaccine was made. After the classes were over, the health stations sent their teams to the work units under their jurisdiction to distribute vaccines.[33]

The involvement of community-level organizations spoke to the broadening scope of immunization programs as well as the integration of health into a new structure of employment that arose in the 1950s. The work unit was an urban administrative division organized around a state-owned workplace, such as a factory or a school. It provided employment, housing, medical care, and welfare subsidies for its members and exerted extensive social and political control over them. By 1957, over 90 percent of city dwellers belonged to a work unit. David Bray argues that because the work unit provided a mechanism for the production of knowledge about urban populations, it became a central site for the exertion of biopower in modern China as the locus of disciplinary activities that made citizens "productive proletarian subjects."[34]

Immunization directly contributed to this construction of urban biopower. In 1953, the clinics at work units across Kunming were sending yearly work reports to the municipal bureau of hygiene. Clinic staff recorded the numbers of people they immunized and how close they were to attaining vaccination rates of 100 percent against typhoid fever. These statistics noted that the clinic workers sought to inoculate employees and their dependents, reflecting the growing intervention of the work unit in the lives of entire families. For instance, the health work report for the Yunnan Cigarette Factory stated that smallpox vaccination work specifically targeted children who had previously missed immunization (*louzhongzhe*) as well as those who simply had not yet been vaccinated (*weizhongzhe*).[35]

Identifying those who evaded vaccination became a critical priority for inoculation teams during the 1950s. To do so, they took advantage of new administrative systems then coalescing across the country. While the work unit was taking shape as an urban social division, the *hukou* ("household registration") system was becoming a primary mechanism by which the state exerted power over citizens. Various forms of mandatory enrollment with local authorities had existed throughout the late imperial era and were associated with traditional systems of collective responsibility among households in a community. After its founding in 1911, the Republic of China legally institutionalized the *hukou*, and the CCP built upon this foundation in mandating registration of households.[36]

The *hukou* was more than a means of keeping track of people. It also provided mechanisms for social stratification, differentiation of resource provision, and governmental control—most infamously in the divisions this system created and enforced between urban and rural residency. Those whose *hukou* identified them as city dwellers were, and are, entitled to voting rights, employment, school enrollment, and various welfare benefits provided by the government. These benefits were and are seriously reduced or nonexistent for rural *hukou* holders, who were generally encouraged to practice self-reliance in the absence of state support. Guo Zhonghua suggests that the *hukou* system is "indispensable" to concepts and institutions of Chinese citizenship because of the dichotomy that it created between urban and rural communities and the rights associated with them. Citizenship and membership in the Chinese political community were constituted through these parameters as well as through nationality and ethnicity.[37]

As the *hukou* system evolved and consolidated over the course of the 1950s, public health organizations used it to structure activities and recordkeeping of mass immunization. In doing so they took advantage of the social control that the *hukou* system facilitated. The national regulations for smallpox vaccination promulgated in 1950 specified that smallpox vaccinations were to be recorded in household register books (*huji ce*) and carried out through door-to-door surveys.[38] In Kunming, this was known as the "smallpox vaccination household registration" (*zhongdou hukou*). Health administrations used these registration systems to identify and target people who had previously escaped the reach of inoculators.

A report from the Ninth District Station to the Kunming Bureau of Hygiene on February 12, 1955, suggests some of the logistical complexities of establishing vaccination registration. Station representatives explained that in a recent survey of the rural Fenghua Township Distribution Cooperative, they had sought to make use of previous paperwork recording inoculation status. However, the cooperative had used these forms in a disorderly fashion and the report condemned it for "not taking official documents seriously."[39] Another report articulates the literal identification of individuals with their records. In 1953, the Eighth District Station explained that they had improved vaccination rates in their relatively rural jurisdiction by sending small teams to liaise with township and village cadres and identify the "epidemic prevention *hukou* table." From this document, they identified "blank-space households" (*kongbai hu*) and "blank-space people" (*kongbai ren*)—those who had not yet been vaccinated. A list of "blank spaces" was handed over to local authorities, who arranged for these individuals to get vaccinated.[40]

The disorganization of preexisting paperwork impressed upon health administrators the need to produce better records. A 1959 handbook for inoculators, distributed nationwide by the Ministry of Health, stressed that registration and statistics were important tasks that "could not be neglected."[41] Kunming inoculation teams therefore sought to document immunizations to an unprecedented extent, recording a variety of information about the people they vaccinated. Teams also issued immunization papers, verifying the name, age, date, and agent of immunization, which were usually necessary for most forms of travel outside the village or work unit. In planning to implement certification as a means of controlling travel, the PRC standardized and nationalized processes that had previously been adopted in the wartime southwest and Japanese occupation zones—although CCP propaganda cited Soviet precedent for the practice. One radio broadcast noted that those without vaccine certificates would be subject to "certain restriction."[42]

The number and variety of documents produced by local health administrations raise important questions about their reliability. The CCP employed the quota system in its command economy, and because this typically mandated punishment for work units that did not meet their production goals, many units were incentivized to misrepresent data in reporting to their superiors.[43] Although vaccination was not a form of economic production, it is not unreasonable to assume that falsification may have occurred with vaccination statistics as well. Quotas did exist for immunization work in Kunming. Municipal health administrators typically set targets for district health stations to vaccinate a certain number of people in the following year. And in an April 1953 report, the staff of the Red Cross Hospital resolved to immunize 100 percent of hospital workers within the year.[44]

Although immunization programs produced a wealth of records, reports, and certificates that testify to the extent of campaigns against smallpox, tuberculosis, and typhoid fever, this paperwork was complicated by revisions and elisions.

Despite the neat, clean forms that the Ministry of Health might have sent out to provinces and cities, individual vaccinators had very different ideas about what information mattered. Perhaps for this reason, the 1959 national handbook for inoculators encouraged local health organizations to train workers how to take notes and gather data, treating immunization as "scientific work."[45] In Kunming, mass-produced forms for reporting immunization statistics were often marked up, and items scratched out. While some noted the size of the populations they were vaccinating and broke down their records in terms of age and gender of the people they vaccinated, others did not. This complicates the ability to compare data from different regions, but it also suggests that recordkeeping mattered enough for individual vaccinators to make their own notes.

The details of vaccination reports help illustrate how knowledge about immunization was produced in the early PRC. Compared to reports before 1949, which merely tended to list the number of vaccines distributed in a region, reports from the early 1950s contain much more demographic data. Some reports tracked immunizations by age, gender, and/or place. Many also recorded the number of individuals who were vaccinated multiple times against the same disease. Before 1949, it was common to just note counts of immunizations, so it was difficult to distinguish the original vaccination from repeat inoculations of the same person. But in documents from the early 1950s, there was an emphasis on understanding how many people were inoculated and how many times. This distinction demonstrated the greater attention that vaccinators paid to recording the statuses of individuals.

Statistics reported by vaccination teams suggest that age, gender, and location all helped determine the course of immunization drives in Kunming. For example, age and location were the most critical factors in determining smallpox immunization status in Kunming. In November 1953, in Wujing Township, the Third District Health Station vaccinated about half the people (93 of 181) against smallpox for the first time, and most of these were juveniles under the age of thirty (114 of 181). In nearby Linjiang, about half were vaccinated against smallpox for a second time (365 of 678), and 433 of these were also under thirty. A survey that took stock of how many people were vaccinated for the first time across the district divided the population into three categories: people who lived in private or semiprivate housing overseen by police stations, in rural areas, or in public housing. This last category represented the largest proportion of those surveyed—1,698 of 2,952 in total—followed by the first (1,098 of 4,910).[46]

The biggest improvement in vaccination rates occurred in public housing areas, where every single unvaccinated public housing resident was immunized. Those who lived in communities served by local police stations saw substantial gains: 90 percent to 99 percent of residents were vaccinated or revaccinated. The vaccinators found that from 21 percent to 85 percent of people in these communities had previously received a smallpox vaccine, so their 1953 work represented a substantial improvement on previous vaccination rates in many neighborhoods. Similarly, in rural areas, only about 25 percent of the population had been vaccinated before a November 1953 drive. After its completion, 94 percent were vaccinated or revaccinated. Police stations tracked the gender of the people they vaccinated, whereas the rural and public housing immunization teams did not. The police station data suggested no significant difference in vaccination rates between males and females.[47] Vaccination trends varied across the city. For example, the Seventh District Health Station, which covered Longtou, a village northeast of Kunming city, simply recorded the age and gender of those vaccinated from November 21 to December 10, 1953. Their collected figures suggest that male and female individuals were vaccinated and revaccinated in about equal numbers; the vast majority of those vaccinated for the first time (a total of 2,029) were infants, whereas most of those vaccinated for a second time were above the age of twenty.[48]

Statistics for vaccination against typhoid fever suggest that gender and workplace, unsurprisingly, affected vaccination rates. Immunizations were typically recorded by site of vaccination (usually either organizations—schools, factories, and so forth—or residential neighborhoods). In summer 1953, the Third District Health Station gave typhoid fever immunizations and recorded that the majority of those immunized, 21,220 of 32,537, had received the vaccine for the first time.[49] In 1954, the Eighth District Health Station gave 22,122 vaccinations against typhoid fever. Notably, it inoculated many fewer females than males (8,469 to 18,511 in neighborhoods and 418 as opposed to 3,193 in organizations).[50] The Third District Health Station reported a similar trend in its summer 1954 typhoid fever inoculations. Although the 18,034 people vaccinated in residential areas were fairly evenly distributed between male and female adults and children (9,022 to 8,314), the station only vaccinated 4,385 females in organizations, as opposed to 12,242 males.[51] Without population statistics on gender distribution by workplace and district, it is difficult to ascribe this phenomenon to any one cause. Pregnant women were exempt from immunization mandates, but this explanation seems insufficient for such a wide disparity.

The records of BCG immunization suggest particular difficulties that vaccination teams encountered in attempting to distribute this vaccine in Kunming. A May 1953 report of city-wide immunizations suggests that most who received the vaccine were infants under three months of age. As age increased, children were more likely to test positive for a reaction to tuberculin, indicating that they had already contracted tuberculosis and that the BCG vaccine would therefore be ineffective.[52] A September 1953 vaccination drive operated by the Eighth District Health Station appeared to focus on older children, testing 824 boys and 828 girls for a reaction to tuberculin, but again many were found to have already contracted tuberculosis. Only 344 boys and 344 girls were vaccinated, yielding immunization rates of about 42 percent for each gender (and a remarkably even gender distribution).[53] These figures emphasize the necessarily slow rate at which BCG vaccination progressed in Kunming due to the pervasiveness of tuberculosis in the city.

The reports from Kunming held more than just numbers. They discussed problems that arose in the process of immunization. For example, sometimes vaccinators made mistakes when they did not sterilize needles, and some people had to go to the hospital to be treated for infections after their immunizations.[54] One controversy that arose in a 1954 antityphoid campaign was a disagreement over preferred methods of immunization. During the campaign, some medical personnel refused to use intradermal injection (in the upper layers of the skin). They worried that this method would not be effective compared to subcutaneous injection (beneath the dermis and epidermis). But the workers who were receiving the immunizations feared subcutaneous injection because of the pain. As administrators attempted to explain to their vaccinators, the efficacy of this vaccine actually did not rely on the injection style. The result of the conflict was a chart counting separate totals of people vaccinated using two different methods. Only people in factories and the countryside received intradermal injection, suggesting that their resistance to the subcutaneous method outweighed vaccinators' resistance to the intradermal.[55] This dispute suggested that vaccinators, as well as people receiving vaccines, could misunderstand the proper use of immunizations: both intradermal and subcutaneous injection worked, but each group believed that only one method was acceptable. Moreover, both groups resisted the mandates of higher authorities, who merely wanted the maximum number of people possible to receive a vaccine. The health workers who gave vaccines thus had their own fears and worries about the procedure.

In a 1956 guide to immunization, Tang Feifan himself noted the misgivings of vaccinators as one of the greatest perils to the success of vaccination work. After providing detailed guidance on the manufacture and delivery of commonly used vaccines, Tang admitted that although mass immunization had largely succeeded in controlling infectious diseases since 1949, some flaws in its implementation were still common. Most notable was a misunderstanding of the tendency for many vaccines to provoke a temporary local reaction. Tang suggested that the fear of this reaction was one reason that people resisted immunization, writing, "Many people, and even some medical workers themselves, sometimes demonstrate a tendency to be too concerned to act" (literally *shushou shujiao*, "bind one's hands and feet").[56]

The metaphor is striking, given that it uses violent imagery to stress the danger of inaction. It is hard to resist seeing a connection, in this juxtaposition of force and fear, to the language that described the broader relationship between medical workers and "the masses." If we accept that the state inoculated close to five hundred million people against smallpox and other diseases in the span of a decade, using mechanisms that enacted new and extensive power over individual lives, and that it specifically mandated the use of force to accomplish mass immunization, then questions about coercion and resistance naturally arise. It is telling that in 1953, one unit specifically reported that it had not yet resorted to forcible methods in its typhoid immunizations and stressed this point as a major positive outcome.[57]

Reports from Kunming dwell not on dramatic scenes of coercive injections, however, but rather on the messy arena in which the threat of violence was always present but not always employed and in which people voiced fears and concerns about immunization as part of a dialogue with inoculators. For instance, a 1953 report from the Patriotic Hygiene Campaign listed some common excuses cited for not getting a vaccine: "I can't get vaccinated this time, my store doesn't have someone to look after it," or "The baby hasn't slept." In these cases, vaccinators claimed they had volunteered to hold the baby, watch the shop, or otherwise directly remove impediments to immunization.[58] Another report from a more rural area notes, "Some people said, 'It is an unlucky year for my child.'" And lingering concerns about the season of immunization encouraged some to ask autumn inoculators to come back in the spring. Yet these objections were dismissed as feudal superstition.[59] Exchanges between inoculation teams and those they targeted did not necessarily change the reported outcome of such encounters, which usually ended with the protestor getting vaccinated. The health workers writing these reports would have been keen to stress the success of their work and their harmonious relations with the masses, in keeping with the values of Maoism. Yet these narratives do indicate that citizens could, and did, protest or question the process of immunization. They also suggest why people might have opposed it.

Vaccination in Service of the State

The state articulated the political role of immunization most clearly in its propaganda. Especially after the Patriotic Hygiene Campaign began, health administrations across the nation distributed posters, sponsored radio broadcasts, and held meetings to promote immunization. Promotional materials do not accurately represent conditions of public health in China in the early 1950s. Propaganda about medicine was necessarily anticipatory, presented only the perspective of the central state, and was of dubious educational value.[60] However, a careful reading of posters, radio broadcasts, and articles can partially recover information about the problems that state agents encountered in immunization work and can shed light on the social and political forces that resulted in the production of these texts and images. An examination of the rhetorical strategies that the party employed in publicizing immunization complements archival documentation because it helps articulate how central policymakers understood vaccines as tools of government. Promotional materials discussed vaccination in three important contexts: to educate Chinese about immunity and identify the state with the authority of modern science, to favorably contrast Communist with Nationalist rule, and to address prevalent fears. Each strategy helped articulate a new dynamic of public health in which the central state took direct responsibility for the health of citizens.

Posters, songs, and radio broadcasts sought to persuade citizens to get vaccinated by teaching them about the production of bodily immunity. These materials invoked the authority of scientific medicine using a technical vocabulary that repeatedly referenced the equipment and theories of experimental microbiology. This strategy suggested that the goal of such propaganda was the construction of popular trust in science, more than getting large numbers of people to understand complex scientific theories. For instance, in a 1950 radio broadcast in Chongqing, the microbiologist Wang Liang said, "What we are now injecting is the combined cholera and typhoid fever vaccine of the National Epidemic Prevention Bureau. It has the differentiated cultures of the curved cholera bacterium and the typhoid fever bacillus which reproduced many times." Wang explained in greater detail the methods of manufacturing, noting that the pathogens were killed with heat and diluted in solution.[61] Listeners did not need to know all of these details about the official manufacture of vaccines, but describing their production in precise terms, using the language of bacteriology, indicated that these representatives of the state possessed medical authority and expertise.

Education about immunization using the terminology and iconography of Western medicine enforced a broader power: that of the central Communist state over the health of the people. For instance, in a public health journal article about BCG immunization, Ren Kangcai cautioned, "Before giving vaccinations, one must first go through ideological mobilization, and make sure that the parents of children receiving the vaccine understand the idea of immunization." The use of a term such as "ideological mobilization" (*sixiang dongyuan*) at a time when the same vocabulary described more prominent movements, such as "thought reform" (*sixiang gaizao*) of intellectuals, reinforces the point that educating Chinese parents about vaccination was a fundamentally political act.[62] Regardless of whether these materials succeeded in teaching people about the shots they were receiving, using the language of Western medical science to promote immunization suggested a new relationship between the people and the state in which the state asserted control over health education as well as research.

Educational materials responded to particular fears and beliefs about vaccines, suggesting that these concerns were significant—or at least widespread enough to justify the development of propaganda to counter them. In a 1950 radio broadcast encouraging cholera-typhoid vaccination in southwestern China, narrator Wang Huiyin discussed two apparently widespread fears: first, that it would be painful, and second, that it would cause a more serious adverse reaction.[63] The latter fear was not unfounded, given that fevers, rashes, and malaise were often typical reactions to the cholera-typhoid vaccine. Another 1950 broadcast did not deny that vaccines hurt but claimed that it was the duty of citizens to get vaccinated for the good of the people, using politically loaded language. "The hygienic organizations at every level . . . are assuming responsibility for the masses," said narrator Lu Zhijun. "For our safety, it is worth bearing bitterness for a short time. Otherwise, when one contracts illness and suffers, it can still affect other people."[64] Party rhetoric claimed that the importance of immunization justified both individual suffering and the intervention of the central state in their everyday lives—implying that substantial numbers of people feared the "bitterness" of getting a shot. The term "masses" (*guangda renmin*), pervasive in political discourse of the time, evoked Maoist populism. By submitting to immunization, Lu suggested, people could demonstrate cooperation with the goals of the party—even if it hurt at the time.

Aside from these fears, many people appear to have resisted vaccination because they thought it unnecessary. Wang Huiyin denounced prevailing attitudes, especially among older people, that contracting cholera or typhoid was unlikely, even if one was unvaccinated.[65] Alternatively, some had too much faith in the preventive power of immunization. During a 1950 antismallpox campaign in Chengdu, inoculators encountered many locals who believed that since they had been vaccinated once, they were protected from smallpox for the rest of their lives.[66] State propaganda attempted to counter such "indifference" by invoking the fear of epidemic catastrophe and again asserting the responsibility of Chinese to submit to vaccination, and revaccination, for the sake of the masses. "We all should get vaccinated, in order to prevent the kind of tragedy that resulted from the spread of cholera in the past," said Wang. "We must understand that if one person becomes ill, it can spread to every place, and affect the safety of many people. This pervasive spread of disease does not pay mind to any random Zhang or Li."[67]

Reminding listeners of past epidemics provided a means to critique health administration before 1949. In asserting the safety and efficacy of state-provided vaccines, party propaganda politicized immunization by favorably comparing its own work to that conducted under Nationalist rule. The Nationalist state had produced ineffective vaccines and administered them badly, claimed broadcasts and articles, while in contrast the PRC produced safe vaccines and distributed them efficiently. "Because the Nationalist reactionary faction did not emphasize the people's health, they did not have equipment for vaccinations; when they did immunize, the shots were mediocre and ineffective, so when [cholera] came, they gave away many people's lives," said Wang Huiyin.[68]

The new regime sought to demonstrate its benevolence in providing effective—and free—immunizations. In discussing cholera and typhoid fever vaccination, Wang wrote, "These immunizations are equivalent to the government maintaining the people's health and holding a campaign." It was the central state—not the Ministry of Health or local health brigade—that, Wang claimed, "goes and hangs signs in public health offices" to promote immunization.[69] And it was the state that funded these vaccinations. In a 1950 radio play discussing cholera and typhoid fever, one character, a doctor, said, "Our people's government spent a lot of money, expended a lot of effort, and mobilized many in order to give the people vaccines."[70] Such ham-fisted dialogue may not have made for riveting drama, but it did convey official narratives of the benevolence and success of the CCP in vaccination work.

The rhetoric of vaccine promotion in the early 1950s demonstrates that the CCP quickly made immunization an overtly political act. Miriam Gross has argued that the party used antischistosomiasis campaigns during the late 1950s to establish itself as a mediator of political life and scientific knowledge. Mass immunization campaigns in the early 1950s provided an important precedent for this process of "scientific consolidation."[71] To get immunized was to acknowledge and receive a service provided by the state and therefore to enter a particular relationship with the government, as a citizen submitting to its mandates. Educating citizens about vaccines, addressing their fears, and presenting the party as a viable and preferable alternative to the old Nationalist regime were all strategies that the CCP employed in an effort to legitimize its assumption of power over the health of the Chinese people.

In 1953, the Number Eight Public Health Station in Kunming reported a success story in its autumn smallpox vaccination campaigns. There was a man in the household of a family named Lin, who, since the founding of the new PRC in 1949, had refused to accept a vaccine against smallpox. "For three years we had not been able to persuade him," read one of the reports from Kunming, "but this time we explained to him over and over again, and after the team leader . . . persuaded him, finally he was vaccinated."[72] This short anecdote omits key details. What precisely did the leader say to the man? And why had he resisted for so long? The episode demonstrated the new ability of health authorities in a small city like Kunming to reach individual citizens. It also suggested some of the problems inherent in keeping track of such a rapidly expanding project. And the incident emphasized the intermediary role of vaccinators in persuading a man who had stubbornly resisted the public health work of the new government to comply with its policies. The success or failure of immunization campaigns in the early PRC hinged on personal, individual choices like the long-awaited vaccination of Mr. Lin. These small-scale actions not only added concrete figures to the sum of those vaccinated but also gradually reinforced the legitimacy of the state that claimed responsibility for each immunization.

MASS IMMUNIZATION IN EAST ASIA AND GLOBAL HEALTH, 1960–80

Zhao Kai never expected to find himself in Lhasa. A virologist trained at Shanghai's elite Fudan University, in the late 1970s Zhao held a senior position at the National Vaccine and Serum Institute overseeing the national production and testing of vaccines. When, in 1979, the WHO requested a report from the PRC on its claim to have eradicated smallpox, Zhao was involved in the efforts of the Ministry of Health to prepare the necessary documentation. In a 2003 interview with the Chinese television station CCTV-1, Zhao explained that this seemed like a straightforward task, in part because of the lack of direction from organization officials. He said, "Reports on the epidemic situation were coming up from below, and [the ministry] did not understand what documentation the WHO expected, so it was relatively easy to write a report."[1]

It was a surprise to Zhao and his colleagues, then, when the WHO expressed dissatisfaction with the resulting sixteen-page paper, which summarized the policies, administrative structures, and reported final cases of smallpox vaccination in China.[2] Organization officials pressed the PRC for more information, particularly because of a conflicting set of accounts that had arisen along the contested China-India border. During the course of a survey in India, WHO representatives had encountered a community of Buddhist political exiles living in Dharamsala, in northern India, who had fled the PRC after the 1959 Tibetan uprising. Two people among them claimed to have caught smallpox in China in 1962.[3] How could this have happened if the PRC had indeed eradicated the disease within its borders two years beforehand?

To disprove the Tibetans' story, Zhao and two colleagues were sent to the Xizang Autonomous Region to conduct a survey that Zhao described as "little short of fishing for a needle in the ocean" (*dahai laozhen*), in order to verify that China really had eliminated smallpox in 1960. Because of the altitude sickness they experienced upon arrival—Lhasa has an elevation of 3,656 meters—Zhao and his colleagues could only work half days at first, conducting surveys to determine which government organizations might have dealt with the cases in question. In its communications, the WHO had cited English terms for health organizations that had a bewildering variety of possible Chinese translations. These difficulties of translation and poor local documentation meant that the team from Beijing was stymied, even after making use of a local geological exploration team's extensive map collection to identify potential sites of smallpox infection. They claimed that they simply could not find a trace of the cases.[4] This failure of record keeping presented a serious risk to the historical narratives that propaganda organs of the PRC had articulated over the past two decades, which stressed the development of effective, efficient rural health in China.

The public success of mass immunization in China, as determined by the eradication of smallpox and the "control" of other infectious diseases such as measles and cholera, contributed crucial evidence for the success of Chinese public health more broadly—an idea that state agents sought to promote around the world in the 1970s and that shaped the course of global health. After a period of new vaccine development and distribution in the early 1960s, mass immunization in China continued throughout the turmoil of the Cultural Revolution from 1966 to 1976, albeit administered by new groups of people and in different structures. By the 1970s, immunization was comfortably entrenched in the rural health system that the PRC promoted on a global scale. It exported goods, personnel, and funds as a form of medical diplomacy from the 1960s onward. It also cultivated the goodwill of Western observers who traveled to China after 1971. These international activities contributed to the prominence of the PRC in discussions of global health policy, culminating in the WHO's Alma-Ata Declaration of 1978 and its major policy shift toward promoting "primary health care": interventions meant to provide basic clinical services for many people, including those in rural areas. The PRC became famous for its "barefoot doctors," semiprofessional medical workers who received minimal training in Chinese and Western medicine and were then sent into the countryside to both work in the fields and provide basic clinical and preventive care to peasants, as the human faces of the rural health system it promoted. However, the state's eradication and control of infectious diseases—a consequence of mass immunization—provided key evidence that helped consolidate its position as a leading national model of public health.

A variety of sources illuminate this point. They include histories of medicine in the Cultural Revolution, accounts by American and European travelers to China who wrote about their impressions of medicine there in the 1970s, and discussions of primary health care by international health officials and experts. There are significant issues with treating any of these sources as unproblematic, faithful representations of their time. As discussed in the previous chapter, the narratives that propaganda materials promote tend to obscure lived experiences in favor of serving state interests, official statistics are subject to the same dangers, and Western visitors' perceptions of China were often carefully shaped and mediated by their hosts. In her work on agriculture in the Cultural Revolution, Sigrid Schmalzer provides a model of how to use visual materials, educational texts, and other propaganda as historical sources. She points out that at the time, the people who produced these narratives took seriously the political ideologies that they reflect, and these materials gave expression to understandings and approaches that exerted global influence even as they diverged from Western models of scientific practice. Revolutionary sources may be biased, she suggests, but they can still tell us useful information about the experiences of people who lived through this time and the kinds of concerns that shaped the state creation of propaganda.[5]

The global success of the PRC health model depended on active efforts to promote it abroad. Chinese officials engaged in medical diplomacy, or processes by which one state provides medical aid to another, with the goal of improving the broader economic and political relationship between the two nations.[6] During the 1960s and 1970s, the PRC intervened in global politics through transnational exchanges in public health. Recently, historians have suggested that the PRC actively promoted its health achievements in the developed West as well as the Global South, so that the Chinese state itself was instrumental in the adoption of its health-care system as a model for rural health care by international health authorities.[7] This chapter investigates the role of mass immunization in these medical diplomacy programs during the 1960s and 1970s. While most scholarship has stressed the influence of barefoot doctor and other paraprofessional training programs in the emergence of the PRC as a global model for rural health services, mass immunization programs in China had measurable results—in terms of lowered incidence of disease—that helped legitimize these training efforts and the nation's program of rural health care more broadly.

The global popularization of Chinese public health was a consequence of regional competition within East Asia. During the Cold War era, the PRC used medical aid to foreign countries to compete for power and influence with the Republic of China on Taiwan, where institutions and personnel that the Nationalist Party brought to the island after 1948 built upon practices established during the period of Japanese colonial rule (1895–1945). Historians have posited that because Taiwan and South Korea shared similar experiences of governance—first on the periphery of the Qing Empire, then incorporated into the Japanese Empire, and finally as American protectorates during the Cold War—their modern medical systems were "highly contingent, contested, and pluralist," not reflecting any one colonial modernity or developmental model.[8] The legacy of Japanese imperial rule and health administration meant that after 1945, the Republic of China on Taiwan inherited infrastructure for mass vaccination and assumed control over a population that was both already free of smallpox and also accustomed to regular immunization campaigns. The involvement of Taiwan in medical diplomacy reflected the expansionist agendas of its Western allies in the Cold War as well as competition with the PRC for recognition as the legitimate government of mainland China.

This chapter's focus on Chinese medical diplomacy during the 1960s and 1970s contributes a new perspective to histories of Cold War science and medicine, which have been traditionally characterized by a focus on binary relationships between the Communist Soviet Bloc and the capitalist West.[9] Recently, anglophone scholars in science and technology studies have attempted to deprovincialize the Cold War by examining the history of science in decolonized states and nonaligned territories.[10] They have suggested that the influence of Soviet advisers, as well as the movement between the United States and China of American-educated Chinese scientists, resulted in significant exchanges and influences. Yet in socialist China, ideology was more important to science policy than the United States *or* the Soviet Union by the 1950s, so that policymaking emphasized self-reliance and the production of a distinctively Chinese science.[11] Building on this work, an analysis of transnational public health programs that investigates the PRC's involvement in South-South relations and its use of rural health interventions to create diplomatic goodwill reminds us that Cold War diplomacy was not the sole province of Soviet and Western states and their allies. The PRC promoted its vision of a self-reliant, uniquely Chinese medical science around the world.

New Vaccines and a Return to Old Patterns of Public Health, 1961–66

The model of rural health that became a hallmark of CCP medical diplomacy took shape in the 1960s. It drew upon the mass immunization programs of the 1950s described in the previous chapter as well as programs that emerged after the upheaval of that decade's end. In 1958, the Great Leap Forward was launched, with its goal the massive and rapid industrialization of the Chinese state. The consequences for public health were disastrous. This set of ambitious, overreaching central policies, with its harsh demands and high quotas for grain production alongside wildly flawed plans for industrialization, lasted for three years and resulted in widespread famine, disease, and hardship. As many as thirty-six million died. After the Leap ended in 1961, the PRC went through a period of readjustment in which the Ministry of Health regained policymaking power from CCP organs, inheriting a failing rural health system in the process. Many laborers who had assumed positions as part-time medical workers returned to farming full-time, resulting in a reduction in numbers of medical personnel by about five hundred thousand. Moreover, the construction of hospitals and employment of medical workers in cities rapidly and disproportionately exceeded that in rural areas, leading to the decentralization and collapse of the rural commune health system that had been established in the 1950s. During the economic retrenchment of these years, many medical schools closed.[12] And in the wake of the Sino-Soviet split, after 1960, Soviet advisers who had provided instruction in health administration and clinical practice were withdrawn to the Soviet Union.

Despite these challenges, the 1960s were years of relative productivity for state immunological work, when a number of diseases were successfully eliminated or "controlled" (reduced to very low incidence rates). In 1962, the Ministry of Health established a protocol that employed a "ring vaccination" strategy against smallpox. In addition to the mandate that every newborn receive a vaccine after reaching six months of age, each province, city, and autonomous region was to be divided up into six parts, and each year revaccination work was to be carried out in one of the six, so that the entire nation would be totally covered in the course of six years. This was the procedure throughout the 1960s and 1970s. It appeared to succeed. A 1979 survey of Yunnan and Tibet found no one under the age of twenty with smallpox pockmarks. Further census work revealed that about 90 percent of the population in each province bore smallpox vaccination scars, lending credence to the assertion that China had eradicated smallpox.[13]

Progress in developing immunizations against other diseases continued. In 1959, the Ministry of Health issued an order specifying its expectations for implementation of the diphtheria-tetanus combined vaccine, as well as those for diphtheria, typhoid, paratyphoid, cholera, and plague. This policy was followed by a 1963 nationwide order to strengthen the organization, leadership, and planning of immunization work. Infectious diseases continued to break out, belying the effectiveness of these orders. Most notably, in 1961, cholera erupted in Guangdong and quickly spread to nine other provinces as part of the El Tor global pandemic.[14] Nevertheless, it was in the early 1960s that vaccination against measles and Japanese encephalitis began. In 1957, at the National Vaccine and Serum Institute, Tang Feifan followed John Enders's protocol to successfully isolate and attenuate the measles virus and produce a live vaccine. During the early 1960s, researchers at the Chinese Academy of Medical Sciences worked with colleagues in Hebei and Tianjin to test a vaccine using viral strains from China and the Soviet Union in Beijing schoolchildren. The first large-scale trial took place in 1963 and 1964, immunizing six million children, and by the mid to late 1970s, measles incidence had fallen to less than one per hundred thousand people. In 1950, this figure had been roughly nine hundred per hundred thousand. Although the National Vaccine and Serum Institute had distributed a killed vaccine for Japanese encephalitis from 1952 to 1957, the continued incidence of the disease led researchers to isolate new strains of the virus, although a new vaccine was not developed until the late 1970s.[15]

The introduction of polio vaccination in 1960 illustrates state capacities for vaccine production, even as the Great Leap Forward was commencing. Poliomyelitis had a relatively low incidence in China until a 1955 outbreak in Jiangsu Province, after which regular episodes occurred in major cities. The National Vaccine and Serum Institute and the Department of Virology at the Chinese Academy of Medical Sciences (Zhongguo yixue kexueyuan, formerly PUMC) were tasked with developing a vaccine. Their team was led by Gu Fangzhou, who had trained at Peking University Medical School and the Russian Academy of Medical Sciences Department of Virology before assuming a position as a researcher at the Chinese Academy of Medical Sciences.[16]

Gu first experimented with inactivated vaccines grown on tissue cultures from monkey kidneys, following procedures developed by Jonas Salk in the United States. But he and his colleagues were not able to figure out how to industrialize the process on a large scale or how to streamline the distribution of the vaccine given that it would require multiple injections over an extended period of time. The team then switched to the live, attenuated vaccine developed by Albert Sabin, Mikhail Chumakov, and others. Although Soviet aid to the PRC was rapidly decreasing during this period, the PRC received samples of the vaccine from the Soviet Union and commenced trial production in 1959.[17]

Gu later reflected on the risks his team took in using a Soviet product, saying, "The experience of other countries and the material they had published were assurance enough that the vaccine would be safe to use." A 1960 trial of four million children in fifteen cities, setting up city-specific groups under a central committee, was successful. Several thousand medical staff volunteered for the campaign and "cooperated with residents' committees to make door-to-door visits and explain to mothers the benefit of having their children take the vaccine."[18] In 1963 and 1964, the vaccine was popularized in the cities and countryside and drastically reduced morbidity rates. By 1963, fifty million had been vaccinated against polio.[19]

In an article for the magazine *China Reconstructs*, Gu described one problem in particular: the liquid Sabin vaccine had to be shipped "at sub-freezing temperatures and must be carefully diluted and repacked in smaller units for use in the localities. This is not easy to arrange in rural areas."[20] While the context of Gu's account, an English-language propaganda organ, would have incentivized emphasis on the hardships and challenges that PRC scientists overcame in their efforts to produce polio vaccines, it is clear that the material requirements of the Sabin vaccine for refrigeration would have been very difficult to fulfill in the infrastructural vacuum that still characterized most of rural China in the early 1960s.

In 1962, Gu's research team collaborated with Shanghai's Xinyi Pharmaceutical Plant to produce oral polio vaccines as a type of candy with a hard shell and soft center. This meant the immunizations could be transported without refrigeration in the winter, when temperatures were normally between four and eight degrees Celsius across much of the country, and they could last for several months—an achievement unmatched in the West (see fig. 1). After the success of this initial campaign, Gu set up a laboratory for further experimentation in Kunming. In 1971, researchers there completed development of an attenuated

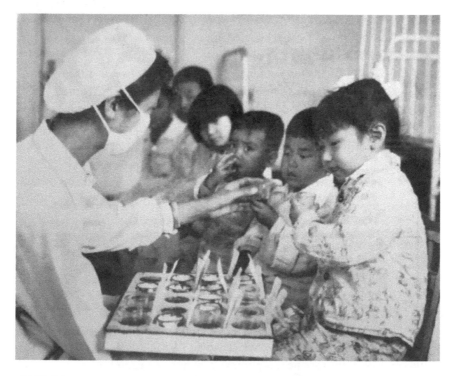

FIGURE 7.1   Candied polio vaccines being distributed to schoolchildren, 1963. Gu, "Mass Vaccination against Polio," 28.

live vaccine using indigenous viral strains.[21] Yunnan thus continued to play a key role in vaccine development and research.

Barefoot Doctors and Revolutionary Medicine

Polio was an urban disease in China, but by the mid-1960s the focus of health policy was moving away from the cities. The dramatic expansion of rural health had significant precedents in the rural reconstruction movements of the 1930s and the medical training initiatives that began in the 1950s, but most narratives attribute the impetus for its large-scale expansion to a specific moment in 1965, at the very top of the PRC leadership. On June 26, Mao Zedong issued a directive on public health in which he famously criticized the elite, urban focus of the Ministry of Health, finally instructing health administrators to focus their efforts on rural populations. Even before this speech, in the early 1960s, the ministry had already implemented a hierarchical, integrated network of institutions in which county clinics connected rural health services to elite urban hospitals.[22]

These developments in rural health care took on greater significance after the outbreak of the Cultural Revolution, when Mao launched a mass movement that incited urban Chinese youth to rise up against older, more senior party authorities—some of whom were attempting to limit Mao's personal power. The revolution is remembered today largely as a decade of terror and upheaval, only ending with Mao's death in 1976. During the movement, almost all medical schools closed their doors to advanced training. And with the rise of young "Red Guards" who attacked elders and experts for being counterrevolutionary, many physicians with advanced training, professors at medical schools, and other experts in the health sciences were politically persecuted and sent to the countryside.[23]

Yet the revolutionary era was also a period when China's health-care system was widely acknowledged as a remarkably efficient and successful means of providing medical care to the countryside. Recently, Sigrid Schmalzer and Miriam Gross have called for a rethinking of science and medicine in the Cultural Revolution, suggesting that despite the persecution and hardship experienced by many experts, it was a productive period for agricultural development and antischistosomiasis campaigns.[24] The history of mass immunization during the Cultural Revolution presents a complex picture. Major research developments did not occur in the late 1960s and early 1970s. Yet as a regular part of rural health work, large-scale vaccination did contribute fundamentally to the success of a public health system that attracted increasing attention from political leaders and the outside world.

After the Cultural Revolution launched in 1966, political directives to uplift the rural proletariat meant that barefoot doctors became highly visible providers of health care. One of the key responsibilities of these medical workers was to undertake vaccination and other epidemic prevention methods alongside implementing revolutionary thought, encouraging family planning, and demonstrating self-reliance.[25] Barefoot doctors' manuals provided instructions on how to give the kinds of intradermal injections typically required in vaccination. A section on preventive inoculations from one manual published in Hunan Province gave a brief overview of the significance of immunization to the mandate to focus on preventive health and the different kinds of active and passive immunity. The piece instructed, "Plan a vaccination program for the production team (brigade), based on the size of the team and prevailing epidemic conditions. When vaccinations are given, it is best to adopt a centralized mass approach, supplemented by individual vaccinations. Keep records."[26] A sample vaccine schedule mandated vaccination of infants and young children against tuberculosis, smallpox, pertussis, poliomyelitis, diphtheria, Japanese encephalitis, and typhoid.[27]

By the early 1970s, vaccines were a visible and substantive part of the work of barefoot doctors and rural health more broadly.[28] Medical propaganda emphasized immunization activities throughout this period. For instance, a poster of the Beijing Tuberculosis Prevention and Treatment Office from around the year 1965 displayed a woman with a peasant's straw hat shouting into a megaphone with the Red Cross emblazoned on it (see fig. 2). Large red characters proclaimed underneath, "Children must prevent tuberculosis! Quickly get the BCG vaccine!"[29] Insets presented a series of images displaying the immunization process in detail. And a *People's Daily* article from 1975 on vaccination work in Shaanxi Province began with the note, "Since the Cultural Revolution began, most of the medical workers and barefoot doctors in our county have followed the guidance of Chairman Mao to 'put prevention first' and carried out rural health work, vigorously implementing every kind of vaccination."[30]

While immunization constituted one of the activities expected of barefoot doctors, it is less clear how assiduously individual workers obeyed this mandate or how strictly they followed the guidance set forth in handbooks and manuals. Certainly the 1979 struggles of Zhao Kai to identify potential sites of smallpox infection in Tibet suggest that record keeping in the 1960s and 1970s was often imperfect. Yet many infectious diseases came under "control" during this period, meaning that their incidence was lowered dramatically. Standard narratives of medical history in China state that from the 1950s onward, plague, cholera, leishmaniasis, and measles were, by this definition, controlled. When WHO representatives Frank Fenner and Joel Breman traveled to China in 1979, they attributed

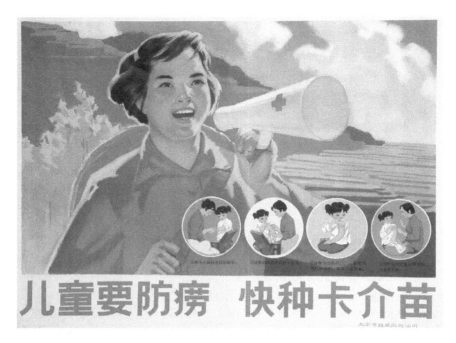

FIGURE 7.2   "Children must prevent tuberculosis! Quickly get the BCG vaccine!," circa 1965. Beijing shi jiehebing fangzhi suo, "Ertong yao fanglao." Courtesy of United States National Library of Medicine.

the control of these diseases in part to the "careful planning, organization and execution" of immunization programs.[31]

The Role of Vaccines in Chinese Medical Diplomacy

The PRC promoted a model of public health in which mass immunization explicitly contributed to rural disease prevention. It publicized this model on a global stage via medical diplomacy. This strategy was part of a longstanding tradition in the PRC of using cultural and social media to improve international relations. From the early 1950s on, the CCP had established cultural cooperation with other Soviet-aligned states that included student exchanges, tours of music and dramatic arts groups, participation in international competitions and festivals, and translation of literature for circulation around the Soviet Bloc.[32] In the 1960s, after the Sino-Soviet split, the PRC continued to engage in programs of cultural diplomacy but with a new geographic and strategic focus: the nonaligned "Third World," where the CCP sought to exert power and influence. These transnational interventions reflected the mainland regime's competition with a rival across the Taiwan Strait. The PRC used medical diplomacy to compete fiercely with the Republic of China on Taiwan for influence, goodwill, and—most of all—recognition as the legitimate ruling government of "one China" that included both the mainland and Taiwan.

In the PRC, this form of diplomacy consisted of the provision of medical aid to other non-Western states as well as the extension of invitations to physicians and researchers from foreign countries to visit China. These efforts ranged around the globe, from Southeast Asia to Latin America. The most robust programs, however, were established in Africa. There, representatives of the PRC presented their country as a provider of aid lacking the imperialist motivations that had characterized European interventions on the continent. Like many recently decolonized African states, the PRC had undergone its own anticolonial conflicts. Its diplomats emphasized this shared experience and their interest in building equitable relationships that would assist African nations but not interfere in their domestic affairs. Chinese medical aid typically took the form of teams of physicians, supplies, educational materials, and occasionally student-exchange programs. It was often concomitant with other forms of military, economic, and agricultural assistance. For instance, in 1962, the PRC sent twenty-one tons of medical supplies along with wheat and rolled steel to Algeria, which had just declared its sovereignty after an eight-year war with France for its independence. And on July 31, 1964, representatives of the PRC signed a treaty agreeing to medical cooperation with North Vietnam during a period when China was also providing Hanoi with military assistance in resisting the US-backed South Vietnamese government.[33]

In establishing programs of medical diplomacy, the PRC promoted the system of rural medical care its Ministry of Health had instituted. For instance, starting in 1964, the PRC sent teams of physicians to the newly formed United Republic of Tanzania. These groups helped establish a health program based on the Chinese barefoot doctor model and funded the construction of a laboratory for manufacture of vaccines and other biological products. In addition to providing clinical care, teams' work in supporting rural medical services included training medical personnel, administering hospitals, and conducting health demonstrations in villages. One of the impacts of Chinese intervention on Tanzanian health policy was the latter's adoption of a policy of free mass vaccination alongside expanded health education programs and the commune clinic model.[34]

Vaccines, sera, and drugs were critical to the success of Chinese medical aid abroad. They were an important part of the model of rural health that the PRC sought to promulgate because they were quantifiable, portable materials that could produce rapid results in disease prevention and treatment. For instance, in February 1961, China sent one hundred cases of drugs to the newly independent Republic of Guinea, along with forty-five hundred tons of rice, cinema projectors, an x-ray machine, and electrical generators. In February 1965, it sent aid to drought-stricken Somalia that included 438 cases of medical drugs and equipment as well as twelve hundred tons of rice. In 1966, the Chinese Red Cross Society sent fifty thousand milliliters of unspecified vaccine to its sister society in Nepal after an earthquake struck the country. And in 1971, the PRC donated cholera vaccines as well as the equivalent of $2.5 million to the nation of Chad after an outbreak of cholera there. A year later, that country recognized the CCP as the legitimate ruler of mainland China. In similar fashion, five months after the PRC sent three hundred thousand doses of measles vaccine and large quantities of antibiotics to the government of famine-stricken Upper Volta (now Burkina Faso) in 1973, the latter recognized the regime in Beijing.[35]

Even after the Cultural Revolution broke out in 1966, then, China continued to send medical aid abroad. From 1963 to the early 2000s, over fifteen thousand Chinese medical workers went to forty-seven different African nations.[36] Insofar as it was meant to improve overall relationships between the PRC and these countries, medical diplomacy worked. It was at least a contributing factor in African states' recognition of the PRC, and disavowal of the Republic of China on Taiwan, as the legitimate authority of China. Throughout the 1950s and 1960s, a succession of African states established formal relations with the PRC—nineteen in total.[37] Yet formal recognition by other states was not the only purpose of Chinese medical diplomacy. The PRC also promoted its system of rural medical care as a model for the future of global health governance.

Chinese Health Care in Western Eyes

The PRC sent medical teams and equipment to Africa, Southeast Asia, and other parts of the decolonized world. It also sought to disseminate the ideologies underlying its public health programs on a global stage. Throughout the 1960s and 1970s, the CCP promulgated texts and images that described and praised in English and other Western languages the activities of Chinese barefoot doctors and other medical workers. After relations with the United States resumed in 1971, China invited delegations from the US and Western Europe to witness firsthand the achievements of the nation's public health programs—albeit in highly controlled settings designed to impress these selected foreign visitors. It succeeded in selling them a model of medical care for impoverished rural populations. Upon return to their home countries, delegates promoted Chinese medical administration as a model for the ideal of primary health care then arising in spheres of international health governance. Analysis of these Chinese engagements with Western audiences and their roles in discourses of international health shows that mass immunization and the eradication of smallpox played key roles in the promotion of China as a model for primary care because they provided verifiable evidence of the effectiveness of China's medical system.

In the 1960s, the Western world started hearing about developments in public health in China, largely via English-language periodicals that the PRC published and circulated. During the Cultural Revolution, the *Chinese Medical Journal*— the official publication of the Chinese Medical Association, which had been published in English and Chinese—was renamed *China's Medicine* and published under this name from 1966 to 1968. In addition to the requisite speeches and writings of Mao Zedong, it printed occasional research articles as well as a "News and Notes" section that discussed Chinese medical work abroad. Other foreign-language periodicals that published articles related to medicine included the widely circulated *China Pictorial* and *China Reconstructs*, which specifically aimed at encouraging the sympathies of readers in the capitalist West and its former and remaining colonies. The China International Bookstore distributed these magazines abroad; by 1964, it had contracted with 738 companies in ninety-one countries.[38]

In addition to official propaganda organs, other publications found their way outside China's borders and into non-Chinese languages. The barefoot doctors' manual from Hunan Province mentioned above was translated into English and published in 1974 by the John E. Fogarty International Center for Advanced Study in the Health Sciences in Bethesda, Maryland. Part of the National Institutes of Health and established in 1968, this institute was the only branch of the NIH dedicated exclusively to promoting global health, supporting the interests of its namesake, a Democratic representative from Rhode Island. Several years later Cloudburst Press, a small independent press based in British Columbia and affiliated with the counterculture movement, republished the manual. It sold well, going through two reprintings in 1977 and 1978.

The manual was an instructive plan, not a report of the work actually done by barefoot doctors. Likewise, propaganda organs had every motivation to present a rosy view of medical care in China. Yet from the 1960s onward, Americans tended to agree that the PRC had experienced a rapid and remarkable transformation in health since 1949. William Chen, a medical officer at NIH, used *Chinese Medical Journal* articles and English translations of other Chinese journal articles by the US Department of Commerce to produce a survey of health in China in 1961. "Since the Communist Party took over China, greater strides have been made in the improvement of sanitation, health education and prevention and control of common infectious and parasitic diseases," he wrote in glowing tones. "Hand in hand with public health work, clinical medicine is claimed to have contributed to the total disappearance of cholera in China. Plague and smallpox are said to have been eradicated. Typhus, relapsing fever and other 'notifiable' or 'reportable' infectious diseases have been brought under control." Chen attributed this success in large part to the Four Pests Campaign to eradicate vectors of disease during the Great Leap Forward and—rather vaguely—to the "effectiveness of Chinese Communist organizational techniques."[39]

A report by the Fogarty Center was more reserved in its praise, describing the 1950s and early 1960s as a period of stable pharmaceutical manufacturing "with serums and vaccines of acceptable quality being mass-produced, and mass-inoculation campaigns carried out" and noting the development of vaccines against Japanese encephalitis and trachoma as being "of potential interest to Western medicine." James Chen, director of medical research at the California Medical Group, stressed the equivalence of Chinese biomedical work with that of Euro-American contemporaries. "The pharmaceutical industry has kept pace with modern technology including drug synthesis," he noted, going on to say that "regarding biological agents, all common antibiotics and biologicals currently used in the West have reached the production stage in China today."[40] Chen did not specify his sources, but his assertion that Chinese pharmaceutical production was "modern" and "Western" belied an assumption that it had undergone great change to become so since 1949.

Some firsthand accounts complemented these reports of transformative governance. The authors were all individuals who had demonstrated loyalty to the Communist cause before 1949 and who correspondingly had little to criticize about the PRC or its public health. Most notable was the narrative of Joshua Horn, a British physician and Communist who was welcomed to the PRC as a health consultant and lived there from 1954. In a book published after his return to Britain in 1969, he praised China's rural medical service system. "In accordance with policy," he wrote of local medical brigades, "preventive work is given priority. All children are immunized against infectious diseases by a travelling inoculation team which visits the villages whenever primary immunization or 'booster' doses become due" (see fig 7.3). Horn made an explicit comparison to pre-1949 conditions, adopting characterizations of radical change that also appeared in Chinese magazines and other propaganda. "Before Liberation only vaccination against smallpox was available for the rural population and this involved a journey to the country town and the payment of about ten pounds of grain. Now," he claimed, "immunization is free and, to express their appreciation and also to encourage the children to regard the doctors as friends rather than enemies, the villagers make the inoculation team's visit a festive occasion." Horn also repeated prevalent claims about rapid and effective disease control.

"Smallpox, typhoid, diphtheria, infantile paralysis [polio] and whooping cough have now practically disappeared from this area and recently Chinese medical scientists have developed a method of active immunization against measles which has greatly reduced its incidence and severity."[41] The representativeness of Horn's experience is debatable. Yet again we see a key claim for the efficacy of Chinese health care premised upon the control of epidemic diseases using mass vaccination, as well as quarantine, disinfection, and other methods.

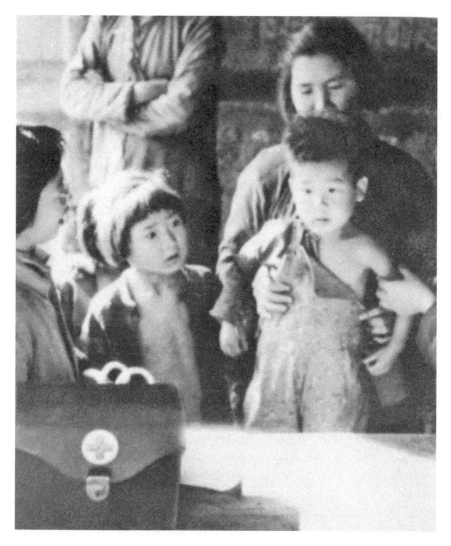

FIGURE 7.3   "A village inoculation team at work." Horn, *Away with All Pests*, 89. Reproduced courtesy of Monthly Review Press.

Popular accounts joined those written by medical specialists. The American journalist Edgar Snow had received international acclaim for *Red Star over China*, an account of his time embedded among CCP troops in Yan'an during the Second Sino-Japanese War. The book heavily praised the Communist regime, and the PRC invited Snow to return to the country in 1960. Snow's account of this trip described his experiences with China's health-care system, in part through the eyes of Lebanese American doctor George Hatem. Hatem had come to China to aid the CCP during the war, then remained in the PRC as a sympathizer who consulted on medical affairs and consequently received Chinese citizenship. At an airport, Snow discovered he had lost his immunization card and was given new vaccinations on the spot for a perfunctory charge of one yuan (forty cents). "Control of preventable and communicable diseases combined with state protection and care of mothers has sharply reduced the adult death rate while increasing live births," wrote Snow, repeating a familiar line.[42] The implication was that disease control had contributed to a demographic transition, a theoretical shift from higher to lower birth and death rates in a population as a consequence of its industrialization. This observation tacitly linked epidemic control to family planning: in such a transition, both the birth and death rates fell. Vaccination could lower death rates, but it was the task of reproductive controls to lower fertility rates.

PRC officials were incentivized to stress China's successful control of infectious diseases as a sign of its transition not just to a new demographic stage but also to economic and technological modernity. After 1971, political change brought new opportunities for foreigners to observe medicine in China directly. Yet the China that they observed was typically carefully mediated to showcase the accomplishments of the socialist state. *New York Times* journalist James Reston gave a very public, and positive, view of Chinese health care in 1971 when he covered President Richard M. Nixon's historic visit to the country. After developing appendicitis, Reston underwent an appendectomy at the Beijing Anti-Imperialist Hospital, formerly PUMC. His subsequent article in the *Times*, "Now, about My Operation in Peking," lauded the surgeons who treated him and the doctors of Chinese medicine who gave him pain relief with acupuncture and herbal drugs.[43] A few months after Reston's experience, in September 1971, an American delegation comprising four physicians and their wives traveled to the PRC at the invitation of the Chinese Medical Association. More visits followed, and as Zhou Xun has demonstrated, their members became exponents of China's public health systems. These delegates were often sympathetic to the Communist cause and predisposed to praise China. In general, state agents carefully managed their observations and interactions.[44] The veracity of their experiences, however, is less interesting than the evidence these visitors cited in support of their advocacy for

Chinese medical achievements. The eradication of smallpox and control of many infectious diseases was a particular achievement that many of them cited in their promotion of the Chinese model.

Victor and Ruth Sidel, a physician and a psychiatric social worker, respectively, who went to China as part of the initial 1971 delegation, are perhaps the most famous of these exponents. Already sympathetic to the Communist cause before their visit, they were so impressed by their Chinese hosts that after their return to the United States, they published numerous works and gave public lectures praising health care in China, especially the barefoot doctor programs.[45] The Sidels specifically stressed the responsibility that rural health workers took for distributing vaccines. "Immunizations are an important responsibility of the barefoot doctor, but again are often done by the 'health workers'" who had been trained by the former, Victor explained. "At the health center of the Mai Chia Wu production brigade of the West Lake People's Commune near Hangchow [Hangzhou], for example, Mai Jen-chai, one of the two barefoot doctors, showed us the detailed immunization records for each child in the 251 families of the brigade." He claimed that the Chinese rural healthcare program was a system the United States ought to emulate. "There are, I believe, a number of lessons for us in the Chinese experience with barefoot doctors and other health workers."[46]

Philip Lee, a professor of social medicine at the University of California, San Francisco, traveled in China as part of a delegation of American physicians in June and July 1973. Like the Sidels, Lee noted the steep decline in infectious diseases, writing, "Major epidemic diseases have been controlled, and in some cases apparently eradicated." Praising preventive medicine in the PRC, he wrote, "Stress has been placed on environmental sanitation, health education, immunization, maternal and child health and the control of communicable diseases. The results have been impressive by any standard." And like the Sidels, Lee praised the organizational capabilities of the CCP as the key factor enabling the success of hygiene campaigns in the PRC. "The mass inoculation and clean-up campaigns depend more on efficient organization and widespread propaganda (or publicity) than on large expenditures of money and highly trained personnel," he wrote.[47] Lee's account, like others, consistently referenced immunization and the eradication of smallpox as landmark achievements of the PRC alongside the barefoot doctor system and cooperative medical services.

Such high praise attracted broader attention to mainland China as a potential model for new strategies in public health. A 1975 documentary film titled *Barefoot Doctors of Rural China* by the United States Agency for International Development, the primary American government organization responsible for administering civilian foreign aid, set forth this idea with some force.[48] Narrator Diane Li noted, "Cholera and other waterborne diseases have been controlled by the paramedics through mass immunization campaigns. But the lasting success of their efforts can also be attributed to an increased concern for sanitation."[49] Like visitors and analysts, Li balanced consideration of the barefoot doctor system with an assertion of the competence of the Chinese Ministry of Health. "Although they join the largest population that China has ever known, in terms of health and medical care this generation will be the most privileged in China's history," said Li at the end of the film. "These young children receive regular checkups and vaccinations administered by barefoot doctors who will attend to their medical needs for the rest of their lives." One of the closing scenes of the film is a queue of schoolchildren waiting to receive inoculations from medical workers.[50]

The efficacy of mass immunization lent credibility to the other claims that these authors discussed, from the practical value of the barefoot doctors to the efficacy of acupuncture anesthesia. The latter programs and therapies were new, unusual endeavors in a distant land that few foreigners had visited, but in the eyes of Americans and Europeans, mass vaccination was reliable and, in the case of smallpox, demonstrably effective in controlling diseases. Although the previous chapters have shown the substantial work of Chinese actors in developing, producing, and distributing vaccines, the observers discussed here saw immunization as a technology with thoroughly Western origins. The Chinese state's adoption of large-scale vaccination, in their eyes, was therefore an indication of its modernization and successful adoption of Western practices.

The CCP itself promoted this view, most notably in the case of a dispute over vaccination requirements for travel. In July 1967, the Soviet Union began requiring Chinese citizens entering its borders to produce certificates of vaccination against smallpox and cholera. The PRC responded with a statement of protest, describing the move as a "grave step taken by the Soviet revisionist ruling clique in uniting with the United States to oppose China." The PRC objected, too, to the Soviet Union's announcement of this requirement through the WHO, which it described as "an agency of the United Nations which is a tool of US imperialism."[51] For the Soviets to impose such a condition—after a 1960 agreement with China specifically ending any such requirement—constituted an implicit claim that China had not, in fact, eradicated smallpox or controlled cholera. If vaccination served as a transnational standard of public health, imposing a requirement for Chinese travelers crossing borders to show vaccination certificates reflected a lack of trust in the Chinese ability to vaccinate. The Chinese protest of the Soviet policy suggested that the successful—and public—control of infectious diseases was a valuable, even critical benchmark for national modernization. It provided a basis for trust between nations, or the lack thereof, that had larger ramifications in the broader sphere of Cold War politics.

The PRC as a Model for Health-Care Reforms

The PRC opened its doors to foreign delegations just as the field of international health experienced a backlash against the technocratic, top-down approaches that had characterized the work of the WHO, the Rockefeller Foundation, and allied groups in the 1950s and 1960s. In the wake of failed efforts to eradicate malaria, these agencies were subject to criticism from fellow policymakers, health practitioners, and the governments of developing nations, all of whom tended to favor an alternative focus on "primary health care." The success of rural medical care in the PRC suggested that it could provide a model for this new priority in health governance.

The concept of primary health care has a long history, one that is as Chinese as it is Western or global. The 1937 Bandung Conference by the League of Nations Health Organization had recommended a decentralized approach to health interventions that provided "the greatest benefit to the health of the rural populations, at the smallest cost."[52] The term itself may have first occurred in the early 1970s in a publication of the Christian Medical Commission, a member organization of the World Council of Churches that supported grassroots health movements by training rural health workers and supplying them with basic drugs.[53] The ascendance of primary health care as a specific goal for WHO policymaking began in the late 1960s, after a number of Western health administrators and policymakers published condemnations of the kind of "vertical" approach, using highly technological, non-context-specific methods and characteristically employing mass vaccination, that the WHO had exemplified in its failed malaria-eradication program. The global economic recessions of the 1970s and the famines that resulted from the withdrawal of aid to places such as sub-Saharan Africa provided patent evidence that these interventions had failed to provide for the basic needs of populations. One critic, the physician and Rockefeller Foundation consultant John Bryant, wrote, "The most serious health needs [of the developing world] cannot be met by teams with spray guns and vaccinating syringes."[54]

The result was a widespread movement for a different, more "horizontal" approach to public health, one that sought to promote a kind of public health that prioritized the needs of local communities and the attainment of social equality, which took as its goal the principle of "Health for All by the Year 2000." The then director general of the WHO, Halfdan Mahler, and others promoted primary health care. A number of other models for health care were suggested to articulate such a policy. WHO consultant Carl Taylor suggested that Indian rural medicine could be such a model. The American biologist and health worker David Werner published a public health manual, *Donde No Hay Doctor* (*Where There Is No Doctor*), which championed the cause of community participation in health provision and provided basic clinical advice drawn from the experiences of health workers in rural Mexico. It sold over three million copies. *Health by the People*, a volume edited by WHO officer Kenneth Newell and published in English, Japanese, Nepali, French, Russian, and Spanish, provided a range of examples of primary health care. In addition to a piece by Victor and Ruth Sidel on the PRC, contributions discussed public health in Cuba, Guatemala, Iran, Niger, Venezuela, and other nations.[55]

Yet China was an especially prominent archetype of primary health care. Historian Marcos Cueto cites the barefoot doctor programs and their concomitant "massive expansion of rural medical services in Communist China" as an "important inspiration for primary health care." Sung Lee makes a similar claim that China's rejoining the WHO in 1973 provided a model for health care that challenged the prevailing ideology that WHO should diffuse the practices and standards of Western professional medicine around the world. A 2008 WHO publication itself claimed, "China's barefoot doctors were a major inspiration to the primary health care movement leading up to the conference in Alma Ata."[56] The Chinese experience provided a model for the expansion of rural health in which primary health care was defined as a program that combined strong local leadership, grassroots labor, mass education, and "affordable, low-tech prevention activities."[57] But a relatively high-tech strategy typically allied with vertical health interventions—mass immunization—legitimized that experience and model.

Alma-Ata and the Legacy of Mass Immunization in Primary Health Care

From the sixth to the twelfth of September 1978, the World Health Assembly held an International Conference on Primary Health Care. The meeting convened in Alma-Ata, capital of the Kazakh Soviet Socialist Republic. This location was no accident: after the PRC suggested the need for a meeting that would establish WHO commitment to the cause of primary health care and as a result of competition between Soviet states and Maoist-aligned states, the Soviet Union offered $2 million in support, on the condition that the meeting take place within the Soviet Bloc. The result was the Alma-Ata Declaration—a document that articulated an imperative for primary health-care services, designed with community input to meet local needs, to be the means of attaining the WHO goal of "health for all" by the year 2000. If health was indeed a fundamental human right and one that underlay economic development, then only by understanding it as a state of well-being, and not the absence of disease, could an international organization like the WHO achieve such an aim. The declaration suggested that global health organizations ought to focus on new strategies, such as "appropriate technologies" and the creation of local clinics in rural areas, rather than the highly targeted interventions and urban hospital centers of the vertical approach.[58]

Chinese contributions to the adoption of primary health care as a global health strategy have been underrecognized. The Chinese delegation had originally proposed the idea for the Alma-Ata conference. Yet it was not present at the conference because it was held on Soviet territory and Sino-Soviet relations were at a low point following the border conflicts of 1969.[59] Its delegation therefore did not participate in the sessions of the conference and was not one of the signatories of the declaration. Moreover, despite active Chinese involvement in medical diplomacy around the world, the PRC proved uncooperative in dealing with the major international health organization, the WHO. On September 26, 1977, the WHO regional office sent a telegram to Beijing asking for the date of the last case of smallpox, the current state of epidemiological surveillance, what legislation and policies governed vaccination, and what laboratory stocks of variola were held and where. The reply from Beijing to Geneva, on October 24, 1977, simply stated that various government institutions held stocks of *Variola* virus. "The reaction of the Chinese seemed to be one of indifference to the opinion of the rest of the world," reads a retrospective account published by the WHO. "They seemed to feel that no one need doubt their word that smallpox had been eliminated from China many years earlier."[60] Until, that is, surveys in India suggested that Tibetans had caught smallpox in China in the early 1960s, casting doubt on official narratives. And so we return to the mission of the virologist Zhao Kai in Lhasa, where he and two colleagues sought unsuccessfully to determine the source of rumors that smallpox persisted.

Faced with a dearth of documentation and no clear source for these accounts, Zhao ultimately turned to astronomy to explain the discrepancy between Tibetan and Chinese narratives. Zhao suggested to his superiors that the Tibetans may have given the WHO a date based on the Tibetan calendar, which is lunisolar rather than solar, "so that it was thought to be 1962 and actually wasn't," and that Tibetan methods of age reckoning, which add a year to actual ages, might have also led to the misunderstanding that smallpox had broken out in 1962.[61]

WHO officials accepted this explanation and the work of Chinese authorities in investigating smallpox in Tibet. The date of smallpox eradication was thus fixed as 1960, with the final case of Hu Xiaofa. But as Zhao himself says of this explanation: "It's not totally proven, it's speculation."[62] Retrospective accounts now note that there had been one case of smallpox in Rikeze, Tibet, following importation from Nepal in 1962 and five cases there in 1964. The 2003 documentary includes close-up images of a report confirming that smallpox had been eliminated in China by 1960. It reads, "Zhao Kai recommends that if anyone doesn't believe this, then who can, amidst the crowded masses, find one youth of around twenty years of age with a pockmarked face?"[63]

The politics of smallpox reflected a larger geopolitics. China could disavow the Tibetan exiles as not under its jurisdiction but only at the cost of giving up the authority over them that it claimed. The government was so unwilling to do this that it sent three employees of the National Vaccine and Serum Institute to Tibet to conduct an exhaustive survey. This incident demonstrates that smallpox eradication in China happened around 1960, but it was more or less arbitrary; that epidemics and borders signaled a critical intersection of state and biological security that could have significant consequences on the global political scene during the Cold War, even as a matter of history; and that staff from the former National Epidemic Prevention Bureau continued to play a critical role in the determination of health politics. Public health was an arena in which the broader political authority of the PRC could be confirmed or contested. Trust played a key role here. The PRC asked the WHO to accept its eradication of smallpox on faith, and it did.

Epilogue

By the end of the socialist period in 1978, a new generation of immunologists and bacteriologists was beginning to rise to prominence, although the Cultural Revolution had broadly impeded and delayed education in this field. Many founding figures in modern Chinese immunology were by this time retired or dead. In 1957, Wei Xi took up a position as researcher at the Chinese Academy of Medical Sciences, eventually becoming head of the microbiology research group there. He had a long and productive career, publishing a variety of clinical textbooks on bacteriology and immunology before passing away in 1989 at the age of eighty-six.[1] Xie Shaowen had a similarly productive career. After a stint in the military at the PLA's Academy of Medical Sciences, Xie returned in 1962 to his old post at PUMC, then called the China Medical University. He also held a research post at the Chinese Academy of Medical Sciences. Aside from a brief period during the Cultural Revolution, Xie seems to have escaped major political persecution during the upheavals of the later twentieth century. He was elected to the Chinese Academy of Sciences in 1980 before dying in 1995 at the age of ninety-two.[2]

Tang Feifan did not share in the fates of his colleagues. He died in 1958, a few years after making the discovery that would define his career. Before the Second Sino-Japanese War broke out, Tang had focused his research on trachoma, a disease that was estimated to have affected over one third of the population of Republican China.[3] After the founding of the PRC, Tang resumed this work. Identifying the cause of trachoma had become a major goal of microbiology researchers around the world, and Tang is largely remembered as the first scientist to successfully do this in 1955, when he identified, isolated, and cultivated the bacterium *Chlamydia trachomatis*.[4] In 1981, the International Organization against Trachoma posthumously awarded Tang a gold medal for this research. A bronze statue of Tang has been erected in front of the National Vaccine and Serum Institute in Beijing, and in 1992, the PRC issued a postage stamp to commemorate his achievement.[5]

But in the late 1950s, success in the laboratory did not correlate with political invulnerability. Tang was labeled as a rightist "white flag" (an enemy of the state who ideologically opposed the CCP), probably because of his foreign connections—but also, perhaps, his time in Kunming. During the later years of the Second Sino-Japanese War, the capital of Yunnan had become a hotbed of political activity for intellectuals who opposed the coming civil war between Nationalist and Communist Parties. These antiwar activists were persecuted—and in some cases, assassinated—by the Nationalist Party, and when the CCP came to power, it also denounced these activists for not supporting it. Tang's time in Yunnan, and more significantly his status as the son-in-law of the Nationalist official He Jian, may have contributed to his uncertain ideological position. In 1955, he was rejected for membership in the Chinese Academy of Sciences on political grounds, although he was eventually appointed two years later.[6]

In 1957, the CCP launched a national antirightist campaign, and Tang fell prey to its persecutions. Following the "Hundred Flowers" movement, which encouraged academics and intellectuals to voice their political opinions freely, the CCP initiated a crackdown on these elements of society.[7] In late September, the party secretary at the National Vaccine and Serum Institute made a visit to Tang's office and advised him to submit to a self-criticism session in which he would confess to anti-Communist thoughts and invite denunciation from his colleagues. The session was held over two days on September 28 and 29 and became increasingly heated. Tang's biographer Liu Juanxiang reports that by the second day, Tang was forced to stand with his head lowered as people shouted at him, "All your experiments were done by other people for you, and you exploited the labor of other people to win fame and fortune for yourself!" and "Why did you share the trachoma virus with foreigners? Why did you tell foreigners about the methods of isolating the virus? How many scientific secrets have you sold? What benefits have you gotten from it? Confess and tell us the truth!"[8] The following morning, September 30, 1958, Tang hung himself at his home in Beijing. A year later, C. E. Lim, a professor at PUMC, wrote that instead of committing suicide, Tang "should have faced the music!" If Tang had lived, Lim implied, he would have been rehabilitated, with his reputation restored, rather than died under a cloud of political suspicion.[9]

Tang died at a pivotal moment in the history of the PRC. In 1958, China was descending into the fearsome grip of famine—and so, even though the biological production Tang oversaw at the National Vaccine and Serum Institute may have preserved lives, it was only for the short term. The Great Leap Forward began, provincial officials declared record reaping rates for harvests they had never sown, and thirty-six million people perished. How many people were saved from epidemic disease and a swift end at the hands of cholera or plague, only to die a slow and agonizing death from hunger or edema? It is this bleak calculus that ultimately characterizes our understanding of mass immunization and its role in the demographic transformations of twentieth-century China.

Historians have argued that emphases on eradicating disease in the early PRC arose from recent experiences of total war, environmental disaster, and anticolonial revolutionary sentiment.[10] Yet the history of vaccination in China shows that the adoption of mass immunization to eradicate disease entailed longer, more complex processes of institutionalization, cooperation, and organization. China became the focus of increasingly comprehensive epidemic-control programs in the first decades of the twentieth century. When the war with Japan broke out, vaccination became a central focus for research, manufacturing, and clinical testing during outbreaks of cholera, typhoid fever, and plague. Researchers and physicians who gathered in the wartime hinterlands developed a novel vaccine production-and-distribution system that sought to vaccinate all members of the public in both rural and urban areas against a host of diseases.

This book has shown that the rise of mass vaccination against multiple diseases in China contributed new methods, materials, and manpower to the global development of immunology. Kunming, the capital of Yunnan Province, was a major center of research and development, but we have seen that it was not the only site of its kind. The research and production of vaccines was a common endeavor that linked many cities across the wartime hinterlands. International biomedical interest groups facilitated Chinese development of a variety of vaccines and brought cholera vaccines from Buenos Aires, Bucharest, and Cairo to Chongqing. The links between Chinese researchers and colleagues working with the League of Nations, ABMAC, and other international organizations facilitated Chinese contributions to immunology, making the field more transnational in character long after the end of war.

After 1949, the widespread distribution of vaccines in the early PRC was a state-building process as much as a health intervention. It required massive governmental investment, not only in the production of vaccines but also in the training of teams to persuade—and compel—individuals to get immunized. Vaccination came to characterize the experiences of people under the CCP alongside other, more explicit forms of defining citizenship in the PRC, such as being issued a household registration booklet or being assigned to a work unit.

And for most people, a direct experience of the Chinese state, in addition to the aforementioned registrations and work units, was its insistence on immunizing their bodies. Mass immunization thus provided a key opportunity for the party to use discourses of health and biology to consolidate state power and authority. Even though the party defined its new universal, free vaccination policies in opposition to the previous Nationalist state, these policies built upon the foundations that that Republican state had established to accomplish comprehensive immunization work against smallpox and other diseases.

The mass vaccination programs that the PRC sponsored were consonant with broader interests in eradicating disease that emerged in the field of international health during the mid-twentieth century. While the WHO fixed its efforts on eliminating malaria in developing countries, the PRC sought to stamp out infectious diseases, inadvertently anticipating the WHO's eventual focus on smallpox eradication in the 1970s.[11] Chinese mass immunization contributed to this global focus on disease eradication—not just insofar as it permitted the elimination of smallpox in the world's most populous nation but also because the success of this practice contributed to its consolidation as a top-down, highly technological, ultimately successful strategy for international health, even as the PRC used its successful control of infectious diseases to promote an alternative vision of global health governance that focused on local needs and primary health care.

Despite the erosion of many programs that had delivered vaccines and other health services to large rural populations, mass immunization has continued after the economic reforms of the 1980s as a mandatory, regular practice of childhood health in China. A baby born in the PRC, much like her counterparts in the United States and Europe, is given a battery of mandatory shots by the age of two that provides protection against diphtheria, tetanus, pertussis, measles, mumps, rubella, and other illnesses—and including the BCG and oral polio vaccines.[12] These vaccinations are administered against a backdrop of growing environmental crisis and rising pharmaceutical safety concerns. The ailments that will concern her parents are no longer infectious diseases such as plague or cholera but rather environmentally triggered diseases such as allergies and asthma. By 2010, cancer, respiratory disease, cardiovascular disease, and other chronic illnesses replaced infectious diseases as the primary causes of death.[13] China's twentieth century thus saw a remarkable transformation in causes and scales of mortality. The establishment of a universal, mandatory immunization system in the mid-twentieth century helped make that transformation, and its surveillance, possible.

Notes

The following abbreviations are used in the notes:

ABMAC Collection of the American Bureau for Medical Aid to China, Columbia
       Rare Books and Manuscripts Library, Columbia University, New York
AH   Academia Historica, Taipei, Taiwan
AS   Institute of Modern History Archives, Academia Sinica, Taipei, Taiwan
CADN   Centre des archives diplomatiques, Nantes, Pays de la Loire, France
CAOM   Centre des Archives d'Outre-mer, Aix-en-Provence, France
CMA   Chongqing Municipal Archives, Chongqing, China
CUA   Papers and Correspondence of Joseph Needham, CH, FRS, Cambridge
       University Archives, Cambridge, United Kingdom
KMA   Kunming Municipal Archives, Kunming, Yunnan, China
KMT   Kuomintang Archives, Taipei, Taiwan
LON   Archives of the League of Nations, United Nations, Geneva
NRI   Needham Research Institute, Cambridge, United Kingdom
RAC   Rockefeller Archive Center, Tarrytown, New York
RG   Record group
YPA   Yunnan Provincial Archives, Kunming, Yunnan, China

INTRODUCTION

1. Elgert, *Immunology*, 641; Fine, "Herd Immunity," 266, 295–98.

2. Chen and Chen, "China's Exceptional Health Transitions," 19; "The Sick Man of the Far East," *New York Times*, August 16, 1905.

3. Rogaski, *Hygienic Modernity*; Lei, *Neither Donkey nor Horse*; Andrews, *Making of Modern Chinese Medicine*; Core, "Tuberculosis Control in Shanghai," 128.

4. Leung, "Variolisation et vaccination"; Leung, "Business of Vaccination," 31.

5. For an example of medical histories that give scant attention to the wartime southwest, see Yip, *Health and National Reconstruction*, 176–78.

6. Lampton, *Health, Conflict*; Lucas, *Chinese Medical Modernization*; Lei, *Neither Donkey nor Horse*, 224.

7. Campbell and Sitze, "Introduction," 22.

8. Foucault, "Right of Death," 45; Foucault, "Society Must Be Defended"; Campbell and Sitze, "Introduction."

9. Cohen, *Body Worth Defending*, 3–6; Martin, *Flexible Bodies*, 3–19; Anderson, "Getting Ahead," 606–16.

10. Esposito, "Biopolitics," 317, 340–42.

11. Greenhalgh, "Chinese Biopolitical," 207–8; Greenhalgh, "Governing Chinese Life," 148–49; Winckler and Greenhalgh, *Governing China's Population*; Salter, "Biomedical Innovation"; Chen, "Cord-Blood Banking"; Zhan, "Human Oriented?"; Thompson, "'Living Capital'"; "Beijing Bets on Facial Recognition in a Big Drive for Total Surveillance," *Washington Post*, January 7, 2018.

12. Gross, *Farewell*; Fang, *Barefoot Doctors*; Rogaski, *Hygienic Modernity*; Iijima, *Pesuto to kindai Chūgoku*.

13. Hughes, "Evolution of Large Technological Systems," 52–53.

14. See also Brazelton, "Engineering Health."

15. Lam, *Passion for Facts*, 1–18.

16. Rose and Novas, "Biological Citizenship," 439–440; Petryna, "Biological Citizenship," 250–51, 261–65; Huisman and Oosterhuis, "Politics of Health and Citizenship."

17. Walker, "Early Modern Japanese State," 121–29; Durbach, *Bodily Matters*; Conis, *Vaccine Nation*; Colgrove, *State of Immunity*.

18. Culp, *Articulating Citizenship*; Morris, *Marrow of the Nation*; Harrison, *Making of the Republican Citizen*.

19. Culp, "Synthesizing Citizenship."

20. Liu, "From Five 'Imperial Domains,'" 20–30.

21. Guo, "Translating Chinese Citizenship," 374–75; Yu, "Citizenship, Ideology"; Shih, "Ethnic Economy"; Woo, "Law and the Gendered Citizen."

22. Silverstein, *History of Immunology*; Moulin, *Le dernièr langage de la médicine*; Arnold, *Colonizing the Body*, 61–115; Chakrabarti, *Bacteriology in British India*.

23. Arnold, *Colonizing the Body*; Anderson, "Immunization and Hygiene," 1–20; Pelis, *Charles Nicolle*; Hodges, "Global Menace."

24. To give just a few examples: Needham et al., *Science and Civilisation in China*; Elman, *On Their Own Terms*; Fan, *British Naturalists in Qing China*.

25. *Report to the International Sanitary Conference*, 9.

26. Packard, *History of Global Health*, 242.

27. Hoch, "Social Consequences of Soviet Immunization," 1; Vargha, "Between East and West."

28. Brown, Cueto, and Fee, "World Health Organization," 66.

29. Giersch, *Asian Borderlands*; Mullaney, *Coming to Terms*, 1–17.

30. Bello, "To Go"; Yang, "Zhang on Chinese Southern Frontiers."

31. Mitter, *Manchurian Myth*; Brook, *Collaboration*; Selden, *Yenan Way*; Chen, *Making Revolution*; Mitter, *Forgotten Ally*; MacKinnon, Lary, and Vogel, *China at War*; Barnes, *Intimate Communities*; Soon, "Coming from Afar;" Van de Ven, *China at War*.

32. Pepper, *Civil War*, 7–41; Lary, *China's Republic*, 151–55.

1. JOURNEY TO THE SOUTHWEST

1. Cameron, "Pharmacy in China in 1938," 148. Although the Chinese name of the National Epidemic Prevention Bureau may also be translated as the Central Epidemic Prevention Bureau, I have chosen to use the English title that the bureau itself employed in its English-language publications.

2. Silverstein, *History of Immunology*, 329; Lawrence, "Continuity in Crisis," 312–13.

3. Hardy, *Salmonella Infections*, 140–42; Kupferberg, "History of the International Union," 11–13.

4. Chakrabarti, *Medicine and Empire*, 172–73; Chakrabarti, *Bacteriology in British India*; Palmer, "Beginnings of Cuban Bacteriology"; Stepan, *Beginnings of Brazilian Science*.

5. For an example of a translation, see Zhi, *Jinshi bingyuan weishengwu ji mianyixue*.

6. Long, *Mianyixue yuanli*; "Long Yuying (1900–1983)," 167; Silverstein, "History of Immunology." The authors of "Long Yuying (1900–1983)" date Long's text to 1923, but the Shanghai Library catalogs it as having been published in 1933.

7. Topley and Wilson, *Principles of Bacteriology and Immunity*, 809–36.

8. Xue, "'Tang shi bingdu'"; Cheng, Ming, and Gao, "Recollection"; Wu and Xie, "In Memory of Professor Tang Fei-fan," 512; "Obituary Notices," 318–21. Although National Central University was famously sited in Nanjing, its clinical school of medical instruction was based in Shanghai for a period in the 1930s.

9. Xue, "'Tang shi bingdu'"; Wu and Xie, "In Memory of Professor Tang Fei-fan," 513.

10. Song and Lin, *Xiandai Puxian renwu*, 25–26; Elgert, *Immunology*, 141–42.

11. Lu, "Xie Shaowen," 459; Grove, *Tapeworms, Lice, and Prions*, 412.

12. Vincent, "China Medical Board," 241; Chen, "Experiments"; Chen, "Etiology of Epidemic Poliomyelitis"; Zinsser and Chen, "On Hyperleucocytosis"; *Columbia University Bulletin of Information*, 15.

13. "Yu He," 333; Cao, "Immunology in China," 339; "Lin Feiqing (1904–1998)," 817.

14. Luesink, "Dissecting Modernity," 36, 167–70; Andrews, "Tuberculosis," 148–51; Shanghai shangwu yinshuguan, "Tushu jieshao," 47; "Yu He," 333.

15. Guoli bian yi guan, *Xijunxue mianyixue mingci*; *Xijunxue zonglun, mianyixue, xijun mingcheng*.

16. Ji, "Vaccin yufang jiezhong"; Yuan and Zhai, *Zhongguo gaige da cidian*, 3287; Witebsky, "Ehrlich's Side-Chain Theory."

17. Xie, "Xijunxue ji mianyixue jiaoshou," 6–10.

18. Zhongguo kexue jishu xiehui, *Zhongguo kexue jishu*, 281; Davenport, "Robert Kho-Seng Lim," 288–89; Tang, "Adsorption Experiments"; Lei, *Neither Donkey nor Horse*, 51; Bowers, *Western Medicine in a Chinese Palace*, 83.

19. Yip, *Health and National Reconstruction*; Rogaski, *Hygienic Modernity*.

20. Wu, *Plague Fighter*, 1–102; Lei, "Sovereignty and the Microscope"; Summers, *Great Manchurian Plague*, 12–17, 33–38; Lynteris, "Skilled Natives, Inept Coolies."

21. Yip, *Health and National Reconstruction*, 107–8; Yu, "Epidemics and Public Health," 97–98; Gamsa, "Epidemic of Pneumonic Plague," 156–63; Leung, "Business of Vaccination"; Bretelle-Establet, "French Medicine," 143.

22. National Health Administration and Central Field Health Station, *National Epidemic Prevention Bureau*, 1–2.

23. Yip, *Health and National Reconstruction*, 16; National Health Administration and Central Field Health Station, *National Epidemic Prevention Bureau*, 130.

24. Yip, *Health and National Reconstruction*, 45–50, 107–8; Yu, "Epidemics and Public Health," 98; Deng and Cheng, *Zhongguo yixue tongshi*, 313; Zhang, *Minguo shiqi de chuanranbing*, 200.

25. Yip, *Health and National Reconstruction*, 52, 109; National Health Administration and Central Field Health Station, *National Epidemic Prevention Bureau*, 86–88.

26. National Health Administration and Central Field Health Station, *National Epidemic Prevention Bureau*, 86–88, 101.

27. Lin, "Zhongyang yimiao," 111–13.

28. Chen, "Public Health," 60–68.

29. Letter to Dr. J. Heng Liu, Nanjing, July 22, 1933, National Epidemic Prevention Bureau, record group (RG) 1029.1.51, YPA; National Health Administration and Central Field Health Station, *National Epidemic Prevention Bureau*, 73–74.

30. Yip, *Health and National Reconstruction*, 109.

31. Mitter, *Forgotten Ally*, 79–172.

32. Ye, *Seeking Modernity*; Harrell, *Sowing the Seeds*.

33. Lu, "Xie Shaowen," 457–58; Shen, "Riben zai Manzhou," 143.

34. Yu, "Xiao nei xiaoxi," 145; Watt, "Public Medicine in Wartime China," 42.

35. Eastman, *Seeds of Destruction*, 25–27.

36. Israel, *Lianda*, 13–60; Johnson, *Childbirth in Republican China*, 6–7; Yip, "Health and Nationalist Reconstruction," 402; Watt, "Public Medicine in Wartime China," 33–34.

37. Pei, "Nian ba nian ben shi," 71; Ride, "Test of War," 290.

38. Liu, *Yixue kexue jia*, 53.

39. Cameron, "Pharmacy in China in 1938," 148; Lary, *Chinese People at War*, 63.

40. Yu, "Xiao nei xiaoxi," 145.

41. Zhu, "Medical Education," 18–20.

42. Yang, "Kangri zhanzheng shiqi," 135–40.

43. Benedict, *Bubonic Plague*, 1–48; Bello, "To Go," 283–317; Israel, *Lianda*, 319; Yip, "Disease and the Fighting Men," 174; Borg, "Chinese Health Work," 134.

44. Yip, *Health and National Reconstruction*, 11–12.

2. LEGACIES OF WARLORDS AND EMPIRES

1. Sutton, *Provincial Militarism*; McCord, *Power of the Gun*; Sheridan, *Chinese Warlord*; Lin, "Warlord, Social Welfare and Philanthropy."

2. Arnold, *Colonizing the Body*, 120–21.

3. Gaubatz, *Beyond the Great Wall*, 77–78; Yang, *Between Wind and Clouds*; Giersch, *Asian Borderlands*, 26; Scott, *Art of Not Being Governed*, ix–xiii; Perdue, "Is Pu-er in Zomia?," 6–8.

4. Thompson, "Setting the Stage," 45.

5. Thompson, "Mission to Macau," 194; Thompson, "Nguyễn Initiative."

6. Bello, "To Go"; Giersch, *Asian Borderlands*, 1–14; Atwill, *Chinese Sultanate*, 185–90; McGrath, "Warlord Frontier," 7–11.

7. Yunnan sheng difang zhi bianji weiyuanhui, *Yunnan shengzhi*, 333; Leung, "Business of Vaccination."

8. Walsh, "Yunnan Myth"; Colquhoun, "Exploration"; Eastman, *Throne and Mandarins*.

9. Bretelle-Establet, "Resistance and Receptivity," 173–78; Rocher, "Notes sur la peste."

10. Georges Mouillac, "Rapport sur le fonctionnement du poste médical consulaire de Yunnanfou durant l'année 1921" [Report on the function of the Kunming consular medical post during the year 1921], pp. 2–4, box 559, coll. 513PO/A, CADN.

11. "Aucune précaution n'est prise et il n'est pas rare de voir dans les rues, portés par leurs mères, des enfants encore converts de croûtes varioliques." Ortholan, "Rapport médical," 42.

12. "Devant le succès de cette vaccination, je ne doute pas que les années suivantes, on ne vaccine un beaucoup plus grand nombre d'enfants, mais il faut compter avec la routine et l'indolence des Chinois. Presque tous les enfants vaccinés étaient de familles ayant une position sociale relativement élevée et en général riches. C'est tout le contraire qui se produit pour les consultations ordinaires." Ortholan, "Rapport médical," 43.

13. "Le médecin inspecteur des services sanitaires et medicaux de l'Indochine, à Monsieur le Gouverneur-Général de l'Indochine, Hanoi" [From the inspector-general of the sanitation and medical boards of French Indochina to Monsieur Governor-General of Indochina, Hanoi], March 24, 1910, GGI.dos.25107, CAOM. Translated in Bretelle-Establet, "Resistance and Receptivity," 174.

14. McGrath, "Warlord Frontier," 9–10; Yeung, "Yunnan Province," 1440; Webster, *Gentlemen Capitalists*, 213; Thant, *Making of Modern Burma*, 129; Anderson, *Report on the Expedition*.

15. See Brunero, *Britain's Imperial Cornerstone*, and van de Ven, *Breaking with the Past*.

16. Chand, "Report 1909," 59.

17. Sircar, "Report," 38.

18. Sircar, 38.

19. Chand, "Report 1910," 100.

20. Sircar, "Report," 39.

21. Chand, "Report 1909," 58. Chand's given name on this report varies from that on the 1910 report. It is possible, but unlikely, that two physicians of the same foreign surname were in Tengyueh a year apart.

22. Chand, "Report 1910," 100–101.

23. Clark, "In Consultation," 212. Medical missionaries who worked for the China Inland Mission were typically white men from England and North America.

24. "Editorials," 282–83.

25. Ma, "Peking Union Medical College," 167–68.

26. Sutton, *Provincial Militarism*, 184–261.

27. Shen, *Jindai Zhongguo shiliao congkan*, 113–20; Zhao, *Tang Jiyao yanjiu wenji*; Sutton, *Provincial Militarism*, 141; Remick, "Police-Run Brothels," 443–45.

28. Tao, "Minguo shiqi Kunming," 8.

29. Yunnan sheng difang zhi bianji weiyuanhui, *Yunnan shengzhi*, 333.

30. Yunnan sheng zhi bian zuan weiyuanhui, *Xu Yunnan tongzhi*, 208–9.

31. Bretelle-Establet, "La santé en Chine," 33.

32. "Cela donne une idée de la foule qui peut se presser, par jour de beau temps, dans la cour de l'hôpital et qui, parfois, assiège littéralement la porte de la salle de consultation." Vadon, "Un poste médical," 504–5.

33. "Les médecins variolisateurs deviennent médecins vaccinateurs; beaucoup se servent de vaccins anciens venant du Japon ou de Shanghaï, mais beaucoup aussi viennent s'approvisionner à l'hôpital français, où, au préalable, quelques leçons pratiques de vaccination leur sont données." Vadon, 511.

34. "Dans les premières années de l'existence du poste médical ces vaccinations n'ont pas eu grand succès ; mais depuis ces deux dernières années elles ont suivi une progression constante et très marquée." Vadon, 510.

35. Mouillac, "Rapport 1921," 2–6; Bretelle-Establet, "Resistance and Receptivity," 178–86.

36. "Sa parfaite connaissance de la langue chinoise, des mœurs et habitudes locales ainsi que les amitiés qu'il a su nouer parmi les fonctionnaires et notables en font un très précieux collaborateur." Georges Mouillac, "Rapport sur le fonctionnement du poste médical consulaire de Yunnanfou, année 1922" [Report on the function of the Kunming consular medical post, year 1922], April 2, 1923, 6, box 559, coll. 513PO/A, CADN.

37. Bretelle-Establet, "Resistance and Receptivity," 183.

38. Mouillac, "Rapport 1921," 6–8.

39. Remick, "Police-Run Brothels," 444; Dr. Georges Mouillac, Yunnanfou, to the French Consul, Delegate of the Ministry of Foreign Affairs in Yunnan, Yunnanfou, June 10, 1922, box 559, coll. 513PO/A, CADN.

40. Bretelle-Establet, "French Medicine," 141–42.

41. "Peu après en effet les rôles se trouvèrent reversés et le médecin français prenait la place précédemment donnée aux anglais." Mouillac to the French Consul, June 10, 1922.

42. "J'ai administrai du serum anti-dipthérique, pour en constater d'ailleurs l'inefficacité." Mouillac, "Rapport 1922," 65.

43. Mouillac, "Rapport 1922," 62–75.

44. "Les tablettes portées en grande pompe sur des brancards fleuris accompagnés de musiciens ancien style ont parcouru une partie de la ville avant d'arriver à l'hôpital ou elles ont été aussitôt fixées à la place qui leur était destinés." Georges Mouillac, "Remise de

tablettes d'honneur et de médailles commemoratives au personnel de l'hôpital consulaire de Yunnanfou" [Honorary tablets and commemorative medals awarded to staff of Yunnanfou consular hospital], letter to consul of France, delegate of the Ministry of Foreign Affairs in Yunnan, Yunnanfou, September 6, 1922, box 559, coll. 513PO/A, CADN.

45. "Le choix fait par les Autorités du Yunnan de notre médecin est un hommage rendu à ses connaissances médicales, en même temps qu'un sûr garant du développement de notre influence et de nos méthodes scientifiques dans cette Province chinoise, limitrophe de notre grande Colonie d'Indochine." "Engagement du Dr. Mouillac comme médecin officiel du gouvernement du Yunnan" [Engagement of Dr. Mouillac as an official physician of the government of Yunnan], A. Boulard, delegate of the Ministry of Foreign Affairs in Yunnan, Kunming, to Mr. Fleuriau, minister of the French Republic in China, Beijing, July 21, 1922, box 559, coll. 513PO/A, CADN.

46. "Les vaccinations sont fort appréciées de la population chinoise et l'hôpital français de Yunnanfou non seulement en pratique sur place un grand nombre mais expédie dans l'intérieur de nombreux tubes de vaccins qui lui sont fournis par l'Institut vaccinogène du Tonkin." Mouillac, "Rapport 1922," 45.

47. "Il n'y a aucun intérêt à créer à Yunnanfou un établissement de ce genre. Le voisinage de Hanoi nous permet de recevoir en temps voulu tout le vaccin que nous pouvons utiliser et dans les meilleures conditions possibles de conservation." Mouillac, "Rapport 1922," 45.

48. "C'était un excellent moyen de propagande, qui maintenant nous fait défaut." Georges Mouillac, "Rapport sur le functionnement du poste médical consulaire de Yunnanfou, Année 1923" [Report on the function of the consular medical post of Kunming, 1923], pp. 61–65, box 559, coll. 513PO/A, CADN.

49. Mouillac, "Rapport 1923," 4.

50. "Le Médecin vaccinateur pour réussir doit se bien répèter de ces coutumes qui sont générales en Chine." Mouillac, "Rapport 1922," 46.

51. "Depuis le début des épidémies personne ne s'est présentée à nos séances de vaccinatins [sic], les chinois prétendent que la vaccine attire la scarlatine, chose assez juste d'ailleurs, l'organisme affaibli par la vaccine lutte moins et se laisse facilement attaquer par les germes de la Scarlatine." Mouillac, "Rapport 1921," 72. Please note that this quote is from Mouillac's report for the year 1921, which was written in May 1922 during the scarlet fever epidemic.

52. Georges Mouillac, "Rapport sur le fonctionnement du poste médical consulaire de Yunnanfou, année: 1925" [Report on the function of the Kunming consular medical post, year: 1925], 3, box 559, coll. 513PO/A, CADN.

53. "Les Anglais ont ouvert en grande pompe, en présence du Maréchal Chef de la Province, un grand hôpital moderne, bien construit et bien outillé. . . . Nous nous trouvons de ce fait en état d'infériorité." Georges Mouillac, "Rapport sur le fonctionnement du poste médical consulaire de Yunnanfou, année 1924" [Report on the function of the Kunming consular medical post, year 1924], 115–16, box 559, coll. 513PO/A, CADN.

54. Vassal, *In and Round Yunnan-fou*, 179.

55. Dreifort, *Myopic Grandeur*, 16.

56. "Il laissa—ce qui fut plus grave—pénétrer dans le Consulat une bande d'une cinquantaine de soldats armés de porte charges, briques, bancs, poignards qui se ruèrent sur nos compatriotes surpris et sans arme." "Rapport Politique Juin 1928: Extrait du rapport du délégue du Ministère des Affaires Étrangers au Yunnan à Monsieur Henry Cosme, chargé d'affaires de France en Chine à Pekin" [Political report June 1928: Extract of the report of the delegate of the Ministry of Foreign Affairs in Yunnan to Mr. Henry Cosme, chargé d'affaires of France in China in Beijing], July 1, 1928, box 559, coll. 513PO/A, CADN.

57. February 15, 1929, telegram to Pekin from Hanoi, box 194, coll. 513PO/A, CADN.

58. "Réouverture de l'hôpital chinois de Kokieou à l'influence française" [Reopening of the Chinese hospital at Gejiu to French Influence], letter from the delegate of the Ministry of Foreign Affairs in Yunnan, Kunming, to His Excellency Mr. De Fleuriau, Minister of the French Republic in China, Beijing, July 6, 1922, box 559, coll. 513PO/A, CADN.

59. Eastman, *Seeds of Destruction*, 13–15; Hall, *Yunnan Provincial Faction*, 99.

60. Li, Dray-Novey, and Kong, *Beijing*, 155; Yip, *Health and National Reconstruction*, 89–90; Rogaski, *Hygienic Modernity*, 238–39; Eastman, *Abortive Revolution*; Ferlanti, "New Life Movement," 961–1000; Yip, "Health and Nationalist Reconstruction," 409; Lary, *China's Republic*, 90; Xin shenghuo yundong cujin hui xuanchuan gu, "Xin shenghuo yundong zhuankan," 19.

61. "Sheng shi zhongdou chuanxi suo zhangcheng" [Republican government department of public health: Provincial and city inoculation seminar guidelines], in Weisheng shu, ed., *Weisheng fagui* [Hygiene laws], 1929, National Defense Archives, RG 502/67, KMT; Zhang, *Minguo shiqi de chuanranbing*, 200.

62. *Kunming shizhi*, 133–34; Yunnan sheng difang zhi bianji weiyuanhui, *Yunnan shengzhi*, 333; Rosinger, "Yunnan," 19.

63. *Yunnan sheng min zheng ting*.

64. Hsu, *Transmission of Chinese Medicine*, 89n5; *Kunming shizhi*, 135–36.

65. Yao, *Yunnan xingzheng jishi*, 7.

66. *Yunnan sheng min zheng ting*.

67. Joseph Needham, Kunming, letter to Dorothy Needham, Cambridge, UK, March 18, 1943, Archives of Joseph Needham, RG C.17, CUA.

3. PRODUCING IMMUNITY ACROSS THE HINTERLANDS

1. J. P. Mauclaire, "Enquête épidémiologique sur le trajet routier Yunnanfou-Kweyang-Chungking-Chengtu (1620 km)" [An epidemiological investigation on the Kunming-Guiyang-Chongqing-Chengdu route (1620 km)], December 1939, box 5779, RG 50, ser. 30817, dossier 31655, LON.

2. Cooter, Harrison, and Sturdy, *Medicine and Modern Warfare*; Fan, "Global Turn," 251–53; Secord, "Knowledge in Transit."

3. Watt, *Saving Lives in Wartime China*; Barnes, "Protecting the National Body"; Soon, "Coming from Afar."

4. "League of Nations Council Committee on Technical Co-operation between the League of Nations and China: Report of the Technical Agent of the Council on His Mission in China, from the Date of His Appointment until April 1st, 1934," Geneva, April 30, 1934, document C.157.M.66, Series of League of Nations Publications General No. 1934.1, box 5721, RG 50, ser. 7263, dossier 11248, LON; League of Nations Health Organization, "Anti-Epidemic Work in China," box 5775, RG 50, ser. 30817, dossier 31153, LON; League of Nations–Health Organization, Special Committee of the Health Committee for Technical Collaboration with China, "Statement by Dr. Victor Hoo, Representative of the Chinese Government," Geneva, October 14, 1937, box 5775, RG 50, ser. 30817, dossier 31153, LON; Balińska, "Ludwik Rajchman," 456–60; "Liste des dons de vaccine anti-cholerique obtenus par l'intermédiare de la Société des Nations" [List of cholera vaccine donations obtained through the League of Nations], August 12, 1938, box 5788, RG 50, ser. 30817, dossier 34507, LON.

5. Ludwik Rajchman, personal note, October 28, 1937, box 5776, RG 50, ser. 30817, dossier 31283, LON.

6. Ludwik Rajchman, Geneva, to Borçic, December 3, 1937, box 5776, RG 50, ser. 30817, dossier 31262, LON.

7. League of Nations Health Organization, "War and Epidemics in China," C.H. 1333(1), 3, May 16, 1938, box 5775, RG 50, ser. 30817, dossier 31153, LON.

8. H. Mooser, "Report on the Activities of the League of Nations Epidemic Commission, First Unit, Sian, for the Month of July, 1938," 50, box 5786, RG 50, ser. 30817, dossier 33625, LON.

9. Mooser, "Report . . . July, 1938," 6.

10. H. Mooser and Y. N. Yang, "Report of the First Unit of the League of Nations Epidemic Commission to China for the Month of February 1938," pp. 1, 5, box 5785, RG 50, ser. 30817, dossier 33625, LON.

11. H. M. Jettmar, "Appendix VIII: Report on a Trip to Pingliang to Study There the Sanitary Conditions and to Establish a New Anti-Epidemic Branch," p. 5, in H. Mooser, "Report on the Activities of the League of Nations Epidemic Commission, First Unit, Sianfu, for the Month of November, 1938," box 5786, RG 50, ser. 30817, dossier 33625, LON.

12. "Report: The League of Nations Epidemic Commission Unit II: Book VI, July and August 1938, Changsha," pp. 6–7, box 5787, RG 50, ser. 30817, dossier 33626, LON; League of Nations Health Organization, "War and Epidemics," 8–10; Rajchman to Borçic, December 3, 1937; Mackenzie, Geneva, to Gordon Thompson, London, March 17, 1938, box 5776, RG 50, ser. 30817, dossier 31199, LON.

13. "Guolian xiezhu woguo fangyi," 38; "Guowai zhi bu," 44–45.

14. H. Mooser, "League of Nations Epidemic Commission, First Unit, Report for the Month of April," May 26, 1938, pp. 18–19, box 5786, RG 50, ser. 30817, dossier 33625, LON; Harris, *Factories of Death*.

15. League of Nations Health Organization, "Anti-Epidemic Work in China," 3; C. E. Smets, Geneva, to Hoo Chi-Tsai, Geneva, March 13, 1939, box 5791, RG 50, ser. 30817, dossier 37847, LON; S. G. Xenakis, Geneva, to Hoo Chi-Tsai, Geneva, May 9, 1939, box 5791, RG 50, ser. 30817, dossier 37847, LON; Taylor, Hanoi, to F. C. Yen, Chongqing, January 16, 1939, box 5791, RG 50, ser. 30817, dossier 37847, LON.

16. Liu, "Relocating Pastorian Medicine," 46.

17. League of Nations Health Organization, "War and Epidemics," 6; Mooser and Yang, "Report of the First Unit February 1938," p. 5.

18. H. Mooser and Y. N. Yang, "League of Nations Epidemic Commission Unit No. 1 Report for the Month of March [1938]," May 6, 1938, pp. 10–11, box 5785, RG 50, ser. 30817, dossier 33625, LON.

19. Pan Tai Foh, "Appendix No. 1: January Report on Work Done by Medical Department," in H. M. Jettmar, "Report on the Activities of the League of Nations Epidemic Commission, First Unit, for the Month of January, 1939," box 5786, RG 50, ser. 30817, dossier 33625, LON.

20. Mooser and Yang, "League . . . March [1938]," 8; H. M. Jettmar, "Report on the Activities of the League of Nations Epidemic Commission, First Unit, for the Month of December 1938," p. 1, box 5786, RG 50, ser. 30817, dossier 33625, LON.

21. Mooser, "Activities . . . July, 1938," 12.

22. "League of Nations Epidemic Commission Unit II: Report for September [1938]," p. 15, box 5787, RG 50, ser. 30817, dossier 33626, LON.

23. H. Jettmar, Xi'an, "Report on the Activities of the League of Nations Epidemic Commission, First Unit, Sianfu, for the Month of December 1938," January 26, 1938, 9, box 5786, RG 50, ser. 30817, dossier 33625, LON; H. M. Jettmar, "Report on the Activities of the League of Nations Epidemic Commission, First Unit, for the Month of February 1939," p. 4, box 5786, RG 50, ser. 30817, dossier 33625, LON.

24. League of Nations Health Organization, "War and Epidemics," 8.

25. Ch'i Ta-chih, Senior Health Officer, "Report of the Kiangsi Branch of the 2nd Unit of the League Epidemic Commission," p. 3, June 17, 1938, box 5786, RG 50, ser. 30817, dossier 33626, LON.

26. Mooser and Yang, "League . . . March [1938]," 11; R. Cecil Robertson, "Report of the Activities of the Unit [II] during the Latter Part of December January and February," February 28, 1939, p. 4, box 5787, RG 50, ser. 30817, dossier 33626, LON.

27. P. Dorolle, Kunming, letter to M.D. Mackenzie, Geneva, December 22, 1939, box 5791, RG 50, ser. 30817, dossier 37901, LON.

28. P. Dorolle, Kunming, to P. Hjelt, Health Section, League of Nations, Geneva, December 22, 1939, box 5791, RG 50, ser. 30817, dossier 37901, LON; S. G. Xenakis, Geneva, to P. Dorolle, Hotel du Lac, Kunming, January 13, 1940, box 5791, RG 50, ser. 30817, dossier 37901, LON.

29. League of Nations Health Organization, "Anti-Epidemic Work in China," 1, 5.

30. Mackenzie, Geneva, to Gordon Thompson, London, March 17, 1938, p. 3, box 5776, RG 50, ser. 30817, dossier 31199, LON.

31. League of Nations Health Organization, "Rapport au conseil sur les travaux de la vingt-neuvième session du comité d'hygiène (Genève, 12 au 15 Octobre 1938)" [Report to the council on the work of the twenty-ninth session of the health committee, Geneva, October 12–15, 1938], document C.380.M.226.1938.III [C.H. 1381(I)], box 5788, RG 50, ser. 30817, dossier 37258, LON; "League of Nations Health Organization: Collaboration of the League of Nations in the Control of Epidemics in China," C.H. 1353, July 26, 1938, LON.

32. C. Smets, Secretary of the Council Committee for Technical Collaboration with China, Geneva, to Manager, English Coaling Co. Ltd., Port Said, November 3, 1938, box 5788, RG 50, ser. 30817, dossier 34507, LON.

33. Dr. Asim Arar, sous-secrétaire d'état au Ministère de l'Hygiène et de l'Assistance Sociale, Ankara, to C. Smets, secrétaire du comité du conseil pour la collaboration technique avec la Chine, Société des Nations, Geneva, October 14, 1938, box 5788, RG 50, ser. 30817, dossier 34507, LON.

34. Manager, English Coaling Co., Ltd. (unnamed), Port Said, to C. Smets, Secretary of the Council Committee for Technical Collaboration with China, Geneva, October 20, 1938, box 5788, RG 50, ser. 30817, dossier 34507, LON.

35. J. J. Taylor, Hong Kong, to Smets, Geneva, October 3, 1938, box 5788, RG 50, ser. 30817, dossier 34507, LON.

36. Unnamed representative of Jardine Matheson Co. Ltd., Hong Kong, to Smets, Geneva, September 21, 1938, box 5788, RG 50, ser. 30817, dossier 34507, LON.

37. John J. Taylor, Hong Kong, to Smets, Geneva, September 8, 1938, box 5788, RG 50, ser. 30817, dossier 34507, LON.

38. Smets, Geneva, to Director, Eastern and Australian Line, Melbourne, September 28, 1938, box 5788, RG 50, ser. 30817, dossier 34507, LON; Smets, Geneva, to Director, Compagnie de Navigation K.P.M., Singapore, September 28, 1938, box 5788, RG 50, ser. 30817, dossier 34507, LON; Smets, Geneva, to Director, British India Steam Navigation Company, Rangoon, September 28, 1938, box 5788, RG 50, ser. 30817, dossier 34507, LON.

39. B. Borçic, Zagreb, to Smets, Geneva, August 29, 1938, box 5788, RG 50, ser. 30817, dossier 34507, LON.

40. Li, *Echoes of Chongqing*, 18; Barnes, "Protecting the National Body," 72–73; McIsaac, "City as Nation."

41. Eastman, "Fascism in Kuomintang China," 1–31; Muscolino, "Refugees, Land Reclamation," 453–78.

42. Yip, *Health and National Reconstruction*, 177–78.

43. Watt, *Saving Lives*, 217–19; "Report: Epidemic Prevention and Control Work in China," pp. 1–2, box 20, folder 2, ABMAC.

44. "Weishengshu: Pai Chen Zongxian daili Zhongyang fangyi chu chuzhang suoyou jiaojie shiyi huitong banli er gei daili Zhongyang fangyi chu chuzhang Tang Feifan de xunling [National Health Administration: Sending Chen Zongxian as substitute president of the National Epidemic Prevention Bureau; all handover arrangements to be handled jointly and giving orders to acting NEPB president Tang Feifan]," October 17, 1938, Records of the National Epidemic Prevention Bureau, RG 1029.2.23, document 9, YPA.

45. Barnes, "Protecting the National Body," 77, 80–81, 102–4.

46. "Zhongdou tiaoli," 506; Lary, *Chinese People at War*, 158.

47. Joseph Needham to Mr. W. Bridges-Adams, June 25, 1943, Papers of Joseph Needham, RG C.22, CUA; Needham, *Science Outpost*, 16–17, 87.

48. Joseph Needham, "Report to His Excellency President and Generalissimo Chiang Kai-shek on the Position and Prospects of Science and Technology in China," *Chinese Papers 1942–1946*, vol. 2, Chungking, winter 1945, 26, NRI.

49. Joseph Needham, "Lists of Orders of Scientific Supplies for Chinese Universities and of 'Missing Orders,'" RG Needham C.142, CUA.

50. Dorothy Needham, "Manuscript Notes on Visits to Institutions," RG Needham C.63, CUA.

51. Needham, *Science Outpost*, 287–94.

52. Watt, *Friend in Deed*, 1–6; Soon, "Blood, Soy Milk, and Vitality."

53. Elvin, *Retreat of the Elephants*, 216–17.

54. Watt, *Saving Lives*, 123–29.

55. Joseph Needham and Dorothy Needham, "Report on a Journey in the South-West of China, Occupying August, September and October, 1944," report submitted to the Foreign Office of the United Kingdom, in *Chinese Papers 1942–1946*, vol. 1, p. 18, NRI.

56. Watt, *Saving Lives*, 116, 163; Guiyang shi zhengfu xinwen bangongshi, *Guoji huanhua*, 9, 44; Needham, *Science Outpost*, 209; Mitter, *Forgotten Ally*, 274.

57. Needham, *Science Outpost*, 209; Monath, "Yellow Fever Vaccines," 116; Needham and Needham, "Report on a Journey," 22.

58. "Report: Epidemic Prevention," 12; Mitter, *Forgotten Ally*, 212.

59. "Report on the Chinese Army," pp. 2, box 2, folder 1, ABMAC; "Report: Epidemic Prevention," 12; "JN name cards.xls," Excel file containing digitized contents of Joseph Needham's business card collection, courtesy John Moffett, NRI; Needham and Needham, "Report on a Journey," 20.

60. "The Emergency Medical Service Training Schools of the Ministry of War, First Report, May 1938–June 1942," pp. 23–24, 46, box 2, folder 2, ABMAC; Soon, "Coming from Afar," 109; "What Is the EMSTS?," box 2, folder 2, ABMAC; "Field Units Report (1): EMSTS Units with 'Y' Force in Yunnan, February–August 1944," p. 8, box 2, folder 2, ABMAC.

61. Needham, *Science Outpost*, 209; Wei Xi (Hsi), Guiyang, to Dr. George W. Bachman, Chungking, July 6, 1943, box 20, ABMAC.

62. Needham and Needham, "Report on a Journey," 22–23; Needham, *Science Outpost*, 209; Plotkin, Orenstein, and Offit, *Vaccines*, 7.

63. Jia, "Guizhou weisheng shiye gaishu," 2–3.

64. Needham and Needham, "Report on a Journey," 28–29.

65. Gaubatz, *Beyond the Great Wall*, 47–54.

66. Needham, *Science Outpost*, 134–35; "A Brief Report of the Northwest Epidemic Prevention Bureau, Lanchow, Kansu, from January 1939 to December 1942," box 20, ABMAC.

67. "Zhongyang fangyi chu: Zhongyang fangyichu Lanzhou zhizao suo caichan qingce (National Epidemic Prevention Bureau: Detailed list of the property of the National

Epidemic Prevention Bureau's Lanzhou branch)," April 19, 1938, Records of the National Epidemic Prevention Bureau, RG 1029.2.43, file 3, YPA; "Brief Report," ABMAC.

68. Needham, *Science Outpost*, 134; Chinese Ministry of Information, *China Handbook*, 703.

69. "Brief Report," ABMAC; Joseph Needham, "Report on a Journey in the North West, Occupying Aug., Sept., Oct., Nov. 1943," pp. 13–14, report submitted to the Foreign Office of the United Kingdom, in *Chinese Papers 1942–1946*, vol. 1, NRI; Needham, *Science Outpost*, 134.

70. "Brief Report," ABMAC, 6.

4. THE EMERGENCE OF MASS IMMUNIZATION IN WARTIME KUNMING

1. Rosinger, "Yunnan," 19.

2. Anderson, Jackson, and Rosenkrantz, "Toward an Unnatural History," 587; Löwy, *Between Bench and Bedside*; Kroker, Keelan, and Mazumdar, *Crafting Immunity*.

3. Feng, *Hall of Three Pines*, 111–12.

4. Tang, "National Vaccine and Serum Institute," 179.

5. Australian Associated Press, "Japanese Bomb Burma Road: Attack on Kunming," *Sydney Morning Herald*, October 15, 1940.

6. "Student Describes Bombing," 35–36.

7. Watt, "Public Medicine in Wartime China," 41–42.

8. Tang Feifan and P. Z. King, "A Request for Subsidies for Increased Production of Vaccines and Sera and Their Distribution," folder 2, box 2, ABMAC; Tang Feifan, Kunming, copy of letter to P. Z. King, Chongqing, November 24, 1944, folder 2, box 2, ABMAC.

9. Needham, *Science Outpost*, 86.

10. Needham and Needham, "Report on a Journey in the South-West," NRI, 32–33.

11. Zhu, "Medical Education," 19.

12. Zhu, 19.

13. "Plague on Great Road: Sickness at 'Back Door' of China," *Straits Times*, November 17, 1939; "Dian xi fa sheng shu yi (Plague occurs in Yunnan)," *Kunming zhongyang ribao*, July 11, 1940; Tian, *Yunnan yiyao weisheng*, 150.

14. "Weisheng shiyan chu: Jia jin fang yi gong zuo" [Experimental health station: Intensifying disease prevention work], *Kunming zhongyang ribao*, August 14, 1940); Tian, *Yunnan yiyao weisheng*, 154–55, 159, 162–63.

15. "Yunnan sheng san shi yi nian," 7.

16. Wang and Ding, "Zhongyang fangyi chu," 154.

17. "Zhongyang fangyi chu," *Yunnan Yikan*.

18. "Zhongyang fangyi chu zhizao xueqing," 45–46.

19. Borg, "Chinese Health Work," 133.

20. Jin, "Chang qi kang zhan," 46; Jin, "Zuijin de weisheng jianshe."

21. Tang, "National Vaccine and Serum Institute," 180; Yan Wai, Xishan, Kunming, to Dr. Tang Feifan, October 28, 1941, Records of National Epidemic Prevention Bureau, RG 1029.2.51, YPA.

22. MacPherson, "Invisible Borders," 32.

23. Guo, "Dijun shiyong xijun zhan," 9.

24. Guo, 11. The broadcast likely referred to antidysentery serum rather than vaccination.

25. Pang, "Duiyu zhongyang fangyi chu"; Tang and Wei, "Morphological Studies"; Cheng, Ming, and Gao, "Recollection," 349.

26. P. P. Laillau, London, to Dr. F. F. Tang, Changsha, June 10, 1938, Records of National Epidemic Prevention Bureau, RG 1029.1.51, YPA; Yip, "Disease and the Fighting Men," 175.

27. Wei, "Preparation of Simple and Dried Smallpox."

28. Wang, "Chuxi Zhonghua yixuehui," 1; "Di wu jie da hui," 603–11.

29. "Fifth General Conference," 4.

30. Tang, Chu, and Wong, "Study of *Vibrio Cholerae*," 1; "Yunnan sheng san shi yi nian," 1.

31. Wu, *Cholera*, 80; Carpenter and Hornick, "Killed Vaccines," 90–92.

32. Gardner and Venkatraman, "Antigens of the Cholera Group," 262–77.

33. Tang, Chu, and Wong, "Study of *Vibrio Cholerae*."

34. Tang, Chu, and Wong, table I, 3–4. Four *X* marks in the rightmost two columns of the final two rows indicate that Tang and colleagues did not carry out the agglutination test on Inaba and Ogawa stock strains. This control measure would have indicated that the agglutination test was working properly.

35. Barenblatt, *Plague upon Humanity*, 164–69; Yang, Zhang, and Ng, *Historical Treasures of China*, 162; Li, "Japan's Biochemical Warfare," 295–96.

36. Harris, *Factories of Death*; Tian, *Yunnan yiyao weisheng*, 154.

37. National Health Administration to Dr. F. F. Tang, Kunming, August 15, 1941, Zhongyang fangyi chu (National Epidemic Prevention Bureau), RG 1029.1.51, YPA; Davis, *Boy's War*, 222–23; Wei Xi, Kunming, to Chinese Red Cross Society Medical Relief Corps, Guiyang, April 3, 1942, Zhongyang fangyi chu (National Epidemic Prevention Bureau), RG 1029.1.51, YPA; Huang Youwei to Dr. Marshall Balfour, November 10, 1943, Zhongyang fangyi chu (National Epidemic Prevention Bureau), RG 1029.1.51, YPA; telegram from Central Bank, Kunming branch, to Foreign Exchange Control Committee, Chongqing, in reference to "Zhongyang fangyi chu jizheng Shen Ding[hong] fengming fu Yindu kaocha zhizao shuyi junmiao" [National Epidemic Prevention Bureau senior specialist Shen Dinghong traveling under orders to India to investigate the production of plague vaccine], April 3, 1942, RG 0286-0001-00773, CMA.

38. "Report of Anti-Epidemic Activities for 1942–43, National Health Administration, Jan 1 1942 to June 30, 1943," 5, box 20, ABMAC; Needham, *Science Outpost*, 88–89.

39. "Yunnan sheng san shi yi nian," 2.

40. "Yunnan sheng san shi yi nian," 4.

41. "Yunnan sheng san shi yi nian," 4; "Kunming shi huoluan yufang zhushe," 146; Israel, *Lianda*, 198; Wang, "Chuxi Zhonghua yixuehui," 6.

42. "Yunnan sheng san shi yi nian," 10.

43. "Yunnan sheng san shi yi nian," 3.

44. "Yiqing," 14–15.

45. Shih, *China Enters the Machine Age*, 20.

46. Barnes and Watt, "Influence of War," 236–38; "Yunnan sheng san shi yi nian," 5.

47. Tian, *Yunnan yiyao weisheng*, 154.

48. Kuo, *Yün-nan sheng*, 3–4, 14; "Yunnan sheng san shi yi nian," 15; Rosinger, "Yunnan," 19.

49. Wu, *Cholera*, 83–84.

50. Yunnan sheng difang zhi bianji weiyuanhui, *Yunnan shengzhi*, 333.

51. Carpenter and Hornick, "Killed Vaccines," 92–93.

52. National Health Administration and Central Field Health Station, *National Epidemic Prevention Bureau*, 37–42; Clasener and Beunders, "Immunization."

53. Pier, "Vaccines and Vaccination," 515–16.

54. Serrie, "Obituaries," 168–71.

55. Hsu, *Magic and Science*, 3–4, 6–7, 31.

56. Hsu, 8, 11; Katz, *Demon Hordes and Burning Boats*, 39–75.

57. Wu, *Cholera*, 80; Hsu, *Magic and Science*, 19–21, 26–27.

58. Hsu, 28; Barnes, "Protecting the National Body," 275–76.

59. Hsu, *Religion, Science and Human Crises*, 80–81.

60. Hsu, 81.

61. Strong, *Protective Inoculation*, 9–10.

62. Hsu, *Magic and Science*, 28, 39–45.

63. Hsu, *Exorcising the Trouble Makers*, 1–7; Hsu, *Religion, Science, and Human Crises*, 114. Quote from *Religion, Science, and Human Crises*.

64. Hsu, *Magic and Science*, 46.

65. "Weisheng, biao san," 38:18, 41:9, 42:5, 48:22, 55:26, 73–74:32; "Weisheng, biao er," 39:7.

66. "Report of Anti-Epidemic Activities for 1942–43"; Yunnan sheng difang zhi bianji weiyuanhui, *Yunnan shengzhi*, 333.

67. Yip, *Health and Reconstruction*, 108; National Health Administration and Central Field Health Station, *National Epidemic Prevention Bureau*, 96.

68. Wei and Wen, "Experimental Infection of Silkworm," 171–73.

69. Needham, *Science Outpost*, 74.

70. "Zhongyang fangyi chu," *Yunnan yikan*.

71. "Zhongyang fangyi chu," *Gonggong weisheng yuekan*.

72. "Niudou bixu," 7. See also Xu, "Xiao'er ke zhong chang jian."

73. Peng Shuchang to National Epidemic Prevention Bureau, RG 1029.1.51, YPA.

74. Wang and Ding, "Zhongyang fangyi chu," 153.

5. NATIONALIZING MASS IMMUNIZATION AMID CIVIL WAR AND REVOLUTION

1. Tang, "National Vaccine and Serum Institute," 180.

2. Eastman, *Seeds of Destruction*; Westad, *Decisive Encounters*; Pepper, *Civil War*.

3. McMillen, *Discovering Tuberculosis*; Andrews, "Tuberculosis"; Elvin and Zhang, "Environment and Tuberculosis," 523–30.

4. Elvin and Zhang, "Environment and Tuberculosis," 524, 539.

5. Tang, "National Vaccine and Serum Institute," 181. Although the name of the organization technically translates to the "Beijing Biological Products Office," its staff have used the name "National Vaccine and Serum Institute" in English-language publications.

6. Tang, 181.

7. Tang, 181; "Medical News," 926; "Program for the Formal Opening of the New Laboratories of the National Vaccine and Serum Institute (National Epidemic Prevention Bureau), Temple of Heaven, Peiping, China, January 1, 1947," box 20, ABMAC.

8. Fu and Deng, "Jiu weishengbu zuzhi," 273–74.

9. Shen, "Riben zai Manzhou," 144–46; Rogaski, *Hygienic Modernity*, 254–84; Rogaski, "Vampires in Plagueland," 141–42.

10. Harris, "Japanese Biomedical Experimentation," 480–81; Martin, Christopher, and Eitzen, "History of Biological Weapons," 3–4.

11. Shen, "Riben zai Manzhou," 145; Harris, *Factories of Death*, 59–63; Rogaski, *Hygienic Modernity*, 272–73; Liu, "'Qingjie,' 'weisheng,' yu 'baojian,'" 41–88.

12. Paine, *Wars for Asia*, 240–41; Harris, *Factories of Death*, 235–38.

13. Cui, *Zhongguo dangdai yixuejia*, 314.

14. Lucas, *Chinese Medical Modernization*, 91–100; Yen, "Differential Medium"; Qiao, "Project on BCG Vaccination"; Deng, Zhu, and Wu, "Immunization against Whooping Cough."

15. "Zao niudoumiao"; "Wei Xi (1903–1989)," 402–3; "Xie Shaowen," 88–98 at 91, a section of Liu, Li, and Weng, *Xiangya renwu*; Song and Lin, *Xiandai Puxian renwu*, 25; Cheng, "Wo guo fangshe."

16. F. F. Tang to ABMAC, January 13, 1947, box 9, ABMAC; Tang in Beijing to Helen Kennedy Stevens, executive director, ABMAC, NY, January 13, 1947, box 20, ABMAC.

17. Westad, *Decisive Encounters*, 73.

18. Fu and Deng, "Jiu weishengbu zuzhi," 275.

19. "Xialing weisheng yundong shishi banfa," 604–5.

20. "Shanghai shi weishengju gongzuo baogao" [Shanghai city health department work report], January–August 1946, p. 5, file 028000003061A, AH; "Chongqing shi weisheng ju gongzuo baogao" [Chongqing city health department work report], October 1946, p. 1, file 028000003062A, AH; "Guangzhou shi weisheng ju san shi si nian jiu yue zhi san shi wu nian ba yue gongzuo baogao shu" [Guangzhou city health department work report, September 1945–August 1946], 1946, file 028000003063A, AH; "Qingdao shi weisheng ju gongzuo baogao, zi sanshiwu nian san yue zhi san shi wu nian ba yue" [Qingdao city health department work report, from March 1946 to August 1946], 1946, p. 5, file 028000003064A, AH.

21. Wu et al., "Kunming," 326; Wang, "Renmin yiyuan," 6. In 1950, Kunming's population was reported to be 337,200.

22. Shen, "Riben zai Manzhou," 119.

23. "Zhongguo hongshizi hui Kunming fenhui yiyuan: Fangyi zhengshu" [Chinese Red Cross Kunming Branch Hospital: Epidemic prevention certificate], file 93, "Kunming shi zhengfu: Hongshizi hui, sheng shiyan chu hanjian, xunling he shi gonggong weisheng weiyuanhui de hanjian ji yi jiu si yi nian ge yiyuan fangzhi huoluan de zhunbei wenjian sheng youguan yao guanli zhangcheng de" [Kunming city government: Correspondence of the Red Cross Society and the provincial experimental station, instruction with correspondence of the municipal hygiene committee, and 1941 preparations of each hospital to control cholera with procedures to supervise medicine], RG 32-31 (Minguo Kunming shi hongshizi hui), KMA.

24. "Ministry of Health Shanghai Quarantine Service Quarantine Notification No. 25 of 1947 (English Translation): Anti-cholera inoculation of in-coming passengers," and "Ministry of Health Shanghai Quarantine Service Circular Letter to all Shipping Companies and Agents, 20 September 1947," file 102, "Kunming shi zhengfu: Weishengju; Fangyi an juan di yi ce" [Kunming city government: Bureau of health; records of epidemic prevention, vol. 1], RG 32-39 (Minguo Kunming shi weisheng ju), KMA.

25. "Fujian sheng weisheng chu gongzuo baogao" [Fujian provincial health department work report], p. 13, file 028000003058A, AH; Ho, *Studies on the Population of China*, 94.

26. "Weisheng xingzheng huiyi Guangdong sheng weisheng gongzuo baogao" [Health administration meeting Guangdong province health work report], October 1946, pp. 8–9, file 028000003059A, AH.

27. Israel, *Lianda*, 376.

28. "Gongzuo baogao yu gongzuo yijian," 6–11.

29. Chen, "Baoshan shuyi shicha baogao," 6; Miao and Chen, "Yunnan yi xi qu," 6–7.

30. Chen, "Baoshan shuyi shicha baogao," 6.

31. Wang, "Dianxi shuyi fangzhi," 9.

32. Qi, "Xibei fangyi chu"; Cui, *Zhongguo dangdai yixuejia*, 314; Luo, *Gansu renwu cidian*, 205; Qi, "Jiefang qian xibei," 85–92.

33. Zhongguo renmin, *Lanzhou wenshi ziliao xuanji*, 109–15.

34. Cai, "Huoluan yimiao," 11.

35. Tang, "National Vaccine and Serum Institute," 179; Lynch, *Chinese Civil War*, 36–37; "Jia Lianyuan," 83.

36. "Guanyu xiaji fangyi" [Summer disease prevention], *Renmin ribao*, July 19, 1949.

37. "Weisheng ju fangyi gongzuo zhushe da sa qi wan ren bu ying er qian yu wan tou" [The Public Health Department's disease prevention work has vaccinated 37,000 people and exterminated over 20,000,000 flies], *Renmin ribao*, August 10, 1949.

38. Pepper, *Civil War*, 385.

39. Elvin and Zhang, "Environment and Tuberculosis," 526.

40. Elvin and Zhang, 521.

41. Core, "Tuberculosis Control in Shanghai," 128.

42. Tomes, *Gospel of Germs*, 5–10; Rothman, *Living in the Shadow of Death*; Condrau and Worboys, *Tuberculosis Then and Now*.

43. Andrews, "Tuberculosis"; Rogaski, *Hygienic Modernity*; Core, "Tuberculosis Control in Shanghai," 128–30; Honig, *Sisters and Strangers*, 155, 267n97.

44. Mitter, *Forgotten Ally*, 366–67; Pepper, *Civil War*, 95, 121–22, 424–25.

45. Gheorgiu, "Antituberculosis BCG Vaccine," 47–50; Liu et al., "Review," 71; Fine, "BCG Story," S353.

46. Flower, *Bioinformatics for Vaccinology*, 45; Petroff and Branch, "Bacillus Calmette-Guérin"; Feldberg, *Disease and Class*, 145–52; Plotkin, Orenstein, and Offitt, *Vaccines*, 808.

47. Liu and Guo, "B.C.G. Vaccination"; Chen, Wei, and Zhu, "BCG in China," 437.

48. Wang, "Lun BCG," 16.

49. Liu and Guo, "B.C.G. Vaccination," 275–77; Chen, Wei, and Zhu, "BCG in China," 437.

50. Comstock, "International Tuberculosis Campaign," 528–35; Plotkin, Orenstein, and Offitt, *Vaccines*, 797.

51. Chen, Wei, and Zhu, "BCG in China," 437–38.

52. Wu, "Guest Editorial," 383.

53. Qiao, "Project on BCG Vaccination," 568.

54. Liu, "B.C.G. yimiao jiezhong," 209.

55. Qiao, "Project on BCG Vaccination," 572–73.

56. Wang, "Lun BCG," 15–16.

57. Song, "Guest Editorial," 287–90.

58. Qiao, "Project on BCG Vaccination," 570–71; Wang, "Lun BCG," 15–16.

59. Abolnick, "BCG Vaccination in the U.S.S.R."

60. Wang, "Lun BCG," 13–16.

61. Aronson, Parr, and Saylor, "Specificity and Sensitivity"; Aronson and Palmer, "Experience with BCG"; Aronson, "Protective Vaccination."

62. Liu and Guo, "B.C.G. Vaccination," 276.

63. "The Present Status of the NEPB Penicillin Laboratory," December 1948, box 24, ABMAC.

64. Xie, *Xie Shaowen lun zhu xuanji*, 1.

65. J. Heng Liu, ABMAC China office, Shanghai, to Magnus Gregersen, New York (ABMAC president), December 21, 1948, box 24, ABMAC.

66. Xie, "Guest Editorial."

67. Wu, *Zhongguo xiehe yike daxue*, 24.

68. Liu, *Yixue kexue jia*, 5.

69. "Wei Xi (1903–1989)," 403.

70. Liu, *Yixue kexue jia*, 2–4.

71. Liu, 3.

72. Tang, "National Vaccine and Serum Institute," 181.

6. VACCINATION IN THE EARLY PRC, 1949–58

1. Brown and Pickowicz, *Dilemmas of Victory*; Rogaski, "Nature, Annihilation, and Modernity," 388; Ai, "Xin zhongguo chengli," 146; Xu and Jiang, "Eradication of Smallpox"; Banister, *China's Changing Population*, 80.

2. Banister, *China's Changing Population*, 55–56, 80–85; Eggleston, "Health, Education," 153–54; Bloom and Williamson, "Demographic Transitions," 424–25; Lavely, Lee, and Wang, "Chinese Demography," 812–13.

3. Mullaney, *Coming to Terms*; Ghosh, "Accepting Difference," 68–69; Ghosh, "Making it Count."

4. "Di yi jie quanguo weisheng huiyi tuanmu yi zhi tongyi yi 'mianxiang gong nong bing,' 'yufang weizhu,' 'tuanjie zhong xi yi' wei weisheng gongzuo sanda yuanze" [First National Health Conference concludes, all agree on 'serve the workers, rural people, and soldiers,' 'put prevention first,' and 'unite Western and Chinese medicine' as the three great principles of health work], *Renmin ribao*, August 20, 1950; Kaple, "Soviet Advisors in China," 121.

5. Weishengbu and Renmin geming junshi, "Guanyu kaizhan junmin chunji," 830–31; Lei, *Neither Donkey nor Horse*, 224; Taylor, *Chinese Medicine*.

6. Zhou, "Zhengwu yuan," 841–42.

7. "Zhongdou zanxing banfa," 843–44.

8. Luo, *Mianyi yufang*, 4; Lucas, *Chinese Medical Modernization*, 100; Liu, *Yixue kexue jia*, 91–92.

9. Cowdrey, "'Germ Warfare,'" 169–70; "Wo xijunxue zhuanjia Wei Xi, Liu Weitong qinshen zhengshi meiguo xijunzhan zuixing: Fennu zhi huan meiguo zhengfu guoqu suo shouyu de xunzhang jiangzhuang" [Our bacteriology experts Wei Xi and Liu Weitong personally confirm the American crime of germ warfare: Angrily throwing away the Medal of Commendation once received by the American government], *Renmin ribao*, May 19, 1952.

10. "Report of the International Scientific Commission"; Andreen et al., *Report of the International Scientific Commission*; Peking Film Studio of China and the National Film Studio of Korea, *Oppose Bacteriological Warfare*; *U.S. Crime of Bacteriological Warfare*.

11. Leitenberg, "New Russian Evidence," 186–87.

12. Wu, *Yi ming jun yi*, 40–41; Leitenberg, "China's False Allegations," 10–14.

13. Wei and Zhong, "Peace and Pestilence," 8.

14. Tang Feifan, "Women yao yong shiji xingdong lai kangyi mei diguozhuyi de baoxing" [We must take action to resist the atrocities of American imperialism], *Renmin ribao*, March 9, 1952; Tang Feifan, "Guoji kexue weiyuanhui chedi jiechuan mei diguozhuyi jinxing xijunzhan de zuixing" [An international scientific committee thoroughly exposes the American imperialists' crime of conducting germ warfare], *Renmin ribao*, September 19, 1952; Tang Feifan, "Xijunxue zhe yao xianchu yiqie liliang, baowei renmin, baowei zuguo" [Bacteriologists give everything in their power to defend the people and the motherland], *Renmin ribao*, February 23, 1952; Xie Shaowen, "Women you kexue shang de tiezheng" [We have iron-clad scientific proof], *Renmin ribao*, April 4, 1952; Tang, "International Scientific Commission," 26–27.

15. "Shoudu xijunxue gongzuozhe duiyu Koulan he du Bosi er shi fouren meiguo jinxing xijunzhan de yanlun de shengming" [The capital's bacteriological workers' voices against the claims of the two American scientists Coughlin and Du Bois denying that America conducted germ warfare], *Renmin ribao*, June 9, 1952.

16. Cowdrey, "'Germ Warfare,'" 169–70; Chen, "History of Three Mobilizations," 222–28; Andreen et al., *Report of the International Scientific Commission*, 53–60.

17. Peking Film Studio of China and the National Film Studio of Korea, *Oppose Bacteriological Warfare*, 27:00–28:00.

18. Strauss, "Morality, Coercion and State Building," 897; Chen and Chen, "'Three-Anti' and 'Five-Anti' Movements," 4–5.

19. Lu, "Fan tanwu, fan langfei"; Taylor, *Chinese Medicine*, 171n64.

20. Lu, "Fan tanwu, fan langfei," 2; Gao, *Communist Takeover of Hangzhou*, 159–60; Lieberthal, *Revolution and Tradition*, 125.

21. Bai Sheng, "Zhongguo xiehe yixueyuan jiji kaizhan fan tanwu yundong" [The China Union Medical College actively undertakes the anticorruption movement], *Renmin ribao*, March 12, 1952.

22. Mao, "Guanyu Fushun," 303.

23. Zhu, Gao, and Gong, *Zhongguo junshi yixue shi*, 481–82.

24. Cowdrey, "'Germ Warfare,'" 164–65; Rogaski, "Nature, Annihilation, and Modernity," 405–10; "Zhengwu yuan," 258–59.

25. Peking Film Studio of China and the National Film Studio of Korea, *Oppose Bacteriological Warfare*, 45:38–45:47.

26. Ye, "Renren fangyi."

27. Government of PRC, "Smallpox Eradication in China," 6–9.

28. Olson, *Ethnohistorical Dictionary*, 356–59; World Health Organization, *Bugs, Drugs, and Smoke*, 7; World Health Organization, "Special Report on Smallpox," 4–8.

29. Yang, Zhang, and Ng, *Historical Treasures of China*, 208.

30. Ai, "Xin zhongguo chengli," 47.

31. Ai, 115.

32. He with Chik, *Mr. China's Son*, 52, 67n4; Joseph, *Politics in China*, 520.

33. "Kunming shi yi jiu wu er nian tuixing kajiemiao jiezhong de mubiao he gongzuo buzhou" [Kunming city 1952 promotion of BCG vaccine goals and work procedures], RG 85-1-1969, KMA.

34. Lü and Perry, "Introduction," 3–8; Bray, *Social Space and Governance*, 8, 95–122; Henderson and Cohen, *Chinese Hospital*, 45–46.

35. "Yunnan zhiyan chang 1953 niandu weisheng gongzuo zongjie" [Yunnan Cigarette Factory 1953 hygiene work summary], RG 85-1-1884, KMA; "Yunnan fangzhi chang baojian suo yi jiu wu san nian quan niandu gongzuo baogao" [Yunnan Textile Mill Health Center 1953 annual work report], RG 85-1-1884, KMA; "Guangkuang yiwu shi 53 nian weisheng fangyi gongzuo zongjie (1953) zhongyang ranliao gongye bu Yunnan dianye ju weisheng shi yi jiu wu san niandu weisheng gongzuo zongjie" [Clinic of the Yunnan Electric Power Bureau, Central Fuel Industry Department 1953 hygiene report and summary], RG 85-1-1884, KMA.

36. Wang, *Organizing through Division*, xii–xiii, 40–45.

37. Guo, "Nationality, *Hukou*, and Ethnicity," 8–10; Cheng and Selden, "China's *Hukou* System," 645.

38. "Zhongdou zanxing banfa," 843.

39. "Kunming shi renmin zhengfu weisheng ju di jiu qu weisheng suo" [Kunming City People's Department of Hygiene Station No. 9 hygiene office report], February 12, 1955, p. 18, RG 85-1-1813, KMA.

40. "Ba qu weisheng suo: Wu san nian qiuji zhongdou gongzuo zongjie" [Number 8 District Hygiene Station: Autumn 1953 smallpox vaccination work summary], file 20, pp. 106–10, RG 85-1-2076, KMA.

41. Zhonghua renmin gonghe guo, *Yufang jiezhong shouce*, 20.

42. Gonggong weisheng chu, "Da fangyi zhen," 16.

43. Perkins, *Market Control*, 42; Chai, *Economic History of Modern China*, 126.

44. "Kunming shi aiwei hui: Kunming hongshizi fenhui guanyu 51 nian shangbannian de gongzuo zongjie, xiaji yufang zhushe gongzuo zongjie (1951); Tiaozhanshu" [Kunming Patriotic Hygiene Campaign Committee: Kunming Red Cross Branch work summary for early 1951, summer immunization work summary (1951); Written challenge], April 16, 1953, RG 97-1-97, KMA.

45. Zhonghua renmin gonghe guo, *Yufang jiezhong shouce*, 20.

46. "Kunming shi renmin zhengfu weisheng ju di san qu weisheng suo: Kunming shi renmin zhengfu weisheng ju di san qu weisheng suo 1953 nian qiuji pucha buzhong niudou gongzuo zongjie" [Kunming City People's Government Department of Health District 3 Health Station: Kunming City People's Government Department of Health District 3 Health Station 1953 Autumn Standard Revaccination Work Summary], 1954, document 18, pp. 70–73, RG 85-1-1228, KMA. Private or semiprivate ownership of urban residences continued into the mid-1950s in many Chinese cities, including Kunming; the

transition to state ownership of property was often not immediate. Zhang, *In Search of Paradise*, 29–30.

47. "Kunming shi renmin zhengfu weisheng ju di san qu."

48. "Qi suo weisheng suo: Wu san nian zhongdou gongzuo zongjie" [District Seven Hygiene Station: 1953 smallpox vaccination work summary], document 15, pp. 88–92, RG 85-1-2076, KMA.

49. "San qu weisheng suo: Nian zhong chu bu zongjie" [District Three Health Station: Preliminary end-of-year summary], document 5, pp. 25–33, RG 85-1-2076, KMA.

50. "Kunming shi di ba qu weisheng suo 1954 nian xia ji shanghan yufang zhushe gongzuo zongjie" [Kunming City District Eight Health Station 1954 summer typhoid fever immunization work summary], pp. 202–5, RG 85-1-1228, KMA.

51. "Kunming shi renmin zhengfu weisheng ju di san qu weisheng suo xia ji shanghan yufang zhen zhushe gongzuo zongjie" [Kunming City People's Government Health Department Number Three Health Station summer typhoid fever immunization work summary], pp. 66–68, RG 85-1-1228, KMA.

52. "Zai Kunming shi tuixing kajiemiao jiezhong gongzuo baogao" [Report of BCG vaccination work carried out in Kunming city], RG 85-1-1950, KMA.

53. "Kunming shi renmin zhengfu di ba qu weisheng suo shi yi yue fen gongzuo zongjie" [Kunming City People's Government Number Eight Health Station November work report], RG 85-1-1950, KMA.

54. "Si qu weisheng ting: Wu san nian shanghan yufang zhushe gongzuo zongjie" [District 4 Hygiene Station 1953 typhoid immunization work summary], 1953, RG 85-1-2076, KMA.

55. Hayes, "Note on B.C.G. Immunisation," 171–72; "Kunming shi renmin zhengfu weisheng ju di san qu weisheng suo xia ji shanghan yufang zhen zhushe gongzuo zongjie" [Kunming City People's Government Health Department District 3 Hygiene Station summer typhoid fever immunization work summary], 1954, pp. 66–68, RG 85-1-1228, KMA.

56. Tang, *Yufang jiezhong*, 39.

57. "Si qu weisheng ting."

58. "Wu qu weisheng suo: Aiguo weisheng yundong yufang zhushe gongzuo zongjie" [District 5 Hygiene Station: Patriotic Hygiene Campaign immunization work summary], 1953, file 13, RG 85-1-2076, KMA.

59. "Ba qu weisheng suo."

60. Gross, *Farewell*, 98.

61. Wang, "Da fangyi zhen," 7.

62. Ren, "Yong kajiemiao," 13.

63. Wang, "Yufang zhushe," 23.

64. Lu, "Zenyang duguo weixian," 5–6.

65. Wang, "Yufang zhushe," 23; Wang, "Zenyang cai neng," 2–4.

66. Ai, "Xin zhongguo chengli," 87.

67. Wang, "Yufang zhushe," 23.

68. Wang, 23.

69. Wang, 24.

70. Chen, "Da zhen hou," 11.

71. Gross, *Farewell*, 10–12.

72. "Ba qu weisheng suo."

7. MASS IMMUNIZATION IN EAST ASIA AND GLOBAL HEALTH, 1960–80

1. Wang, *Beijing weisheng zhi*, 618; *Wusheng de jiaoliang* (transcript).

2. Government of the PRC, "Smallpox Eradication in China."

3. Deng, *Zhongguo fangyi shi*, 598; Fenner et al., *Smallpox and Its Eradication*, 1250–54.

4. *Wusheng de jiaoliang* (transcript).

5. Schmalzer, *Red Revolution, Green Revolution*, 14–21.

6. Feinsilver, *Healing the Masses*, 1–7.

7. Youde, "China's Health Diplomacy," 153–55; Altorfer-Ong, "Old Comrades"; Zhou, "From China's 'Barefoot Doctor.'"

8. Chiang, "From Postcolonial to Subimperial," 470.

9. Krige, *American Hegemony*; Wolfe, *Competing with the Soviets*; Van Dongen, *Cold War Science*.

10. Heyck and Kaiser, "Introduction to Focus"; Hecht, *Entangled Geographies*; Oreskes and Krige, *Science and Technology*; Hecht, *Being Nuclear*.

11. Wang, "Transnational Science," 369; Schmalzer, "Self-Reliant Science," 77.

12. Yang, *Tombstone*; Lampton, *Politics of Medicine in China*, 129–51; Lucas, *Chinese Medical Modernization*, 109–10, 121–26.

13. Deng, *Zhongguo fangyi shi*, 598.

14. Luo, *Mianyi yufang*, 2–3; Zhang, *Lishi shang de weisheng bu*, 39, 61; Deng, *Zhongguo fangyi shi*, 607.

15. Deng, *Zhongguo fangyi shi*, 608; Huang et al., "Studies on Attenuated Measles Vaccine"; Banister, *China's Changing Population*, 61; Halstead and Yu, "Human Viral Vaccines," 146–48.

16. Hong, *Zhonghua renwu dadian*, 198.

17. Gu, "Mass Vaccination," 28–30; Gu et al., "Large Scale Trial," 131.

18. Gu, "Mass Vaccination," 30. See also Gu et al., "Large Scale Trial."

19. Deng, *Zhongguo fangyi shi*, 608; Banister, *China's Changing Population*, 61.

20. Gu, "Mass Vaccination," 30.

21. Gu, 30; Halstead and Yu, "Human Viral Vaccines," 143; Gu et al., "Poliomyelitis in China," 552.

22. Lucas, *Chinese Medical Modernization*, 110, 137; Deng, *Zhongguo fangyi shi*, 582; Wei, "Barefoot Doctors."

23. Gross, "Between Party, People, and Profession," 339–41.

24. Schmalzer, *Red Revolution, Green Revolution*; Gross, *Farewell*.

25. Sidel, "Barefoot Doctors," 1298.

26. Revolutionary Health Committee, *Barefoot Doctors' Manual*, 51, 58–59; Hunan zhongyi yao yanjiu suo ge wei hui, *Chijiao yisheng shouce*, 115.

27. Revolutionary Health Committee, *Barefoot Doctors' Manual*, 59.

28. Fang, *Barefoot Doctors*, 80–85.

29. Beijing shi jiehebing fangzhi suo, "Ertong yao fanglao."

30. "Jiji gao hao yufang jiezhong" [Actively do a good job in promoting immunization], *Renmin ribao*, January 12, 1975.

31. Jing and Song, *Yixue daolun*, 159; Deng, *Zhongguo fangyi shi*, 605–10; Fenner and Breman, "Report on a Visit," 9.

32. Volland, "Translating the Socialist State."

33. Strauss, "Past in the Present," 779–80; Youde, "China's Health Diplomacy," 154; Larkin, *China and Africa*, 54, 94; Yan, *Zhongguo yu zhoubian*, 128.

34. Altorfer-Ong, "Old Comrades," 244–71.

35. Ogunsanwo, *China's Policy in Africa*, 90, 154; "RCSC Sends Gift," 85; Shinn and Eisenman, *China and Africa*, 244–48.

36. Youde, "China's Health Diplomacy," 159.

37. Shinn and Eisenman, *China and Africa*, 377–80. Ghana, the Democratic Republic of the Congo, Burundi, Tunisia, the Central African Republic, and Benin each temporarily suspended formal relations with the PRC at various points during the 1960s.

38. Fung, "Chinese Journals," 21; Xu, "Translation and Internationalism," 79–84.

39. Chen, "Medicine and Public Health," 158–63.

40. Geographic Health Studies Program, *Topics of Study Interest*, 35–38.

41. Horn, *Away with All Pests*, 130.

42. Snow, *Red China Today*, 301–2.

43. James Reston, "Now, about My Operation in Peking," *New York Times*, July 26, 1971.

44. Zhou, "From China's 'Barefoot Doctor,'" 140–46.

45. Sidel and Sidel, *Serve the People*; Sidel and Sidel, "Health Care."

46. Sidel, "Barefoot Doctors," 1295–98.

47. Lee, "Medicine and Public Health," 431, 433.

48. Zhou, "From China's 'Barefoot Doctor,'" 143.

49. United States Agency for International Development, *Barefoot Doctors*, 11:40–12:00.

50. United States Agency for International Development, 47:00–47:30.

51. "'Statement of the [PRC] Ministry,'" 515.

52. Fleck, "Consensus during the Cold War," 745.

53. Cueto, "Origins of Primary Health Care," 1865.

54. Bryant, *Health and the Developing World*, x.

55. Packard, *History of Global Health*, 240; Werner, *Where There Is No Doctor*; Taylor, *Doctors for the Villages*; Newell, *Health by the People*.

56. Cueto, "Origins of Primary Health Care," 1865; Lee, "WHO and the Developing World," 24–25; Cui, "China's Village Doctors," 914.

57. Gross, *Farewell*, 237.

58. Packard, *History of Global Health*, 227–48; Cueto, "Origins of Primary Health Care," 1867–68.

59. Cueto, "Origins of Primary Health Care," 1866–67; Lüthi, *Sino-Soviet Split*, 340–45.

60. Fenner et al., *Smallpox and Its Eradication*, 1251.

61. Deng, *Zhongguo fangyi shi*, 598.

62. *Wusheng de jiaoliang*.

63. Fenner et al., *Smallpox and Its Eradication*, 1258; *Wusheng de jiaoliang* (film), 7:44.

EPILOGUE

1. "Wei Xi," *Zhongguo jinxiandai gaodeng jiaoyu renwu cidian*, 664.

2. "Xie Shaowen," 916; Lu, "Xie Shaowen," 458–59.

3. Lee and Lo, "Rural Health Care," 148.

4. Tang et al., "Studies on the Etiology of Trachoma."

5. Cheng, Li, and Gao, "Recollection," 350.

6. Hsu, *Wen I-to*, 172–73; Pepper, *Civil War*, 143–45; Cong, *China's Scientific Elite*, 57.

7. For an excellent overview of these movements and how they affected one prominent intellectual, see Cheek, *Propaganda and Culture*.

8. Liu, *Yixue kexue jia*, 140–43.

9. C. E. Lim, Beijing, to an unspecified "Lilian," August 14, 1959, Harold H. Loucks Papers, box 1, folder 14, RAC.

10. Rogaski, "Nature, Annihilation, and Modernity."

11. Packard, *Making of a Tropical Disease*, 150–76.

12. World Health Organization, "WHO Vaccine-Preventable Diseases."

13. Yang et al., "Rapid Health Transition in China," 2012.

Glossary

TABLE G.1 Key terms and organizations

ROMANIZATION	CHARACTERS	ENGLISH
Aiguo weisheng yundong	愛國衛生運動	Patriotic Hygiene Campaign
Beijing daxue yixueyuan	北京大學醫學院	Peking University School of Medicine
Beijing shengwu zhipin yanjiusuo	北京生物製品研究所	National Vaccine and Serum Institute (literally Beijing Biological Products Institute)
chijiao yisheng	赤腳醫生	barefoot doctor
chui hua (also ch'ui-hwa)	吹花	variolation
dahoufang	大後方	"great rear," hinterland
Dalian shengwu zhipin yanjiu suo	大連生物製品研究所	Dalian Biological Products Research Institute
Dalian yixueyuan	大連醫學院	Dalian Medical School
danwei	單位	work unit
Dian xi shuyi fangzhi weiyuanhui	滇西鼠疫防治委員會	Western Yunnan Plague Prevention and Treatment Committee
Donglu Yiyuan	東陸醫院	Donglu Hospital
doumiao xueqing	痘苗血清	smallpox vaccines and sera
Faguo yiyuan	法國醫院	French [consular] hospital
fangyi dui	防疫隊	disease prevention team
fangyi zhan	防疫站	disease prevention station
gong'an ju	公安局	public security office
gonggong hu	公共户	public housing
gongmin	公民	citizen(s)
gongyi	公醫	state medicine
Guandong fangyi jishui bu benbu	關東軍防疫給水部本部	Epidemic Prevention and Water Purification Department (also Kantōgun Bōeki Kyūsuibu Honbu)
Guan dou ju	管痘局	Bureau for the Management of Smallpox

(Continued)

TABLE G.1 (Continued)

ROMANIZATION	CHARACTERS	ENGLISH
guangda renmin	廣大人民	the masses
Guofang yixueyuan	國防醫學院	National Defense Medical College
Guoli bianyi guan	國立編譯館	National Institute for Compilation and Translation
Guoli Shanghai yixueyuan	國立上海醫學院	National Shanghai Medical College
Guoli tongji daxue yixueyuan	國立同濟大學醫學院	National Tongji University Medical College
Guoli xibei yixueyuan	國立西北醫學院	National Northwest Medical School
Guoli xibei yiyuan	國立西北醫院	National Northwest Hospital
Guoli xinan lianhe daxue	國立西南聯合大學	National Southwest Associated University
Guoli zhongshan daxue yixueyuan	國立中山大學醫學院	National Zhongshan Medical College
Guoli zhongzheng yixueyuan	國立中正醫學院	National Zhongzheng Medical College
guomin	國民	people of a nation; citizen(s)
Hongji yiyuan	宏濟醫院	Hongji Hospital
Hongshizi yiyuan	紅十字醫院	Red Cross Hospital
Huidian yiyuan	惠滇醫院	Benevolent Hospital
huji ce	戶籍冊	household register book
hukou	戶口	household registration
jiedao banshichu	街道辦事處	subdistrict office
kajie junmiao or kajiemiao	卡介菌苗 or 卡介苗	BCG vaccine
kexue	科學	science, scientific
kongbai hu/ren	空白戶，空白人	"blank space" household or person
kongzhi	控制	control
Kunhua yiyuan	昆華醫院	Kunhua Hospital
Kunming linshi yiliao fangyi weiyuanhui	昆明臨時醫療防疫委員會	Kunming Temporary Medical Treatment and Disease Prevention Committee
Lanzhou daxue yixueyuan	蘭州大學醫學院	Lanzhou University Medical School
Lanzhou zhongyang yiyuan	蘭州中央醫院	Lanzhou Central Hospital
laobing	癆病	wasting disease (tuberculosis)
louzhongzhe	漏種者	one who missed injection
mianyili or mianyixing	免疫力，免疫性	immunity

ROMANIZATION	CHARACTERS	ENGLISH
minzhong sixiang kexuehua	民眾思想科學化	scientizing the thoughts of the masses
niudou chuanxi suo	牛痘傳習所	cowpox inoculation seminar
qiangpo zhushe	強迫注射	forcible injection
qifa	啟發	persuasive
Renmin ribao	人民日報	*People's Daily*
renmin zhengfu jiedao banshichu	人民政府街道辦事處	local subdistrict office
Renmin yiyuan	仁民醫院	Philanthropic Hospital
Riben dalu kexueyuan mayi yanjiusuo	日本大陸科學院馬疫研究所	Japanese Mainland Academy of Science Equine Disease Research Station
Rijun huabei fangyi chu	日軍華北防疫處	Japanese North China Epidemic Prevention Station
Shanghai fanglao xiehui	上海防癆協會	Shanghai Antituberculosis Association
sheng renmin zhengfu weisheng chu	省人民政府衛生處	provincial people's government hygiene department
shengwu zhipin	生物製品	biological products
shi renmin zhengfu weisheng ju	市人民政府衛生局	municipal bureau of hygiene
shiyan	試驗	experiment
shizheng gongsuo	市政公所	municipal public affairs office
shuofu	說服	persuasion
sixiang dongyuan	思想動員	ideological mobilization
sixiang gaizao	思想改造	thought reform
weisheng	衛生	hygiene
weishengke	衛生科	public health office
weisheng shiyan suo	衛生試驗所	experimental health station
Weishengshu	衛生署	National Health Administration
weishengwu xue	微生物學	microbiology
weishengwu xuejia	微生物學家	microbiologist
weizhongzhe	未種者	one who has not been injected
Xiangya yixueyuan	湘雅醫學院	Xiangya Medical College
Xibei gaoji hushi xuexiao	西北高級護士學校	Northwestern Advanced Nursing School
Xibei yixue yuan	西北醫學院	Northwest Medical School
Xinan yunshu gongsi	西南運輸公司	Southwestern Transportation Company
Xin shenghuo yundong	新生活運動	New Life Movement

(Continued)

TABLE G.1 (Continued)

ROMANIZATION	CHARACTERS	ENGLISH
xiyi	西醫	Western medicine
Yike	醫科	medical sciences
Yixue mingci shenchahui	醫學名詞審查會	Medical Terminology Investigation Committee
Yunnan Lujun Yiyuan	雲南陸軍醫院	Yunnan Army Hospital
Yunnan sheng weisheng chu	雲南省衛生處	Yunnan Provincial Department of Public Health
zhangqi	瘴氣	a group of tropical diseases common in south China
Zhengwu yuan	政務院	Government Administrative Council
zhongdou	種痘	vaccination against smallpox
Zhongguo yaopin shengwu zhipin jianding suo	中國藥品生物製品檢定所	National Institute for the Control of Pharmaceutical and Biological Products
Zhongguo yixue kexue yuan	中國醫學科學院	Chinese Academy of Medical Sciences
Zhongguo lujun zong siling bu weisheng chu	中國陸軍總司令部衛生處	Chinese Army Office of Public Health
Zhonghua renmin gonghe guo weisheng bu	中華人民共和國衛生部	Ministry of Health of the People's Republic of China
Zhonghua yixue hui	中華醫學會	National Medical Association (also Chinese Medical Association after 1932)
Zhonghua yixue zazhi	中華醫學雜誌	National Medical Journal of China (also Chinese Medical Journal after 1932)
Zhongyang fangyi chu	中央防疫處	National Epidemic Prevention Bureau
Zhongyang kangnüe suo	中央抗虐所	Central Antimalaria Office
Zhongyang shengwu xue huaxue zhiyao shiyan chu	中央生物學化學製藥實驗處	Central Biological, Chemical, and Pharmaceutical Production Laboratory
Zhongyang weisheng shiyan suo	中央衛生實驗所	Central Hygienic Laboratory
Zhongyang xibei fangyi chu	中央西北防疫處	Northwest Epidemic Prevention Bureau
Zhongyang yanjiuyuan	中央研究院	Academia Sinica

TABLE G.2 Names of people

ROMANIZATION	CHARACTERS	ENGLISH
Cai E	蔡鍔	
Cai Hongdao	蔡宏道	
Chen Mingguang	陳明光	
Chen Shiguang	陳世光	
Chen Zhengren	陳正仁	
Chen Zongxian	陳宗賢	Also Edgar Tsen and Tsung-Hsien Tsen
Chiang Kaishek	蔣介石	Also Jiang Jieshi
Deng Jinxian	鄧金鎏	Also Teng Chin-hsien
Fang Gang	方剛	
Feng Youlan	馮友蘭	
Gu Fangzhou	顾方舟	
Guo Chengzhou	郭成周	Also C. C. Kouo
Guo Keda	郭可大	
He Lian	何璉	
He Qi	何琦	
Huang Youwei	黃有為	
Hu Xiaofa	胡小发	
Ishii Shirō	石井四郎	
Ji Jilin	計濟霖	
Jin Baoshan	金寶善	Also P. Z. King
Liang Qichao	梁啓超	
Li Guanhua	李冠華	
Lin Feiqing	林飛卿	
Lin Kesheng	林可勝	Also Robert, or Bobby, Lim
Li Tao	李涛	
Liu Juanxiang	劉雋湘	
Liu Sizhi	劉思職	
Liu Xiang	劉湘	
Liu Yongchun	劉永純	Also Y. Ch. Lieou
Liu Zhai	劉摘	
Long Yun	龍雲	
Long Yuying	龍毓瑩	
Luo Yaoxing	罗耀星	
Lu Zhijun	魯之俊	
Mao Zedong	毛泽东	
Miao Ancheng	繆安成	
Pei Cunfan	裴存藩	

(Continued)

TABLE G.2   (Continued)

ROMANIZATION	CHARACTERS	ENGLISH
Qian Nengxun	錢能訓	
Qiao Shumin	喬樹民	Also Chiao Shu-min
Qi Changqing	齊長慶	
Ren Kangcai	任康才	
Rong Dushan	榮獨山	
Shen Dinghong	沈鼎鴻	
Song Jie	宋杰	Also Chieh Sung
Tang Feifan	湯飛凡	
Tang Jiyao	唐繼堯	
Tang Jiyu	唐繼虞	
Tang Peisong	湯佩松	
Usami Uzuhiko	宇佐美 珍彦	
Wang Baoshu	王寶書	
Wang Huiyin	王惠因	
Wang Liang	王良	
Wang Qizong	王啟宗	
Wang Tianzuo	王天祚	
Wang Yuanchen	汪元臣	
Wei Hsi (Xi)	魏曦	
Wei Xihua	魏錫华	
Wu Liande	伍連德	
Wu Ruiping	吳瑞萍	Also Wu Ju-ping
Wu Shaoqing	吳紹青	
Wu Xian	吳宪	
Wu Zhili	吳之理	
Xie Shaowen	謝少文	Also Samuel Zia
Yan Fuqing	顏福慶	Also Jimmy Yen
Yang Yongnian	杨永年	Also Yang Yung-nien
Yao Lianyuan	要连元	
Yao Xunyuan	姚尋源	
Yan Chunhui	顏春輝	

ROMANIZATION	CHARACTERS	ENGLISH
Ye Shanlu	叶善篆	
Yuan Shikai	袁世凯	
Yu He	余贺	
Yu Longsheng	余龍生	
Yu Shufen	俞樹棻	
Zhao Kai	赵铠	
Zhi Hejie	志賀潔	Shiga Kiyoshi
Zhu Futang	諸福棠	Also Chu Fu-tang
Zhu Zongyao	朱宗尧	

TABLE G.3 Names of places

ROMANIZATION	CHARACTERS	ENGLISH
Anshun	安順	
Baoji	寶雞	Also Paochi
Dali	大理	Also Talifu
Gejiu	箇舊	
Geleshan	歌樂山	
Guiyang	貴陽	
Kunming	昆明	Also Yunnanfou and Yunnanfu
Lanzhou	蘭州	
Mengzi	蒙自	
Ruili	瑞麗	
Simao	思茅	Also Pu'er (普洱)
Tengyue	騰越	Also Tengyueh
Tuyunguan	圖雲關	
Yuxi	玉溪	
Zhefang	遮放	Also Chefang

TABLE G.4   Quotations

LOCATION	QUOTE (USING SIMPLIFIED OR TRADITIONAL CHARACTERS ACCORDING TO ORIGINAL TEXT)
Ch1, note 17	"庶幾學成之後，對於各種傳染病之診斷，治療及預防之外，更可督促省縣當局，作普及公共衛生之設施."
Ch1, note 34	"事中經過了千辛萬苦."
Ch1, note 40	"入滇後，以環境關係，校舍頗難覓得相當地址，致各院館教室等分設各處."
Ch1, note 42	"教師方面，因昆明为大后方，人才云集，延聘教师比较容易."
Ch2, note 30	"而边远县，区，偏僻乡村，尚多有相沿旧习，拒绝种痘，专事吹花者，为害婴孩，实非浅鲜."
Ch2, note 65	"各縣執行新法種痘工作醫院方面復於每年春季舉行免費種痘…．除注重實習種痘學術外兼授傳染病及公共衛生之知識以造就普遍之醫務人材."
Ch3, note 46	"第五條：遇有天花流行時，縣市衛生機關得施行強迫種痘，不論兒童或成人，均應一律受種."
Ch4, note 18	"中央防疫處自遷滇以來，即努力進行一切工作，近以前方及各地需要大量各種菌苗及牛痘苗，特積極加工趕製，現痘苗已製出，分發各醫務場所…且售價較廉，不久當可普及各地也."
Ch4, note 20	"（二）預防接種：實施大規模的補種牛痘和注射霍亂傷寒等疫苗."
Ch4, note 24	"第二，是前方的將士們和後方的同胞們應該普遍的每一個人都接受霍亂，痢疾和傷寒疫苗的預防注射，就是打預防針。因為打預防針以後身體裏就有了免疫力，就是偶然被傳染了也不會再有生命的危險的."
Ch4, note 42	"盡量利用文字及口頭宣傳，以期能明瞭重要性而自動注射，必要時得於城門街道強迫施行."
Ch4, note 43	"凡出入境人員，無預防注射証者，不准購買車票及飛機票，並登報通告."
Ch4, note 44	"其有違抗者，由各該地憲警協助，強迫注射."
Ch4, note 46	"本年防疫工作，雖經費種種頗有困難，而進行尚為順利，尚賴各衛生機關同仁之熱心協助，本市注射並未施行強制，均係自動踴躍請求注射."
Ch4, note 70	"仝人等悉心研究，專製各種生物學製品，並參照國際最新方法，嚴密製成."
Ch4, note 72	"一次種痘後，加反應良好，其抗天花之免疫性，約可保持五年."
Ch5, note 18	"结果方刚经服用磺胺类药物及注射抗菌素类药品，竟奇迹般地获得痊愈．其他人员也没有发现续发病例."
Ch5, note 19	"7. 举行霍乱，伤寒，天花，白喉等传染病预防注射与接种."
Ch5, note 23	"茲證明 [blank] 女士/先生 曾在本會醫院接受天花，霍亂，傷寒，及副傷寒，預防疫苗之注射,特給予證明 [blank] 醫師."
Ch5, note 30	"此次預防注射之效果，非僅於臨床統計有明顯之表示，而民眾事後對之亦多有認識。故當本人前往視察時，民眾多迫切希望能得新鮮疫苗之注射."

LOCATION	QUOTE (USING SIMPLIFIED OR TRADITIONAL CHARACTERS ACCORDING TO ORIGINAL TEXT)
Ch5, note 31	"預防注射，用強迫方式者結果反不如用啓發式者能多注射人數."
Ch5, note 34	"常常有人問到關於疫苗過了失效期是否可以注射的問題。其實疫苗瓶上所載的失效期是一個相當抽象的日期。主要的還是要看平日保管得是否適當。而且所謂失效，亦是指其免疫性能慢慢減退，並非說到了某一日期而突然失效毫無用處。假如需要注射而手頭僅有一瓶過期不太久的疫苗，那末仍是可以注射，因為並無害處，何況注射總比不注射要好些."
Ch5, note 36	"从科学医学的进展中，我们知道以人工的方法可以制出疫苗，把此种疫苗注射到人体后，体内即产生一种抵抗此疫苗的抵抗力来；这种抵抗力非但可以抵抗疫苗，并且可以抵抗与这种疫苗相同的传染病."
Ch5, note 37	"解放前注射多用强迫方式，今年则用说服教育方式，故市民皆自动至防疫处所注射."
Ch5, note 48	"念我國防痨之需要，遠遠涉重洋，逕赴巴黎入巴斯德研究院卡爾默特實驗室."
Ch5, note 56	"不能運至遠處施用，即在本地施用，必至拋棄甚多失效菌苗，大不經濟."
Ch5, note 60	"假令卡介苗毫無功效，則早已棄置不用，不至使現今美國學者籌設製造機關以接種美國之小兒矣."
Ch5, note 71	"'离开自己的国家去寄人篱下，我的精神不愉快！'…汤飞凡和夫人已经决定不走，就安下心来等待解放。汤飞凡的情绪好多了，全家人也都好像放下了一付担子，松了一口气."
Ch6, note 7	"第二条：中华人民共和国境内之居民，不分国籍，均须依照本办法之规定种痘."
	第六条：应种痘之居民，因疾病或其他正当理由，未能于规定时间种痘者，于其原因消除后，应即补种．凡无正当理由拒绝种痘，经说服教育无效者，各级卫生行政机关予以强制执行."
Ch6, note 12	"细菌战之事不了了之."
Ch6, note 15	"我们已经完全证实了美国军用机在朝鲜和我国东北境内投下了许多种虫子及其他毒物．各地细菌学家在各不同化验室中，已经由这些虫子及其他毒物分离出了各种致病的细菌."
Ch6, note 19–20	"也還有的人會這樣說：'我是在抗戰期間被趕到大後方來的，我是個外省人，現在解放了也用不着回老家去'…在這樣，就使得應該交給人民國家的財產，就被他們這些所謂'學者'，'科學家'與'技術人員'所瓜分了！"
Ch6, note 22	"请准备在辽东辽西两省全体军民中注射防疫苗．冀东冀中及京津也要作准备."
Ch6, note 23	"供应大批鼠疫，斑疹伤寒等疫苗，对部队进行紧急接种，同时也为驻地附近居民接种疫苗."
Ch6, note 26	"人人防疫，粉碎美帝國主義的细菌战！"
Ch6, note 41	"登記，統計是預防接種中的重要工作，不可忽視."

(*Continued*)

TABLE G.4 (Continued)

LOCATION	QUOTE (USING SIMPLIFIED OR TRADITIONAL CHARACTERS ACCORDING TO ORIGINAL TEXT)
Ch6, note 56	"很多人，甚至一部分医务工作人员本身，对预防接种工作也有时表现得束手束脚."
Ch6, note 58	"'我此刻不能打針，我的鋪子沒有人着' '我的攤子沒收' '娃子沒有睡着'."
Ch6 note 59	"有人說我小孩流年不利."
Ch6, note 61	"我們現在注射的是中央防疫處製造的霍亂傷寒混合疫苗，是把霍亂弧形菌和傷寒桿菌分別培養繁殖很多…."
Ch6, note 62	"在推行接種前，必須先經過一番思想動員，使接受接種兒童的家長，能正確的對接種的意義有所認識，這樣才能達到和我們密切的合作."
Ch6, note 64	"現在西南區各級衛生機關，在各大城市和交通要道，都在進行和佈置這一工作，替廣大人民負責，免費注射…．為了我們的安全，忍受短時的痛苦是值得的，否則自己得了病吃大虧，還要連累到別人."
Ch6, note 67	"我們要曉得，假使有一個人染了病，就可能傳染到整個區域，影響許多人的安全．這種普遍性的疾病流行，是不問張三李四的."
Ch6, note 68	"因為國民黨反動派不重視人民的健康，沒有預防注射設備：就是有，也是馬馬虎虎，不起什麼作用的，所以當這病以來，就送掉了好多人的生命."
Ch6, note 69	"現在人民政府在各級衛生機關，在各個交通要口，都掛了牌子，設了注射站，我們去打預防針，是再方便不過的…我們要曉得，這次預防注射是政府保持人民健康而舉行的一種運動…"
Ch6, note 70	"(醫)：就是因為它兇，所以我們的人民政府，這次花了很多錢，費了很大的力，動員這麼多的人，來給人民打這個防疫針."
Ch6, note 72	"林家院有一人，三年來未曾說服過他，這次我們再三向他解釋，而且經大組長…劝說結果也補種了."
Ch7, note 1	"当时我们卫生部要提供报告，因为根据下面报来的疫情，也不了解世界卫生组织要求什么资料，那么就简单写了一个报告."
Ch7, note 29	"儿童要防痨 快种卡介苗."
Ch7, note 30	"无产阶级文化大革命以来，我县广大医务人员、赤脚医生，遵照毛主席关于'预防为主'的教导，开展了农村卫生工作，大力推行了各种预防接种措施."
Ch7, note 61	"可能是印度的藏民跟世界卫生组织的专家说的时间是藏历年，年龄也可能是虚岁，说的是1962年，实际上不是."
Ch7, note 62	"不是完全证明，是推测."
Ch7, note 63	"赵铠提醒说，如若不信，又有谁能在稠人广众之中找到一个二十岁左右的麻脸青年呢？"
Epilogue, note 8	"试验全是别人替你做，你剥削别人的劳动，自己名利双收！你为什么把沙眼病毒给外国人？为什么把分离病毒的方法告诉外国人？出卖了多少科学秘密？得了什么好处？老实交待！"

Bibliography

A bibliography of the Chinese sources used in this book, with Chinese characters, can be consulted at https://www.people.hps.cam.ac.uk/index/teaching-officers/brazelton.

Abbreviations

SMDRR   Modern Documents Reading Room, Shanghai Library, Shanghai, China
YHMRR   Historical Materials Reading Room, Yunnan Provincial Library, Kunming, Yunnan, China

Archives

Academia Historica, Taipei, Taiwan
Archives nationales d'outre-mer, Aix-en-Provence, France
Archives of the League of Nations, United Nations, Geneva
Centre des Archives diplomatiques, Nantes, Pays de la Loire, France
Chongqing Municipal Archives, Chongqing, China
Collection of the American Bureau for Medical Aid to China, Columbia Rare Books and Manuscripts Library, Columbia University, New York
Institute of Modern History Archives, Academia Sinica, Taipei, Taiwan
Kunming Municipal Archives, Kunming, Yunnan, China
Kuomintang Archives, Taipei, Taiwan
Needham Research Institute, Cambridge, United Kingdom
Papers and Correspondence of Joseph Needham CH FRS, Cambridge University Archives, Cambridge, United Kingdom
Rockefeller Archive Center, Tarrytown, New York
Shanghai Municipal Archives, Shanghai, China
Yunnan Provincial Archives, Kunming, Yunnan, China

Primary sources

Abolnick, S. A. "BCG Vaccination in the U.S.S.R." *Chinese Medical Journal* 66 (October 1948): 564–67.
Anderson, John. *A Report on the Expedition to Western Yunan via Bhamô*. Calcutta: Office of the Superintendent of Government Printing, 1871.
Andreen, Andrea, Jean Malterre, Joseph Needham, Oliviero Olivo, Samuel Pessoa, and Nicolai Nicolaievitch Zhukov-Verezhnikov. *Report of the International Scientific Commission for the Investigation of the Facts Concerning Bacterial Warfare in Korea and China*. Peking: 1952.

Aronson, Joseph D. "Protective Vaccination against Tuberculosis with Special Reference to BCG Vaccination." *American Review of Tuberculosis* 58 (September 1948): 255–81.

Aronson, Joseph D., and C. E. Palmer. "Experience with BCG Vaccine in the Control of Tuberculosis among North American Indians." *Public Health Reports* 61 (June 7, 1946): 802–20.

Aronson, Joseph D., Erma I. Parr, and Robert M. Saylor. "The Specificity and Sensitivity of the Tuberculin Reaction following Vaccination with BCG." *American Journal of Hygiene, Section B* 33 (March 1941): 42–49.

Aspland, W. Graham. "Plague in Harbin." *British Medical Journal* 1, no. 2619 (March 11, 1911): 591.

Baber, E. Colborne. "Travels and Researches in western China," *Royal Geographic Society Supplementary Papers* 1 (1882): 1–201.

Balfour, M. C. "Travels in South-West China: Summary of an Address Given by Dr. M. C. Balfour to the Shanghai Public Health Club at the Y.M.C.A., Blvd. de Montigny, on April 8, 1940," *Shanghai yishi zhoukan* 6, no. 16 (April 15, 1940): 2–3. Accessed via SMDRR.

Beijing shi jiehebing fangzhi suo. "Ertong yao fanglao: Kuai zhong kajiemiao" [Children must prevent tuberculosis: Quickly get the BCG vaccine]. Poster, ca. 1965. National Library of Medicine Chinese Public Health Posters: Prevention of Diseases. https://collections.nlm.nih.gov/catalog/nlm:nlmuid-101561047-img.

"Ben she jin yao qi shi" [This publisher's critical note]. *Tongji yixue jikan* 7, no. 3 (March 31, 1940). Accessed via SMDRR.

Borg, Dorothy. "Chinese Health Work Progressing Despite War." *Far Eastern Survey* 9, no. 11 (May 22, 1940): 132–34.

Bryant, John. *Health and the Developing World*. Ithaca: Cornell University Press, 1969.

Cai Hongdao. "Huoluan yimiao shi zenyang zhizao de" [How the cholera vaccine is made]. *Yichao yuekan* 1, no. 8 (1947): 9. Accessed via SMDRR.

Cameron, John. "Pharmacy in China in 1938." *Chemist and Druggist* 130 (February 11, 1939): 147–148.

Chand, N. "Report on the Health of Tengyueh for the Half-Year Ended 31st March 1910." *China Imperial Maritime Customs II Special Series No. 2: Medical Reports, for the Half-Year Ended 30th September 1904 to the Half-Year Ended 30th September 1910*, no. 68–80: 99–101.

Chand, Wihal. "Report on the Health of Tengyueh for the Year Ended 31st March, 1909." *China Imperial Maritime Customs II Special Series No. 2: Medical Reports, for the Half-Year Ended 30th September 1904 to the Half-Year Ended 30th September 1910*, nos. 68–80: 56–59.

Chen, Lawrence M. (Chen Wentong). "Public Health in National Reconstruction." *Council of National Affairs Information Bulletin* 3, no. 3 (February 1, 1937): 51–82.

Chen Shichang, "Da zhen hou weishenme yao you fanying?" [Why is there a reaction after the injection?]. In Xinan junzheng weiyuanhui, *Guangbo wenji, di er ji*, 10–14.

Chen Shiguang. "Baoshan shuyi shicha baogao" [Report of a survey of the plague in Baoshan]. *Yunnan weisheng* 4, no. 1 (March 1947): 6. Accessed via YHMRR.

Chen, William Y. "Medicine and Public Health." *China Quarterly* 6 (June 1961): 153–69.

Chen Zhengren, Wei Xihua, and Zhu Zongyao. "BCG in China." *Chinese Medical Journal* 95, no. 6 (1982): 437–42.

Chen Zongxian (Tsen, Edgar T. H.). "The Etiology of Epidemic Poliomyelitis." *Journal of Experimental Medicine* 28, no. 3 (September 1, 1918): 269–87.

——. "Experiments on the Production of Anti-Poliomyelitic Serum in Rabbits." *Journal of Immunology* 3, no. 3 (May 1, 1918): 213–17.

Chinese Ministry of Information. *China Handbook 1937–1943*. New York: Macmillan, 1943.

"Chuanranbing guanli fangfa (ze zi Control of Communicable Diseases; A Manual of the American Public Health Association)" [Methods for managing infectious diseases, translated from *Control of Communicable Diseases: A Manual of the American Public Health Association*]. Translated by Wang Baoshu. *Yunnan weisheng* 5, nos. 1–2 (January 1948): 2–20. Accessed via YHMRR.

Clark, W. T. "In Consultation." *China Medical Journal* 24, no. 3 (May 1910): 211–12.

Clasener, H. A. L., and B. J. W. Beunders. "Immunization of Man with Typhoid and Cholera Vaccine: Agglutinating Antibodies after Intracutaneous and Subcutaneous Injection." *Journal of Hygiene* 65, no. 4 (December 1967): 449–56.

Colquhoun, A. R. "Exploration through the South China Borderlands, from the Mouth of the Si-kiang to the Banks of the Irawadi," *Proceedings of the Royal Geographic Society* 4 (1882): 713–30.

Columbia University Bulletin of Information: College of Physicians and Surgeons, Columbia University Announcement, 1917–1918. New York: Columbia University, 1917.

Davis, Paxton. *A Boy's War*. Winston-Salem, NC: John. F. Blair, 1990.

Deng Jinxian (Teng Chin-hsien), Zhu Futang (Chu Fu-t'ang), and Wu Ruiping (Wu Ju-p'ing). "Immunization against Whooping Cough." *Chinese Medical Journal* 64, nos. 5–6 (May/June 1946): 121–28.

Department of Health, Yunnan Province "Special Report on Smallpox and Its Eradication in Yunnan Province, China." World Health Organization report SME/79.10, 1979. http://apps.who.int/iris/handle/10665/68312.

"Di wu jie da hui lun wen timu" [Fifth general conference paper topics]. *Zhonghua yixue zazhi* 26, no. 7 (July 1940): 603–11. Accessed via SMDRR.

"Editorials." *China Medical Journal* 24, no. 4 (July 1910): 281–83.

Feng Youlan. *The Hall of Three Pines: An Account of My Life*. Honolulu: University of Hawaii Press, 2000.

Fenner, Frank, and J. G. Breman. "Report on a Visit to the People's Republic of China to Consider Matters Relating to the Certification of Smallpox Eradication, 14–30 July 1979." World Health Organization document SME/79.11.

"Fifth General Conference of C.M.A." *Shanghai yishi zhoukan* 6, no. 15 (April 8, 1940): 4. Accessed via SMDRR.

The French in Indo-China, with a Narrative of Garnier's Explorations in Cochinchina, Annam, and Tonquin. London: T. Nelson & Sons, 1884.

Gardner, A. D., and K. V. Venkatraman. "The Antigens of the Cholera Group of Vibrios." *Epidemiology and Infection* 35, no. 2 (May 1935): 262–82.

Geographic Health Studies Program, John E. Fogarty International Center for Advanced Study in the Health Sciences. *Topics of Study Interest in Chinese Medicine and Public Health: Report of a Planning Meeting*. Washington, DC: Department of Health, Education, and Welfare, Public Health Service, and National Institutes of Health, 1972.

Gonggong weisheng chu. "Da fangyi zhen weishenme yao fa zhushe zhengming" [Why does vaccination require an injection certificate]? In Xinan junzheng weiyuanhui, *Guangbo wenji, di er ji*, 15–18.

"Gongzuo baogao yu gongzuo yijian" [Work report and work recommendations]. *Yunnan weisheng* 3, nos. 9–10 (October 1946): 6. Accessed via YHMRR.

Government of the People's Republic of China (PRC). "Smallpox Eradication in China." Report submitted to World Health Organization on July 31, 1979. WHO/SE/79.142. http://apps.who.int/iris/handle/10665/68275.

Gu Fangzhou (Ku Fang-chou). "Mass Vaccination against Polio." *China Reconstructs* 12, no. 7 (July 1963): 28–30.

Gu Fangzhou (Ku, F. C.), D. X. Dong, O. S. Jhi, J. T. Niu, and H. H. Yang. "Poliomyelitis in China." *Journal of Infectious Diseases* 146 (1982): 552–57.

Gu Fangzhou (Ku, F. C.), Y. Zeng, C. S. Mao, et al. "Serological Response in Children under Seven Years of Age to Trivalent Sabin's Live Polio Vaccine." *Chinese Medical Journal* 47 (1961): 423–28.

Gu Fangzhou (Ku Fang-chou), Zhang Bingrui (Chang Ping-jui), Zheng Yuanlin (Cheng Yuan-lin), Chen Xisheng (Ch'en Hsi-sheng), Shen Yuzhen (Shen Yü-chen), Wu Mingxing (Wu Ming-hsing), Mao Jiangsen (Mao Chiang-sen), and Li Xuedong (Li Hsüeh-tung). "A Large Scale Trial with Live Polio Virus Prepared in China." *Chinese Medical Journal* 82, no. 3 (1963): 131–37.

Guo Keda. "Dijun shiyong xijun zhan de kenengxing he women ying you de zhunbei" [The possibility of the enemy army's use of biological warfare and the preparations we should make]. *Zhanshi yizheng* 3, nos. 8–9 (October 1941): 9–12. Accessed via SMDRR.

"Guolian xiezhu woguo fangyi" [The League of Nations is aiding our nation's epidemic prevention]. *Yunnan yikan* 1, no. 5 (January 10, 1939): 38. Accessed via YHMRR.

Guoli bian yi guan, ed. *Xijunxue mianyixue mingci* [Dictionary of bacteriology and immunology]. Shanghai: Shangwu yinshuguan, 1937. Accessed via SMDRR.

"Guowai zhi bu, yishi xiaoxi: Guolian daibiao fei yu shang fangyi wenti" [International section, medical news: League of Nations representatives fly to Chongqing to consult on disease prevention problems]. *Yunnan yikan* 1, no. 6 (March 25, 1939): 44–45. Accessed via YHMRR.

He Liyi with Claire Anne Chik. *Mr. China's Son: A Villager's Life.* 2nd ed. Boulder, CO: Westview, 2003.

Horn, Joshua. *Away with All Pests: An English Surgeon in People's China: 1954–1969.* New York and London: Monthly Review Press, 1969.

Hsu, Francis L. K. *Exorcising the Trouble Makers: Magic, Science, and Culture.* Westport, CT: Greenwood, 1983.

——. *Magic and Science in Western Yunnan: The Problem of Introducing Scientific Medicine in a Rustic Community.* New York: Institute of Pacific Relations, 1943.

——. *Religion, Science and Human Crises: A Study of China in Transition and Its Implication for the West.* London: Routledge & Kegan Paul, 1952.

Huang Chenxiang (Huang Chen-hsiang), Jia Bingyi (Chia Ping-yi), Zhu Futang (Chu Fu-t'ang), Guo Kejian (Kuo Ke-ch'ien), Wang Huiying (Wang Hui-ying), Wu Zonglin (Wu Tsung-lin), and Wu Xuexin (Wu Hsueh-hsin). "Studies on Attenuated Measles Vaccine. I. Clinical and Immunologic Response to Measles Virus Attenuated in Human Amnion Cells." *Chinese Medical Journal* 81, no. 1 (1962): 9–22.

Hunan zhongyi yao yanjiu suo ge wei hui, ed. *Chijiao yisheng shouce* [A barefoot doctor's manual]. Changsha: Hunan renmin chubanshe, 1971.

Jia Zhiqin. "Guizhou weisheng shiye gaishu" [A discussion of health work in Guizhou]. *Guoli Guiyang yixueyuan yuankan* (1948), nos. 24–25, 2–3. Accessed via SMDRR.

Ji Jilin. "Vaccin yufang jiezhong zhi mianyixue shang jianjie" [Gaining an understanding of the immunology of vaccinations]. *Yiyao pinglun* 55 (1931): 18–20. Accessed via SMDRR.

Jin Baoshan. "Chang qi kang zhan yu fangyi" [The long war of resistance and preventing disease]. *Xinyun daobao* 14 (1938). Accessed via SMDRR.

——. "Zuijin de weisheng jianshe" [Recent public health establishments]. *Zhandou Zhongguo* 1, no. 5 (1945): 14–19. Accessed via SMDRR.

"Kunming shi huoluan yufang zhushe gongzuo baogao" [Report on preventive injection work for cholera in Kunming city]. *Tongji yixue jikan* 7, no. 3 (March 1940): 146. Accessed via Chongqing Library, Chongqing, China.

Kunming shizhi [Kunming municipal gazetteer]. Kunming: Yunnan sheng Kunming shizheng gongsuo zongwu ke bianzuan, 1924. Accessed via YHMRR.

Kuo Yuan. *Yün-nan sheng ching-chi wen-t'i* [Economic problems of Yunnan Province]. Chongqing: Cheng-chung shu-chü, 1940. Reprinted by Center for Chinese Research Materials, Association of Research Libraries, Washington, DC, 1945.

Lee, Philip R. "Medicine and Public Health in the People's Republic of China." *Western Journal of Medicine*, no. 120 (May 1974): 430–37.

Lee, Wai-Man, and L. Nai-Kwai Lo. "The Rural Health Care Delivery System in the Dingxian Experiment: A Case Study of Educational Transfer in Republican China." *CUHK Education Journal* 16, no. 2 (1988): 145–47.

Lin Zongyang. "Zhongyang yimiao xueqing zhizao jiguan yu chuanranbing zhi yufang" [Central vaccine and sera production organizations and the prevention of infectious disease]. *Zhonghua yixue zazhi* 16, no. 2–3 (1930): 111–13.

Liu Yongchun (Y. Ch. Lieou) and Guo Chengzhou (C. C. Kouo). "B.C.G. Vaccination: Eleven Years of Experience." *Chinese Medical Journal* 67, no. 5 (May 1949): 275–78.

Liu Zhai. "B.C.G. yimiao jiezhong de xiaoguo" [The effectiveness of BCG vaccination]. *Yiyao xinzhi* 1, no. 5 (1948): 209. Accessed via SMDRR.

Long Yuying. *Mianyixue yuanli* [Principles of immunology]. Shanghai: Shangwu yinshu guan, 1933. Accessed via SMDRR.

Lu Zhijun. "Fan tanwu, fan langfei, fan guanliaozhuyi yundong zhuanlan" [Special column on the campaign to oppose corruption, waste, and bureaucratism]. *Xinan weisheng* 5, no. 5 (1952): 2–3.

——. "Zenyang duguo weixian de retian?" [How to endure the dangerous hot days?]. In Xinan junzheng weiyuanhui, *Guangbo wenji, di yi ji*, 4–6.

Mao Zedong. "Guanyu Fushun shijiao faxian da pi kunchong deng de piyu" [Remarks on the city and suburbs of Fushun discovering large amounts of insects, etc.]. In *Jianguo yi lai Mao zedong wengao* [Writings of Mao Zedong at the founding of the nation], vol. 3, 303. Beijing: Zhongyang wenxian chubanshe, 1989.

"Medical News." *British Medical Journal* 2, no. 4484 (December 1946): 926–27.

Miao Ancheng and Chen Shiguang. "Yunnan yi xi qu xian shu yi" [Bubonic plague in western Yunnan]. *Yunnan weisheng* 4, no. 3 (May 15, 1947): 6–7. Accessed via YHMRR.

National Health Administration and Central Field Health Station. *National Epidemic Prevention Bureau: A Report, Being a Review of Its Activities from Its Foundation in March 1919 to June 1934*. Peiping: 1934.

Needham, Joseph, and Dorothy Needham, eds. *Science Outpost: Papers of the Sino-British Science Cooperation Office* (British Council Scientific Office in China), 1942–46. London: Pilot, 1948.

Newell, Kenneth, ed. *Health by the People*. Geneva: World Health Organization, 1975.

"Niudou bixu" [Smallpox inoculation requirements]. *Yunnan Yikan* 1, no. 5 (January 1939): 7. Accessed via YHMRR.

Ortholan, M. le Dr. "Rapport médical sur l'état sanitaire de Szémao pendant le premier semestre 1900" [Medical report on the sanitary conditions of Simao during the first part of the year 1900]. *China Imperial Maritime Customs II Special Series No. 2: Medical Reports, for the Half-Year Ended 30th September 1900*, no. 60: 38–43.

Pang Bin. "Duiyu zhongyang fangyi chu gan yan: Die Seuchenbeknempfung in China" [Impressions of the National Epidemic Prevention Bureau: Fighting disease in China]. *Yi yao xue* (1925): 9–13. Accessed via SMDRR.

Pei Cunfan. "Nian ba nian ben shi kai ye xi yi nianling xiang guan tongji biao" [Table describing the medical staff and equipment in every hospital in this city for the year 1939]. *Kunming shi shizheng tongji* (1939): 71. Accessed via YHMRR.

Peking Film Studio of China. *U.S. Crime of Bacteriological Warfare.* 1952. File ARC 537560 / LI 263.630. National Archives and Records Administration, College Park, MD. https://archive.org/details/gov.archives.arc.1537560.

Peking Film Studio of China and the National Film Studio of Korea. *Oppose Bacteriological Warfare!* 1952. File ARC 1630600 / LI 263.1006. National Archives and Records Administration, College Park, MD. https://archive.org/details/gov.archives.arc.1630600.

Qiao (Chiao) Shumin. "Project on BCG Vaccination for China." *Chinese Medical Journal* 66, no. 10 (October 1948): 568–75.

"RCSC Sends Gift to Nepalese Earthquake Victims." *China's Medicine*, no. 1 (October 1966): 85.

Ren Kangcai. "Yong kajiemiao jiezhong yufang jiehebing" [Using the BCG vaccine to prevent tuberculosis]. *Xinan weisheng*, no. 18 (February 1951): 13–14.

"Report of the International Scientific Commission for the Investigation of the Facts Concerning Bacterial Warfare in Korea and China." *Chinese Medical Journal* 70, nos. 9–12 (1952): 337–651.

Report to the International Sanitary Conference of a Commission from That Body, on the Origin, Endemicity, Transmissibility, and Propagation of Asiatic Cholera. Translated by Samuel Abbot. Boston: Alfred Mudge & Son, 1867.

Revolutionary Health Committee of Hunan Province. *A Barefoot Doctors' Manual: Revised and Enlarged Edition.* Mayne Isle, BC, and Seattle: Cloudburst Press, 1977.

Rocher, Émile. "Notes sur la peste au Yün-nan" [Notes on the plague in Yunnan]. *La Province Chinoise du Yün-nan, deuxième partie* [The Chinese province of Yunnan, second part]. Paris: Librairie de la société asiatique de l'école des langues orientales vivantes, 1880.

Rosinger, Lawrence K. "Yunnan: Province of the Burma Road." *Far Eastern Survey* 11, no. 2 (January 26, 1942): 19–23.

Shanghai fanglao xiehui. "Er tong yao fang lao: Jie zhong ka jie miao" [We must prevent tuberculosis in children: Vaccinate with BCG]. Shanghai: Shanghai fanglao xiehui, 1953. Poster made available online by United States National Library of Medicine. https://collections.nlm.nih.gov/catalog/nlm:nlmuid-101557191-img.

Shih Kuo-heng. *China Enters the Machine Age: A Study of Labor in Chinese War Industry.* Edited and translated by Fei Hsiao-tung and Francis L. K. Hsu. Cambridge, MA: Harvard University Press, 1944.

Sidel, Victor W. "The Barefoot Doctors of the People's Republic of China." *New England Journal of Medicine* 286 (1972): 1292–1300.

Sidel, Victor W., and Ruth Sidel. "The Delivery of Medical Care in China." *Scientific American* 230, no. 4 (April 1974): 19–27.

——. "Health Care in the People's Republic of China." In *Alternative Approaches to Meeting Basic Health Needs in Developing Countries,* edited by V. Djukanovic and E. P. Mach, 35–50. Geneva: World Health Organization, 1975.

——. *Serve the People: Observations on Medicine in the People's Republic of China.* New York: Josiah Macy Jr. Foundation, 1974.

Sircar, Ram Lall. "Report on the Health of Tengyueh for the Two Years Ending 31st March 1908," *China Imperial Maritime Customs II Special Series No. 2: Medical Reports, for the Half-Year Ended 30th September 1904 to the Half-Year Ended 30th September 1910*, nos. 68–80: 35–43.

Snow, Edgar. *The Other Side of the River: Red China Today*. New York: Random House, 1962.

Song Jie (Sung Chieh). "Guest Editorial: BCG Vaccination in China as a Pediatrician Sees It." *Chinese Medical Journal* 67, no. 5 (May 1949): 287–90.

"'Statement of the [PRC] Ministry of Public Health,' NCNA-English, Peking (June 29, 1967), in *FBIS*, no. 127: BBB11–12 (June 30, 1967)." In *People's China and International Law, vol. 1: A Documentary Study*, edited by Jerome A. Cohen and Chiu Hungdah, 515. Princeton, NJ: Princeton University Press, 1974.

Strong, Richard P. *Protective Inoculation against Asiatic Cholera: An Experimental Study*. Publications of the Bureau of Government Laboratories, Department of the Interior, no. 16. Manila: Bureau of Public Printing, 1904.

"Student Describes Bombing of Southwest University." *China at War* 7, no. 4 (October 1941): 35–36.

Tang Feifan. "Adsorption Experiments with the Virus of Vaccinia," *Journal of Bacteriology* 24, no. 2 (August 1932): 133–43.

——. "The International Scientific Commission Discloses the Crimes of the American Imperialists in Waging Bacterial Warfare." *Chinese Medical Journal* 70, supplement (1952): 26–27.

——. "The National Vaccine and Serum Institute: Retrospect and Prospect." *Chinese Medical Journal* 65, nos. 5–6 (May/June 1947): 177–81.

——. *Yufang jiezhong* [Immunization]. Beijing: Kexue puji chubanshe, 1956.

Tang Feifan (T'ang Fei-fan), Chang Xiaolou (Chang Hsiao-lou), Huang Yuantong (Huang Yuan-t'ung), and Wang Keqian (Wang K'o-ch'ien). "Studies on the Etiology of Trachoma with Special Reference to Isolation of the Virus in Chick Embryo." *Chinese Medical Journal* 75, no. 6 (June 1957): 429–47.

Tang Feifan, C. M. Chu, and Y. W. Wong. "A Study of *Vibrio Cholerae* Isolated from the 1942 Kunming Epidemic, with Special Reference to Serological Types." *Indian Journal of Medical Research* 32, no. 1 (May 1944): 1–8.

Tang Feifan and Wei Xi (Hsi). "Morphological Studies on Vaccinia Virus Cultivated in the Developing Egg." *Journal of Pathology and Bacteriology* 45, no. 2 (1937): 317–23.

Taylor, Carl. *Doctors for the Villages: Study of Rural Internships in Seven Indian Medical Colleges*. New York: Asia Publishing House, 1976.

Topley, William W. C., and Graham S. Wilson. *The Principles of Bacteriology and Immunity*. 2nd ed. London Edward Arnold, 1936.

"Tushu jieshao: Zhongwen cankao shu jin kan shi zhong; xijunxue mianyixue mingci (Guoli bianyi guan bianding)" [Introduction to books: Chinese reference works, ten kinds; Bacteriology and immunology terminology (edited by National Institute for Compilation and Translation)]. *Tushu jikan* 1, no. 1 (1939): 47. Accessed via SMDRR.

United States Agency for International Development. *The Barefoot Doctors of Rural China*, 1975. ARC Identifier 46549/local identifier 286.260. Available via PublicResource Org at www.youtube.com/watch?v=1YvwVFC-TJY.

Vadon, M. le Dr. "Un poste médical consulaire en Chine: Yunnan-Fou" [A medical consular post in China: Kunming]. *Annales d'hygiène et de médecine coloniales*, vol. 17. Paris : Doin, 1914. 501–25.

Vassal, Gabrielle M. *In and Round Yunnan-fou*. London: William Heinemann, 1922.

Vincent, George E. "China Medical Board: Report of the General Director." In *The Rockefeller Foundation Annual Report, 1920*, 219–70. New York: Rockefeller Foundation, 1920.

Walsh, Warren B. "The Yunnan Myth." *Far Eastern Quarterly* 2, no 3 (May 1943): 272–85.

Wang Chongji and Ding Xuefeng. "Zhongyang fangyi chu qian kun hou de lishi jiankuang" [A historical profile of the National Epidemic Prevention Bureau after it moved to Kunming]. In *Feng yu yi dang nian: Kunming shizheng xie wen shi ziliao ji cui* [Recalling the storm of that year: Collected historical materials from the Kunming city government], vol. 2, edited by Kunming shizheng xie wenshi ziliao he xuexi weiyuanhui, 150–55. Kunming: Yunnan meishu chubanshe, 1997.

Wang Huiyin. "Yufang zhushe" [Preventive injection]. In Xinan junzheng weiyuanhui, *Guangbo wenji, di yi ji*, 23–26.

——. "Zenyang cai neng bu de huoluan he shanghan?" [How can one avoid catching cholera and typhoid fever?]. In Xinan junzheng weiyuanhui, *Guangbo wenji, di er ji*, 1–5.

Wang Liang. "Lun BCG fanglao yimiao zhi xiaoyong" [Discussion of the efficacy of the BCG vaccine]. *Xin Chongqing* 2, no. 1 (1948): 13–16. Accessed via SMDRR.

——. "Da fangyi zhen zenme hui fangmian huoluan he shanghan?" [How can vaccination prevent cholera and typhoid fever?]. In Xinan junzheng weiyuanhui, *Guangbo wenji, di er ji*, 6–9.

Wang Qizong. "Renmin yiyuan yinan lai gongzuo gaikuang" [A survey of the Philanthropic Hospital's work over one year]. *Gongyi*, no. 1 (December 1, 1949): 4–8. Accessed via YHMRR.

Wang Tianzuo. "Dianxi shuyi fangzhi di san dui gongzuo baogao (xu): Sanshiwu nian liu qi liang yue" [Work report of Western Yunnan Plague Prevention Team No. 3, for the months of June and July 1946]. *Yunnan weisheng* 4, nos. 9–10 (October 15, 1947): 9–11. Accessed via YHMRR.

Wang Yuanchen. "Chuxi Zhonghua yixuehui di wu jie da hui ji canguan dian zhu yiyao weisheng" [Attending the Chinese Medical Association's Fifth General Conference and taking a look at medicine and public health in Yunnan and Guiyang]. *Yiyu* 4, no. 2 (1940): 1–18. Accessed via SMDRR.

"Weisheng, biao er: Zhongyang fangyichu zhipin chanliang" [Public health, chart 2: National Epidemic Prevention Bureau production figures]. *Tongji yuebao*, no. 39 (1939): 7. Accessed via SMDRR.

"Weisheng, biao san: Zhongyang fangyichu zhipin chanliang" [Public health, chart 3: National Epidemic Prevention Bureau production figures]. *Tongji yuebao*, no. 38 (1939): 18. Accessed via SMDRR.

"Weisheng, biao san: Zhongyang fangyichu zhipin chanliang" [Public health, chart 3: National Epidemic Prevention Bureau production figures]. *Tongji yuebao*, no. 41 (1940): 9. Accessed via Accessed via SMDRR.

"Weisheng, biao san: Zhongyang fangyichu zhipin chanliang" [Public health, chart 3: National Epidemic Prevention Bureau production figures]. *Tongji yuebao*, no. 42 (1940): 5. Accessed via SMDRR.

"Weisheng, biao san: Zhongyang fangyichu zhipin chanliang" [Public health, chart 3: National Epidemic Prevention Bureau production figures]. *Tongji yuebao*, no. 48 (1940): 22. Accessed via SMDRR.

"Weisheng, biao san: Zhongyang fangyichu zhipin chanliang" [Public health, chart 3: National Epidemic Prevention Bureau production figures]. *Tongji yuebao*, no. 55 (1941): 26. Accessed via SMDRR.

"Weisheng, biao san: Zhongyang fangyichu zhipin chanliang" [Public health, chart 3: National Epidemic Prevention Bureau production figures]. *Tongji yuebao*, nos. 73–74 (1942): 32. Accessed via SMDRR.

Weishengbu and Renmin geming junshi weiyuanhui weishengbu. "Guanyu kaizhan junmin chunji fangyi gongzuo de zhishi" [Directive on springtime military epidemic prevention work]. In *Zhongyang renmin zhengfu faling huibian, 1949–1950* [Central People's Government Compilation of Laws, 1949–50], edited by Zhongyang renmin zhengfu fazhi weiyuanhui, 829–32. Beijing: Falü chubanshe, 1982.

Wei Xi (Hsi). "Preparation of Simple and Dried Smallpox Vaccine in Gum Acacia." *Chinese Medical Journal* 65, nos. 5–6 (May/June 1947): 163–66.

Wei Xi (Hsi) and Wen Pinwei. "Experimental Infection of Silkworm Pupa with Typhus Rickettsia: A Preliminary Report." *Chinese Medical Journal* 65, nos. 5–6 (May/June 1947): 171–75.

Wei Xi (Hsi) and Zhong Huilan (Chung Huei-lan). "Peace and Pestilence at War." *Chinese Medical Journal* 70, supplement (1952): 8–20.

Werner, David. *Where There Is No Doctor*. Palo Alto, CA: Hesperian Books, 1977.

Witebsky, Ernest. "Ehrlich's Side-Chain Theory in the Light of Present Immunology." *Annals of the New York Academy of Sciences* 59 (September 1954): 168–81.

Wu Liande (Wu Lien-teh), J.W.H. Chun, Robert Pollitzer, and C. Y. Wu. *Cholera: A Manual for the Medical Profession in China*. Shanghai: National Quarantine Service, 1934.

——. *Plague Fighter: The Autobiography of a Modern Chinese Physician*. Cambridge: W. Heffer & Sons, 1959.

Wu Shaoqing (S. C.). "Guest Editorial: BCG Vaccination for Tuberculosis Control in China." *Chinese Medical Journal* 65, nos. 9–10 (September/October 1947): 381–83.

Wu Zhili. *Yi ming jun yi de zishu* [A military doctor's account in his own words]. Beijing: Huaxia chubanshe, 2004.

"Xialing weisheng yundong shishi banfa (1946 nian 8 yue weishengshu gongbu)" [Summer health campaign execution instructions (August 1946 announcement by National Health Administration)]. In *Zhongguo weisheng fagui shiliao xuanbian (1912–1949.9)* [Historical materials and selections from Chinese health laws, 1912–September 1949], edited by Chen Mingguang, 604–5. Shanghai: Shanghai yike daxue chubanshe, 1996.

Xie Shaowen (Samuel H. Zia). "Guest Editorial: A Bacteriologist Looks at Medical Education." *Chinese Medical Journal* 65, nos. 5–6 (May/June 1947): 182–86.

——. *Xie Shaowen lun zhu xuanji: Zhuhe xie lao jiu zhi huadan* [Selected writings of Xie Shaowen: In congratulations upon his retirement at his ninetieth birthday]. Beijing: Beijing yike daxue, Zhongguo xiehe yike daxue lianhe chubanshe, 1993.

——. "Xijunxue ji mianyixue jiaoshou fa zhi shangque" [Discussion of bacteriology and immunology teaching methods]. *Yiyu* 1, no. 7 (1936): 6–10. Accessed via SMDRR.

Xijunxue zonglun, mianyixue, xijun mingcheng, xijun fenlei: Kexue mingci shencha hui yixue mingci shencha ben [Report of the General Committee on Scientific Terminology: Terms in general bacteriology, immunology, names of bacteria, classification of bacteria]: 1918. Accessed via SMDRR.

Xinan junzheng weiyuanhui, ed. *Guangbo wenji, di yi ji* [Collected broadcasts, vol. 1]. Chongqing: Xinan weisheng shubao chubanshe, 1950.

——. *Guangbo wenji, di er ji* [Collected broadcasts, vol. 2]. Chongqing: Xinan weisheng shubao chubanshe, 1950.

Xin shenghuo yundong cujin hui xuanchuan gu, ed. *Xin shenghuo yundong zhuankan* [New Life Movement special issue]. Dali (August 26, 1934). Accessed via YHMRR.

Xu Duanqing. "Xiao'er ke zhong chang jian zhi chuanranbing de yufang" [The prevention of diseases that small children often encounter in the classroom]. *Yunnan yikan* 1, no. 6 (January 1939): 1. Accessed via YHMRR.

Yao Xunyuan. *Yunnan xingzheng jishi 22: Weisheng* [Yunnan administrative report, vol. 22: Public health]. Kunming: 1936. Accessed via YHMRR.

Yan (Yen) Chunhui. "A Differential Medium for the Isolation of *V. Cholerae*." *Chinese Medical Journal* 65, nos. 5–6 (May/June 1947): 133–34.

Ye Shanlu. "Renren fangyi, fensui Mei diguo zhuyi de xijunzhan" [Everybody must take precautions against epidemics to smash the germ warfare of American imperialism]. Beijing: Renmin meishu chubanshe, 1952. IISH/Landsberger Collections. http://chineseposters.net/gallery/e13-964.php.

"Yiqing: Yunnan quansheng weisheng shiyan chu sa yi niandu ba, qi liang yue huoluan fangzhi gongzuo jianbao" [Epidemic situation: Brief report of the work of the Yunnan Provincial Experimental Health Station to control cholera during July and August 1942]. *Yunnan weisheng* 2, no. 8 (November 1942): 13–15. Accessed via YHMRR.

Yu Longsheng. "Xiao nei xiaoxi: Kangzhan hou xuexiao banqian xiaoji" [School news: A short account of the school's wartime relocation]. *Tongji yixue jikan* 7, no. 3 (March 31, 1940): 145. Accessed via SMDRR.

Yunnan sheng minzheng ting, ed. *Yunnan sheng min zheng ting wu nian weisheng gongzuo baogao* [Yunnan Provincial Department of Civil Affairs five-year public health work report], 1932. Accessed via YHMRR.

"Yunnan sheng san shi yi nian huoluan liuxing ji qi fangzhi gongzuo chu (zi wu yue shier ri zhi liu yue san shi ri zhi)" [Cholera's spread in Yunnan in 1942 and early work to prevent and cure it (from May 12 to June 30)]. *Yunnan weisheng* 2, no. 7 (September 30, 1942): 1–16. Accessed via YHMRR.

"Zao niudoumiao zhi chubu baogao" [Initial report of a dessicated smallpox vaccine]. *Yunnan weisheng* 4, nos. 9–10 (October 15, 1947): 11. Accessed via YHMRR.

"Zhengwu yuan guanyu yi jiu wu san nian jixu kaizhan aiguo weisheng yundong de zhishi, yi jiu wu er nian shi er yue san shi yi ri" [Directive of the State Administrative Council regarding the 1953 continuation of the Patriotic Hygiene Campaign, Dec. 31, 1952]. In *Zhongyang renmin zhengfu faling huibian, 1952* [Central People's Government Compilation of Laws, 1952], edited by Zhongyang renmin zhengfu fazhi weiyuanhui, 258–59. Beijing: Falü chubanshe, 1982.

Zhi Hejie (Shiga Kiyoshi). *Jinshi bingyuan weishengwu ji mianyixue* [Modern pathogenic microbes and immunology]. Translated by Tang Erhe. Shanghai: Shangwu yinshuguan, 1928.

"Zhongdou tiaoli" [Rules for inoculators]. In *Minguo fagui jicheng di 59 ce* [Republican law compilation, vol. 59], edited by Cai Hongyuan, 506. Hefei: Huangshan shu she, 1999.

"Zhongdou zanxing banfa: Yi jiu wu ling nian shi yue shi er ri weisheng bu gongbu" [Temporary smallpox vaccination measures: Ministry of Health Public announcement, October 12, 1950]. In *Zhongyang renmin zhengfu faling huibian, 1949–1950* [Central People's Government Compilation of Laws, 1949–50], edited by Zhongyang renmin zhengfu fazhi weiyuanhui, 843–44. Beijing: Falü chubanshe, 1982.

Zhonghua renmin gonghe guo weisheng bu weisheng fangyi si, ed. *Yufang jiezhong shouce* [Handbook for inoculators]. Beijing: Renmin weisheng chubanshe, 1959.

"Zhongyang fangyi chu" [National Epidemic Prevention Bureau]. *Gonggong weisheng yuekan* 1, no. 6 (December 1935). Accessed via SMDRR.

"Zhongyang fangyi chu" [National Epidemic Prevention Bureau]. *Yunnan Yikan* 2, no. 2 (April 1940). Accessed via YHMRR.

"Zhongyang fangyi chu zhizao xueqing" [The National Epidemic Prevention Bureau is producing serum]. *Yunnan Yikan* 1, no. 6 (March 1939): 45. Accessed via YHMRR.

Zhou Enlai. "Zhengwu yuan guanyu fadong qiuji zhongdou yundong de zhishi" [Briefing of the State Administrative Council in relation to launching the autumn smallpox movement]. In *Zhongyang renmin zhengfu faling huibian, 1949–1950* [Central People's Government Compilation of Laws, 1949–50], edited by Zhongyang renmin zhengfu fazhi weiyuanhui, 841–42. Beijing: Falü chubanshe, 1982.

Zhu Hengbi (H. P. Chu) "Medical Education during the Anti-Aggression War." *Chinese Medical Journal* 64, nos. 1–2 (January/February 1946): 17–23.

Zinsser, Hans, and Chen Zongxian (Edgar Tsen). "On Hyperleucocytosis and Its Bearing on Specific Therapy." *Journal of Immunology* 2, no. 3 (April 1, 1917): 247–68.

Zinsser, Hans, Florence Fitzpatrick, and Wei Xi (Wei Hsi). "A Study of Rickettsiae Grown on Agar Tissue Cultures." *Journal of Experimental Medicine* 69, no. 2 (1939): 179–90.

Secondary sources

Ai Zhike. "Xin zhongguo chengli chuqi de chengshi gonggong weisheng yanjiu (1949–1957): Yi huanjing weisheng yu jiyi fangzhi wei zhongxin" [Urban public health research on the early People's Republic of China (1949–1957): Prioritizing environmental hygiene and disease prevention]. PhD diss., Sichuan University, 2010.

Altorfer-Ong, Alicia. "Old Comrades and New Brothers: A Historical Re-examination of the Sino-Zanzibari and Sino-Tanzanian Bilateral Relationships in the 1960s." PhD diss., London School of Economics, 2014.

Anderson, Warwick. "Getting Ahead of One's Self?: The Common Culture of Immunology and Philosophy." *Isis* 105, no. 3 (September 2014): 606–16.

——. "Immunization and Hygiene in the Colonial Philippines." *Journal of the History of Medicine and Allied Sciences* 62, no. 1 (2007): 1–20.

Anderson, Warwick, Myles Jackson, and Barbara Gutmann Rosenkrantz. "Toward an Unnatural History of Immunology" *Journal of the History of Biology* 27, no. 3 (Autumn 1994): 575–94.

Andrews, Bridie. *The Making of Modern Chinese Medicine, 1850–1960*. Vancouver: University of British Columbia Press, 2014.

——. "Tuberculosis and the Assimilation of Germ Theory in China, 1895–1937." *Journal of the History of Medicine* 52 (January 1997): 114–57.

Andrews, Bridie, and Mary Brown Bullock, eds. *Medical Transitions in Twentieth-Century China*. Bloomington and Indianapolis: Indiana University Press, 2014.

Aoki, Masahiko, and Jinglian Wu, eds. *The Chinese Economy: A New Transition*. Basingstoke, UK: Palgrave Macmillan, 2012.

Arnold, David. *Colonizing the Body: State Medicine and Epidemic Disease in Nineteenth-Century India*. Berkeley: University of California Press, 1993.

Atwill, David. *The Chinese Sultanate: Islam, Ethnicity, and the Panthay Rebellion in Southwest China, 1856–1873*. Stanford, CA: Stanford University Press, 2005.

Balińska, Marta Alexandra. "Ludwik Rajchman, International Health Leader." *World Health Forum* 12 (1991): 456–65.

Banister, Judith. *China's Changing Population*. Stanford, CA: Stanford University Press, 1987.

Barenblatt, Daniel. *A Plague upon Humanity: The Hidden History of Japan's Biological Warfare Program*. New York: HarperCollins, 2004.

Barnes, Nicole E. *Intimate Communities: Wartime Healthcare and the Birth of Modern China, 1937–1945*. Oakland: University of California Press, 2018.

——. "Protecting the National Body: Gender and Public Health in Southwest China during the War with Japan, 1937–1945." PhD diss., University of California–Irvine, 2012.

Barnes, Nicole E., and John R. Watt. "The Influence of War on China's Modern Health Systems." In Andrews and Bullock, *Medical Transitions in Twentieth-Century China*, 227–43.

Bello, David A. "To Go Where No Han Could Go for Long: Malaria and the Qing Construction of Ethnic Administrative Space in Frontier Yunnan." *Modern China* 31, no. 3 (July 2005): 283–317.

Benedict, Carol. *Bubonic Plague in Nineteenth-Century China*. Stanford, CA: Stanford University Press, 1996.

Bloom, David E., and Jeffrey G. Williamson. "Demographic Transitions and Economic Miracles in Emerging Asia." *World Bank Economic Review* 12, no. 3 (1998): 419–55.

Bowers, John Z. *Western Medicine in a Chinese Palace: Peking Union Medical College, 1917–51*. Philadelphia: Josiah Macy Jr. Foundation, 1972.

Bray, David. *Social Space and Governance in Urban China: The* Danwei *System from Origins to Reform*. Stanford, CA: Stanford University Press, 2005.

Brazelton, Mary Augusta. "Engineering Health: Technologies of Immunization in China's Wartime Hinterland, 1937–45." *Technology and Culture* 60, no. 2 (2019): 409–37.

Bretelle-Establet, Florence. "French Medicine in Nineteenth- and Twentieth-Century China: Rejection or Compliance in Far South Treaty-Ports, Concessions and Leased Territories." In *Twentieth-Century Colonialism and China: Localities, the Everyday and the World*, edited by Bryna Goodman and David S. G. Goodman, 134–50. New York: Routledge, 2012.

——. "La santé en Chine du Sud à la fin de l'Empire et au début de la République" [Health in the south of China at the end of empire and the beginning of the republic]. PhD diss., Université de Paris VII, 1999.

——. "Resistance and Receptivity: French Colonial Medicine in Southwest China, 1898–1930." *Modern China* 25, no. 2 (April 1999): 171–203.

Brook, Timothy. *Collaboration*. Cambridge, MA: Harvard University Press, 2005.

Brown, Jeremy, and Paul Pickowicz, eds. *Dilemmas of Victory: The Early Years of the People's Republic of China*. Cambridge, MA: Harvard University Press, 2007.

Brown, Theodore, Marcos Cueto, and Elizabeth Fee. "The World Health Organization and the Transition from 'International' to 'Global' Public Health." *American Journal of Public Health* 96, no. 1 (January 2006): 62–72.

Brunero, Donna. *Britain's Imperial Cornerstone in China: The Chinese Maritime Customs Service, 1854–1949*. London: Routledge, 2006.

Campbell, Timothy, and Adam Sitze. "Introduction." In Campbell and Sitze, *Biopolitics*, 1–40.

——, eds. *Biopolitics: A Reader*. Durham, NC: Duke University Press, 2013.

Cao Cong. *China's Scientific Elite*. London: RoutledgeCurzon, 2004.

Cao Xuetao. "Immunology in China: The Past, Present, and Future." *Nature Immunology* 9, no. 4 (April 2008): 339–42.

Carpenter, Charles C. J., and Richard B. Hornick. "Killed Vaccines: Cholera, Typhoid, and Plague." In *Vaccines: A Biography*, edited by Andrew W. Artenstein, 87–103. New York: Springer, 2010.

Chai, Joseph C. H. *An Economic History of Modern China*. Cheltenham, UK: Edward Elgar, 2011.

Chakrabarti, Pratik. *Bacteriology in British India: Laboratory Medicine and the Tropics*. Rochester, NY: University of Rochester, 2012.

———. *Medicine and Empire, 1600–1960*. Basingstoke, UK: Palgrave Macmillan, 2014.

Cheek, Timothy. *Propaganda and Culture in Mao's China: Deng Tuo and the Intelligentsia*. Oxford: Clarendon Press, 1997.

Chen Haidan. "Cord-Blood Banking in China: Public and Private Tensions." *East Asian Science, Technology and Society* 5, no. 3 (2011): 329–39.

Chen, Lincoln, and Ling Chen. "China's Exceptional Health Transitions: Overcoming the Four Horsemen of the Apocalypse." In Andrews and Bullock, *Medical Transitions in Twentieth-Century China*, 17–31.

Chen Shiwei. "History of Three Mobilizations: A Reexamination of the Chinese Biological Warfare Allegations against the United States in the Korean War." *Journal of American–East Asian Relations* 16, no. 3 (2009): 213–47.

Chen, Theodore Hsi-en, and Wen-Hui C. Chen. "The 'Three-Anti' and 'Five-Anti' Movements in Communist China." *Pacific Affairs* 26, no. 1 (March 1953): 3–23.

Chen Yung-fa. *Making Revolution: The Communist Movement in Eastern and Central China, 1937–1945*. Berkeley and Los Angeles: University of California Press, 1986.

Cheng Guangsheng, Ming Li, and George F. Gao. "Recollection: 'A Friend to Man,' Dr. Feifang Tang; A Story of Causative Agent of Trachoma, from 'Tang's Virus' to Chlamydia Trachomatis, to 'Phylum Chlamydiae.'" *Protein Cell* 2, no. 5 (2011): 349–50.

Cheng Tiejun, and Mark Selden. "The Origins and Social Consequences of China's *Hukou* System." *China Quarterly*, no. 139 (September 1994): 644–68.

Cheng Xiaoping. "Wo guo fangshe xue dianji ren: Rong Dushan [A foundational figure in Chinese radiology: Rong Dushan]. Shanghai Municipal Archives. June 25, 2008. http://www.archives.sh.cn/shjy/hsrw/201203/t20120313_6175.html.

Chiang, Howard. "From Postcolonial to Subimperial Formations of Medicine: Superregional Perspectives from Taiwan and Korea." *East Asian Science, Technology, and Society* 11 (2017): 469–75.

Cohen, Ed. *A Body Worth Defending: Immunity, Biopolitics, and the Apotheosis of the Modern Body*. Durham, NC: Duke University Press, 2009.

Colgrove, James K. *State of Immunity: The Politics of Vaccination in Twentieth-Century America*. Berkeley: University of California Press, 2006.

Comstock, George W. "The International Tuberculosis Campaign: A Pioneering Venture in Mass Vaccination and Research." *Clinical Infectious Diseases* 19, no. 3 (September 1994): 528–40.

Condrau, Flurin, and Michael Worboys, eds. *Tuberculosis Then and Now: Perspectives on the History of an Infectious Disease*. Montreal and Kingston, ON: McGill-Queen's University Press, 2010.

Conis, Elena. *Vaccine Nation*. Chicago: University of Chicago Press, 2015.

Cooter, Roger, Mark Harrison, and Steve Sturdy, eds. *Medicine and Modern Warfare*. Clio Medica 55. Amsterdam: Rodopi, 1999.

Core, Rachel. "Tuberculosis Control in Shanghai: Bringing Health to the Masses, 1928–Present." In Andrews and Bullock, *Medical Transitions in Twentieth Century China*, 126–45.

Cowdrey, Albert. "'Germ Warfare' and Public Health in the Korean Conflict." *Journal of the History of Medicine and Allied Sciences* 39 (1984): 153–72.

Cueto, Marcos. "The Origins of Primary Health Care and Selective Primary Health Care." *American Journal of Public Health* 94, no. 11 (November 2004): 1864–74.

Cui Weiyuan. "China's Village Doctors Take Great Strides." *WHO Bulletin* 86, no. 12 (December 2008): 914–15.

Cui Yueli, ed. *Zhongguo dangdai yixuejia huicui di wu juan* [Collected modern Chinese medical experts, vol. 5]. Changchun: Jilin kexue jishu chubanshe, 1991.

Culp, Robert. *Articulating Citizenship: Civic Education and Student Politics in Southeastern China, 1912–1940*. Cambridge, MA: Harvard University Press, 2007.

——. "Synthesizing Citizenship in Modern China." *History Compass* 5, no. 6 (November 2007): 1833–61.

Davenport, Horace. "Robert Kho-Seng Lim": *In Biographical Memoirs*, vol. 15. Washington, DC: National Academies Press, 1980, 280–307.

Deng Tietao. *Zhongguo fangyi shi* [A history of disease prevention in China]. Nanning: Guangxi kexue jishu chubanshe, 2006.

Deng Tietao and Cheng Zhifan, eds. *Zhongguo yixue tongshi: Jindai juan* [A comprehensive history of medicine in China: Modern volume]. Beijing: Renmin weisheng chubanshe, 2000.

Dreifort, John E. *Myopic Grandeur: The Ambivalence of French Foreign Policy toward the Far East, 1919–1945*. Kent, OH: Kent State University Press, 1991.

Durbach, Nadja. *Bodily Matters: The Anti-Vaccination Movement in England, 1853–1907*. Durham, NC: Duke University Press, 2004.

Eastman, Lloyd E. *The Abortive Revolution: China under Nationalist Rule, 1927–1937*. Cambridge, MA: Harvard University Press, 1974.

——. "Fascism in Kuomintang China: The Blue Shirts." *China Quarterly* 49 (January 1972): 1–31.

——. *Seeds of Destruction: Nationalist China in War and Revolution, 1937–1949*. Stanford, CA: Stanford University Press, 1984.

——. *Throne and Mandarins: China's Search for a Policy during the Sino-French Controversy, 1880–1885*. Cambridge, MA: Harvard University Press, 1967.

Eggleston, Karen. "Health, Education and China's Demographic Transition since 1950." In Aoki and Wu, *Chinese Economy*, 150–65.

Elgert, Klaus D. *Immunology: Understanding the Immune System*, 2nd ed. Hoboken, NJ: John Wiley & Sons, 2009.

Elman, Benjamin. *On Their Own Terms: Science in China, 1550–1900*. Cambridge, MA: Harvard University Press, 2005.

Elvin, Mark. *Retreat of the Elephants: An Environmental History of China*. New Haven, CT: Yale University Press, 2004.

Elvin, Mark, and Zhang Yixia. "Environment and Tuberculosis in Modern China." In *Sediments of Time: Environment and Society in Chinese History*, edited by Mark Elvin and Liu Ts'ui-jung, 520–44. Cambridge: Cambridge University Press, 1998.

Esposito, Roberto. "Biopolitics." In Campbell and Sitze, *Biopolitics*, 317–49.

Fan, Fa-ti. *British Naturalists in Qing China: Science, Empire, and Cultural Encounter*. Cambridge, MA: Harvard University Press, 2004.

——. "The Global Turn in the History of Science." *East Asian Science, Technology, and Society* 6 (2012): 249–58.

Fang Xiaoping. *Barefoot Doctors and Western Medicine in China*. Rochester, NY: University of Rochester Press, 2012.

Feinsilver, Julie. *Healing the Masses: Cuban Health Politics at Home and Abroad*. Berkeley and Los Angeles: University of California Press, 1993.

Feldberg, Georgina. *Disease and Class: Tuberculosis and the Shaping of Modern North American Society*. New Brunswick, NJ: Rutgers University Press, 1995.

Fenner, Frank, Donald A. Henderson, Isao Arita, Zdeněk Ježek, and Ivan D. Ladnyi. *Smallpox and Its Eradication*. Geneva: World Health Organization, 1988.

Ferlanti, Federica. "The New Life Movement in Jiangxi Province, 1934–1938." *Modern Asian Studies* 44, no. 5 (September 2010): 961–1000.

Fine, Paul E. M. "The BCG Story: Lessons from the Past and Implications for the Future." *Reviews of Infectious Diseases* 2, supplement 2 (March/April 1989): S353–59.

——. "Herd Immunity: History, Theory, Practice." *Epidemiologic Reviews* 15, no. 2 (1993): 265–302.

Fleck, Fiona. "Consensus during the Cold War: Back to Alma-Ata." *Bulletin of the World Health Organization* 86, no. 10 (October 2008): 745–46.

Flower, Darren R. *Bioinformatics for Vaccinology*. Chichester, UK: John Wiley & Sons, 2008.

Foucault, Michel. "Right of Death and Power over Life." In Campbell and Sitze, *Biopolitics*, 41–60.

——. "'Society Must Be Defended,'" lecture at College de France, March 17, 1976. In Campbell and Sitze, *Biopolitics*, 61–81.

Fu Hui and Deng Zongyu. "Jiu weishengbu zuzhi de bianqian" [Transformations of the old Ministry of Public Health]. In Zhengxie Beijing shi weiyuanhui wenshi ziliao yanjiu weiyuanhui, ed., *Wenshi ziliao xuanbian* [Selected cultural and historical materials], vol. 37, 253–77. Beijing: Beijing chubanshe, 1989.

Fung, Isaac C. H. "Chinese Journals: A Guide for Epidemiologists." *Emerging Themes in Epidemiology* 5 (2008): 1–26.

Gamsa, Mark. "The Epidemic of Pneumonic Plague in Manchuria 1910–1911." *Past and Present*, no. 190 (February 2006): 147–83.

Gao, James Zheng. *The Communist Takeover of Hangzhou*. Honolulu: University of Hawaii Press, 2004.

Gaubatz, Piper Rae. *Beyond the Great Wall: Urban Form and Transformation on the Chinese Frontiers*. Stanford, CA: Stanford University Press, 1996.

Gheorgiu, Marina. "Antituberculosis BCG Vaccine: Lessons from the Past." In Plotkin, *History of Vaccine Development*, 47–56.

Ghosh, Arunabh. "Accepting Difference, Seeking Common Ground: Sino-Indian Statistical Exchanges, 1951–1959," *BJHS Themes* 1 (2016): 61–82.

——. "Making It Count: Statistics and State-Society Relations in the Early People's Republic of China, 1949–1959." PhD diss., Columbia University, 2014.

Giersch, C. Patterson. *Asian Borderlands: The Transformation of Qing China's Yunnan Frontier*. Cambridge, MA: Harvard University Press, 2006.

Goldman, Merle, and Elizabeth Perry, eds. *Changing Meanings of Citizenship in Modern China*. Cambridge, MA: Harvard University Press, 2002.

Goodman, Bryna, and David S. G. Goodman, eds. *Twentieth-Century Colonialism and China: Localities, the Everyday, and the World*. Routledge: London, 2012.

Greenhalgh, Susan. "The Chinese Biopolitical: Facing the Twenty-First Century." *New Genetics and Society* 28, no. 3 (2009): 205–22.

——. "Governing Chinese Life: From Sovereignty to Biopolitical Governance." In *Governance of Life in Chinese Moral Experience: The Quest for an Adequate Life*, edited by Everett Zhang, Arthur Kleinman, and Tu Weiming, 146–62. New York: Routledge, 2011.

Gross, Miriam. *Farewell to the God of Plague: Chairman Mao's Campaign to Deworm China*. Oakland: University of California Press, 2016.

——. "Between Party, People, and Profession: The Many Faces of the 'Doctor' during the Cultural Revolution." *Medical History* 62, no. 3 (2018): 333–59.

Grove, David. *Tapeworms, Lice, and Prions: A Compendium of Unpleasant Infections*. Oxford: Oxford University Press, 2013.

Guiyang shi zhengfu xinwen bangongshi, ed. *Guoji huanhua yiliao dui zai Guiyang: International Medical Team in Guiyang* Beijing: Wuzhou zhuanbo chubanshe, 2005.

Guo Zhonghua. "Nationality, *Hukou*, and Ethnicity: The Institutional Structure of Citizenship in Contemporary Mainland China." *Cambridge Journal of China Studies* 9, no. 4 (2014): 1–19.

——. "Translating Chinese Citizenship." In *Routledge Handbook of Global Citizenship Studies*, edited by Engin F. Isin and Peter Myers, 366–75. New York: Routledge, 2014.

Hall, J. C. S. *The Yunnan Provincial Faction, 1927–37*. Canberra: Australian National University Press, 1976.

Halstead, Scott, and Yu Yong-Xin. "Human Viral Vaccines in China." In *Science and Medicine in Twentieth-Century China: Research and Education*, edited by John Z. Bowers, J. William Hess, and Nathan Sivin, 141–54. Ann Arbor: University of Michigan Center for Chinese Studies, 1988.

Hardy, Anne. *Salmonella Infections, Networks of Knowledge, and Public Health in Britain, 1880–1975*. Oxford: Oxford University Press, 2015.

Harrell, Paula. *Sowing the Seeds of Change: Chinese Students, Japanese Teachers, 1895–1905*. Stanford, CA: Stanford University Press, 1992.

Harris, Sheldon. *Factories of Death: Japanese Biological Warfare, 1932–1945, and the American Cover-up*. New York: Routledge, 1994.

——. "Japanese Biomedical Experimentation during the World-War-II Era." In *Military Medical Ethics*, vol. 2. Washington, DC: Office of the Surgeon General, 2003.

Harrison, Henrietta. *The Making of the Republican Citizen: Political Ceremonies and Symbols in China, 1911–1929*. Oxford: Oxford University Press, 2000.

Hayes, N. "Note on B.C.G. Immunisation." *Irish Journal of Medical Science* 22, no. 4 (April 1947): 171–74.

Hecht, Gabrielle. *Being Nuclear: Africans and the Global Uranium Trade*. Cambridge, MA: MIT Press, 2012.

——, ed. *Entangled Geographies: Empire and Technopolitics in the Global Cold War*. Cambridge, MA: MIT Press, 2011.

Henderson, Gail E., and Myron Cohen. *The Chinese Hospital: A Socialist Work Unit*. New Haven, CT: Yale University Press, 1984.

Heyck, Hunter, and David Kaiser. "Introduction, Focus: New Perspectives on Science and the Cold War." *Isis* 101, no. 2 (June 2010): 362–66.

Hoch, Steven L. "The Social Consequences of Soviet Immunization Policies, 1945–1980." National Council for Eurasian and East European Research Title VIII Program, Washington, DC, 1997. https://www.ucis.pitt.edu/nceeer/1997-812-03g-Hoch.pdf.

Hodges, Sarah. "The Global Menace." *Social History of Medicine* 25, no. 3 (August 2012): 719–28.

Hong Guojing, ed. *Zhonghua renwu dadian, di 1 ji, di 1 juan* [Dictionary of Chinese figures, vol. 1, part 1]. Beijing: Xinhua chubanshe, 1997.

Honig, Emily. *Sisters and Strangers: Women in the Shanghai Cotton Mills, 1919–1949.* Stanford, CA: Stanford University Press, 1986.

Ho Ping-ti. *Studies on the Population of China, 1368–1953, vol. 4.* Cambridge, MA: Harvard University Press, 1959.

Hsu, Elizabeth. *The Transmission of Chinese Medicine.* Cambridge: Cambridge University Press, 1999.

Hsu, Kai-yu. *Wen I-to.* Boston: Twayne, 1980.

Hughes, Thomas. "The Evolution of Large Technological Systems." In *The Social Construction of Technological Systems,* edited by Wiebe Bijker, Thomas Hughes, and Trevor Pinch, 51–82. Cambridge, MA: MIT Press, 1987.

Huisman, Frank, and Harry Oosterhuis. "The Politics of Health and Citizenship: Historical and Contemporary Perspectives." In *Health and Citizenship: Political Cultures of Health in Modern Europe,* edited by Frank Huisman and Harry Oosterhuis, 1–40. London: Pickering & Chatto, 2014.

Iijima Wataru. *Pesuto to kindai Chūgoku: Eisei no "seido-ka" to shakai hen'yō* [Plague and modern China: Hygiene's "systematization" and social change]. Tokyo: Ken bunshuppan, 2000.

Israel, John. *Lianda: A Chinese University in War and Revolution.* Stanford, CA: Stanford University Press, 1998.

"Jia Lianyuan." In *Ha'erbin shi zhi: Renwu fulu* [Harbin city gazetteer: Appendix of personages], edited by Ha'er bin shi difang zhi bianzuan weiyuanhui, 82–84. Harbin: Heilongjiang renmin chubanshe, 1999.

Jing Huiquan and Song Hanjun. *Yixue daolun: Gong jichu, linchuang, yufang, kouqiang yixue lei zhuanye yong* [Introduction to medicine: For professional use in basic, clinical, preventive, stomatological medicine]. Beijing: Beijing daxue yixue chubanshe, 2013.

Johnson, Tina Phillips. *Childbirth in Republican China: Delivering Modernity.* Lanham, MD: Lexington Books, 2011.

Joseph, William A., ed. *Politics in China: An Introduction.* 2nd ed. Oxford: Oxford University Press, 2014.

Kaple, Deborah A. "Soviet Advisors in China in the 1950s." In *Brothers in Arms: The Rise and Fall of the Sino-Soviet Alliance, 1945–1963,* edited by Odd Arne Westad, 117–40. Washington, DC: Woodrow Wilson Center, 1998.

Katz, Paul. *Demon Hordes and Burning Boats: The Cult of Marshal Wen in Late Imperial Chekiang.* Albany: State University of New York Press, 1995.

Krige, John. *American Hegemony and the Postwar Reconstruction of Science in Europe.* Cambridge, MA: MIT Press, 2006.

Kroker, Kenton, Jennifer Keelan, and Pauline Mazumdar, eds. *Crafting Immunity: Working Histories of Clinical Immunology,* Aldershot, UK: Ashgate, 2008.

Kupferberg, Eric. "A History of the International Union of Microbiological Societies, 1927–1990." 1993. https://www.iums.org/images/pdf/IUMS_History.pdf.

Lam Tong. *A Passion for Facts: Social Surveys and the Construction of the Chinese Nation-State, 1900–1949.* Oakland: University of California Press, 2011.

Lampton, David. *Health, Conflict, and the Chinese Political System.* Ann Arbor: Center for Chinese Studies, University of Michigan, 1974.

——. *The Politics of Medicine in China.* Boulder, CO: Westview, 1977.

Larkin, Bruce. *China and Africa, 1949–1970.* Berkeley: University of California Press, 1971.

Lary, Diana. *China's Republic.* Cambridge: Cambridge University Press, 2007.

——. *The Chinese People at War: Human Suffering and Social Transformation, 1937–1945*. Cambridge: Cambridge University Press, 2010.

Lavely, William, James Lee, and Wang Feng. "Chinese Demography: The State of the Field." *Journal of Asian Studies* 49, no. 4 (November 1990): 807–34.

Lawrence, Christopher. "Continuity in Crisis: Medicine, 1914–1945." In *The Western Medical Tradition: 1800 to 2000*, edited by W. F. Bynum, Anne Hardy, Stephen Jacyna, Christopher Lawrence, and E. M. Tansey, 247–390. Cambridge: Cambridge University Press, 2006.

Lee, Sung. "WHO and the Developing World: The Contest for Ideology." In *Western Medicine as Contested Knowledge*, edited by Andrew Cunningham and Bridie Andrews, 24–45. Manchester: Manchester University Press, 1997.

Lei, Sean Hsiang-lin. *Neither Donkey nor Horse: Medicine in the Struggle over China's Modernity*. Chicago: University of Chicago Press, 2014.

——. "Sovereignty and the Microscope: Constituting Notifiable Infectious Disease and Containing the Manchurian Plague, 1910–11." In Leung and Furth, *Health and Hygiene in Chinese East Asia*, 73–106.

Leitenberg, Milton. "China's False Allegations of the Use of Biological Weapons by the United States during the Korean War." *Cold War International History Project Bulletin 78* (2016): 1–82.

——. "New Russian Evidence on the Korean War Biological Warfare Allegations: Background and Analysis." *Cold War International History Project Bulletin 11* (1998): 185–99.

Leung, Angela Ki Che (Liang Qizi). "The Business of Vaccination in 19th-Century Canton." *Late Imperial China* 29, no. 1 (2008): 7–39.

——. "Variolisation et vaccination dans la Chine prémoderne (1570–1911)" [Variolation and vaccination in premodern China]. In *L'aventure de la vaccination* [The enterprise of vaccination], edited by Anne-Marie Moulin, 57–70. Paris: Fayard, 1996.

Leung, Angela Ki Che (Liang Qizi), and Charlotte Furth, eds. *Health and Hygiene in Chinese East Asia*. Durham, NC: Duke University Press, 2011.

Li Danke. *Echoes of Chongqing: Women in Wartime China*. Champaign: University of Illinois Press, 2010.

Li, Lillian M., Alison J. Dray-Novey, and Haili Kong. *Beijing: From Imperial Capital to Olympic City*. New York: Macmillan, 2007.

Li, Peter. "Japan's Biochemical Warfare and Experimentation in China." In *Japanese War Crimes: The Search for Justice*, edited by Peter Li, 289–300. New Brunswick, NJ: Transaction, 2003.

Li Xiaobing and Patrick Fuliang Shan, eds. *Ethnic China: Identity, Assimilation, and Resistance*. Lanham, MD: Lexington, 2015.

Lieberthal, Kenneth G. *Revolution and Tradition in Tientsin, 1949–1952*. Stanford, CA: Stanford University Press, 1980.

Lin, Alfred H. Y. "Warlord, Social Welfare and Philanthropy: The Case of Guangzhou under Chen Jitang, 1929–1936." *Modern China* 30, no. 2 (April 2004): 151–98.

"Lin Feiqing (1904–1998)." In *Tongjian xin Shanghai* [Together building a new Shanghai], edited by Shanghai shi Ningbo jingji jianshe cujin xiehui, Shanghai shi Ningbo tong xiang lian yi hui, and "Ningbo ren zai Shanghai" xilie congshu bian weihui, 817–18. Originally published in Zhang Delong, ed., *Shanghai Gaodeng jiaoyu xitong jiaoshou lu* [Record of professors in the Shanghai higher education system]. Shanghai: Huadong shifan daxue chubanshe, 1988, 431.

Liu, Chien-ling. "Relocating Pastorian Medicine: Accommodation and Acclimatization of Pastorian Practices against Smallpox at the Pasteur Institute of Chengdu, China, 1908–1927." *Science in Context* 30, no. 1 (2017): 33–59.

Liu Juanxiang. *Yixue kexue jia Tang Feifan* [Medical scientist Tang Feifan]. Beijing: Renmin weisheng chubanshe, 1999.

Liu Jun, Vanessa Tran, Andrea S. Leung, David C. Alexander, and Baoli Zhu. "Review: BCG Vaccines; Their Mechanisms of Attenuation and Impact on Safety and Protective Efficacy." *Human Vaccines* 5, no. 2 (February 2009): 70–78.

Liu Shi-yung. "'Qingjie,' 'weisheng,' yu 'baojian': Rizhi shiqi Taiwan shehui gonggong weisheng guannian zhi zhuanbian" ["Sanitation," "hygiene," and "public health": Changing thoughts on public health in colonial Taiwan]. *Taiwanshi yanjiu* 8, no. 1 (2001): 41–88.

Liu Xiaochun, Li Junjie, and Weng Xuedong, eds. *Xiangya renwu* [Figures of Xiangya]. Changsha: Hunan jiaoyu chubanshe, 1994.

Liu Xiaoyuan. "From Five 'Imperial Domains' to a 'Chinese Nation': A Perceptual and Political Transformation in Recent History." In Li and Shan, *Ethnic China*, 3–38.

"Long Yuying (1900–1983)." In *Xiang ren zhu shu biao yi* [A listing of the written works of Hunanese people], edited by Xun Lin and Gong Duqing, 167. Changsha: Yuelu shushe, 2010.

Löwy, Ilana. *Between Bench and Bedside: Science, Healing, and Interleukin-2 in a Cancer Ward*. Cambridge, MA: Harvard University Press, 1997.

Lü Xiaobo and Elizabeth Perry. "Introduction: The Changing Chinese Workplace in Historical and Comparative Perspective." In *Danwei: The Changing Chinese Workplace in Historical and Comparative Perspective*, edited by Lü Xiaobo and Elizabeth Perry, 3–17. Armonk, NY: M. E. Sharpe, 1997.

Lu Xiufang. "Xie Shaowen." In *Zhongguo xiandai kexue jia zhuanji, di si ji* [Biographies of modern Chinese scientists, vol. 4], edited by Lu Jiaxi, 457–62. Beijing: Kexue chubanshe, 1993.

Lucas, AnElissa. *Chinese Medical Modernization: Comparative Policy Continuities, 1930s–1980s*. New York: Praeger, 1982.

Luesink, David. "Dissecting Modernity: Anatomy and Power in the Language of Science in China." PhD diss., University of British Columbia, 2012.

Luo Kangtai, *Gansu renwu cidian* [Dictionary of figures from Gansu]. Lanzhou: Gansu minzu chubanshe, 2006.

Luo Yaoxing. *Mianyi yufang yu jibing kongzhi* [Immunity, prevention, and disease control]. Guangzhou: Guangdong keji chubanshe, 2004.

Lüthi, Lorenz. *The Sino-Soviet Split: Cold War in the Communist World*. Princeton, NJ: Princeton University Press, 2008.

Lynch, Michael. *The Chinese Civil War 1945–49*. Oxford, UK: Osprey, 2010.

Lynteris, Christos. "Skilled Natives, Inept Coolies: Marmot Hunting and the Great Manchurian Pneumonic Plague (1910–1911)." *History and Anthropology* 24, no. 3 (2013): 303–21.

Ma Qiusha. "The Peking Union Medical College and the Rockefeller Foundation's Medical Programs in China." In *Rockefeller Philanthropy and Modern Biomedicine: International Initiatives from World War I to the Cold War*, edited by William Schneider, 159–83. Bloomington: Indiana University Press, 2002.

MacKinnon, Stephen R., Diana Lary, and Ezra Vogel, eds. *China at War: Regions of China, 1937–1945*. Stanford, CA: Stanford University Press, 2007.

MacPherson, Kerrie. "Invisible Borders: Hong Kong, China and the Imperatives of Public Health." In *Public Health in Asia and the Pacific: Historical and Comparative Perspectives*, edited by Milton James Lewis and Kerrie L. MacPherson, 10–54. London and New York: Routledge, 2008.

———. *A Wilderness of Marshes: The Origins of Public Health in Shanghai, 1843–1893*. Oxford: Oxford University Press, 1987.

Martin, Emily. *Flexible Bodies: The Role of Immunity in American Culture from the Days of Polio to the Age of AIDS*. Boston: Beacon, 1994.

Martin, James W., George W. Christopher, and Edward M. Eitzen Jr. "History of Biological Weapons: From Poisoned Darts to Intentional Epidemics." In *Medical Aspects of Biological Warfare*, edited by Zygmunt F. Dembek, 1–20. Falls Church, VA: Office of the Surgeon General, United States Army, 2007.

McCord, Edward. *The Power of the Gun: The Emergence of Chinese Warlordism*. Berkeley and Los Angeles: University of California Press, 1993.

McGrath, Thomas E. "A Warlord Frontier: The Yunnan-Burma Border Dispute, 1910–1937." *Ohio Academy of History Proceedings* (2003): 7–29.

McIsaac, Lee. "The City as Nation: Creating a Wartime Capital in Chongqing." In *Remaking the Chinese City: Modernity and National Identity, 1900–1950*, edited by Joseph Esherick, 174–91. Honolulu: University of Hawaii Press, 2002.

McMillen, Christian W. *Discovering Tuberculosis: A Global History, 1900 to the Present*. New Haven, CT: Yale University Press, 2015.

Mitter, Rana. *Forgotten Ally: China's World War II, 1937–1945*. Boston: Houghton Mifflin Harcourt, 2013.

———. *The Manchurian Myth: Nationalism, Resistance, and Collaboration in Modern China*. Berkeley, CA: University of California Press, 2000.

Monath, Thomas P. "Yellow Fever Vaccines: The Success of Empiricism, Pitfalls of Application, and Transition to Molecular Vaccinology." In Plotkin, *History of Vaccine Development*, 109–36.

Morris, Andrew. *Marrow of the Nation: A History of Sport and Physical Culture in Republican China*. Berkeley and Los Angeles: University of California Press, 2004.

Moulin, Anne-Marie. *Le dernièr langage de la médicine: Histoire de l'immunologie de Pasteur au Sida* [The last language of medicine: History of immunology from Pasteur to AIDS]. Paris: Presses Universitaires de France, 1991.

Mullaney, Thomas. *Coming to Terms with the Nation: Ethnic Classification in Modern China*. Berkeley and Los Angeles: University of California Press, 2011.

Muscolino, Micah S. "Refugees, Land Reclamation, and Militarized Landscapes in Wartime China: Huanglongshan, Shaanxi, 1937–45." *Journal of Asian Studies* 69, no. 2 (May 2010): 453–78.

Needham, Joseph, Lu Gwei-djen, Dieter Kuhn, Donald Wagner, Rose Kerr, Nigel Wood, Peter Golas et al. *Science and Civilisation in China*. Cambridge: Cambridge University Press, 1954.

"Obituary Notices: Sir Henry Dale, O.M., G.B.E., D.Sc., LL.D., M.D., F.R.C.P., F.R.S." *British Medical Journal* 3, no. 5613 (August 3, 1968): 318–21.

Ogunsanwo, Alaba. *China's Policy in Africa, 1958–71*. Cambridge: Cambridge University Press, 1974.

Olson, James Stuart. *An Ethnohistorical Dictionary of China*. Westport, CT: Greenwood, 1998.

Oreskes, Naomi, and John Krige, eds. *Science and Technology in the Global Cold War*. Cambridge, MA: MIT Press, 2014.

Owen, Norman G., ed. *Death and Disease in Southeast Asia: Explorations in Social, Medical and Demographic History*. Southeast Asia Publications Series no. 14. Singapore: Asian Studies Association of Australia, 1987.

Packard, Randall M. *A History of Global Health: Interventions into the Lives of Other Peoples*. Baltimore: Johns Hopkins University Press, 2016.

———. *The Making of a Tropical Disease: A Short History of Malaria*. Baltimore: Johns Hopkins University Press, 2007.

Paine, S. C. M. *The Wars for Asia, 1911–1949*. Cambridge: Cambridge University Press, 2012.

Palmer, Steven. "Beginnings of Cuban Bacteriology: Juan Santos Fernández, Medical Research, and the Search for Scientific Sovereignty, 1880–1920." *Hispanic American Historical Review* 91, no. 3 (August 2011): 445–68.

Pelis, Kim. *Charles Nicolle, Pasteur's Imperial Missionary: Typhus and Tunisia*. Rochester, NY: University of Rochester Press, 2006.

Pepper, Suzanne. *Civil War in China: The Political Struggle, 1945–1949*. 2nd ed. Lanham, MD: Rowman & Littlefield, 1999.

Perdue, Peter C. "Is Pu-er in Zomia? Tea Cultivation and the State in China." Paper presented at the Yale University Agrarian Studies Colloquium, New Haven, CT, October 24, 2008. https://agrarianstudies.macmillan.yale.edu/sites/default/files/files/colloqpapers/07perdue.pdf.

Perkins, Dwight Heald. *Market Control and Planning in Communist China*. Cambridge, MA: Harvard University Press, 1966.

Petroff, S. A., and Arnold Branch. "Bacillus Calmette-Guérin (B.C.G.) Animal Experimentation and Prophylactic Immunization of Children: An Analysis and Critical Review." *American Journal of Public Health and the Nation's Health* 18, no. 7 (July 1928): 843–64.

Petryna, Adriana. "Biological Citizenship: The Science and Politics of Chernobyl-Exposed Populations." *Osiris* 19 (2004): 250–65.

Pier, Gerald B. "Vaccines and Vaccination." In *Immunology, Infection, and Immunity*, edited by Gerald B. Pier, Jeffrey B. Lyczak, and Lee M. Wetzler, 497–528. Washington, DC: ASM Press, 2004.

Plotkin, Stanley A., ed. *History of Vaccine Development*. New York: Springer, 2011.

Plotkin, Stanley A., Walter A. Orenstein, and Paul A. Offit, eds. *Vaccines*. 6th ed. Philadelphia: Elsevier Saunders, 2012.

Qi Changqing. "Jiefang qian xibei fangyi chu yu Zhongyang yiyuan xibei fenyuan jishi" [A record of the pre-liberation Northwest Epidemic Prevention Bureau and the Central Hospital–Northwest Branch]. In *Gansu wenshi ziliao xuanji di 26 ji* [Selected historical materials from Gansu, no. 26], edited by Zhongguo renmin zhengzhi huiyi Gansu sheng weiyuanhui wenshi ziliao yanjiu weiyuanhui, 81–92. Lanzhou: Gansu renmin chubanshe, 1987.

——. "Xibei fangyi chu yu xibei zhiyao chang jianji" [A brief record of the Northwest Epidemic Prevention Bureau and the Northwest Medical Production Factory]. In *Xibei jindai gongye* [Modern industry in the northwest], edited by Zhengxie gansu sheng weiyuanhui wenshi ziliao weiyuanhui, 486–88. Lanzhou: Gansu renmin chubanshe, 1989.

Remick, Elizabeth J. "Police-Run Brothels in Republican Kunming." *Modern China* 33, no. 4 (October 2007): 423–61.

Renshaw, Michelle. *Accommodating the Chinese: The American Hospital in China, 1880–1920*. New York: Routledge, 2005.

Ride, Lindsay. "The Test of War (Part 2)." In *Dispersal and Renewal: Hong Kong University during the War Years*, edited by Clifford Matthews and Oswald Cheung, 289–301. Hong Kong: Hong Kong University Press, 1998. Originally published as "The Test of War" in *The First Fifty Years, University of Hong Kong, 1911–61*, edited by Brian Harrison, 58–84. Hong Kong: Hong Kong University Press, 1962.

Rogaski, Ruth. *Hygienic Modernity: Meanings of Health and Disease in Treaty-Port China*. Berkeley: University of California Press, 2004.

——. "Nature, Annihilation, and Modernity: China's Korean War Germ-Warfare Experience Reconsidered." *Journal of Asian Studies* 61, no. 2 (May 2002): 381–415.

——. "Vampires in Plagueland: The Multiple Meanings of *Weisheng* in Manchuria." In Leung and Furth, *Health and Hygiene in East Asia*, 132–59.

Rose, Nikolas, and Carlos Novas. "Biological Citizenship." In *Global Assemblages: Technology, Politics, Ethics as Anthropological Problems*, edited by Aihwa Ong and Stephen J. Collier, 439–63. Malden, MA: Blackwell, 2005.

Rothman, Sheila. *Living in the Shadow of Death: Tuberculosis and the Social Experience of Illness in American History*. Baltimore: Johns Hopkins University Press, 1995.

Salter, Brian. "Biomedical Innovation and the Geopolitics of Patenting: China and the Struggle for Future Territory." *East Asian Science, Technology, and Society* 5, no. 3 (2011): 341–57.

Schmalzer, Sigrid. *Red Revolution, Green Revolution: Scientific Farming in Socialist China*. Chicago: University of Chicago, 2016.

——. "Self-Reliant Science: The Impact of the Cold War on Science in Socialist China." In *Science and Technology in the Global Cold War*, edited by Naomi Oreskes and John Krige, 75–106. Cambridge, MA: MIT Press, 2014.

Scott, James C. *The Art of Not Being Governed: An Anarchist History of Upland Southeast Asia*. New Haven: Yale University Press, 2009.

Secord, James. "Knowledge in Transit." *Isis* 95, no. 4 (December 2004): 654–72.

Selden, Mark. *The Yenan Way in Revolutionary China*. Cambridge, MA: Harvard University Press, 1971.

Serrie, Hendrick. "Obituaries: Francis L. K. Hsu." *American Anthropologist* 103, no. 1 (2001): 168–74.

Shen Giashan. "Riben zai Manzhou jianli de mianyi jishu yanjiu jigou ji qi fangyi, 1906–1945" [The immune technology research organizations established by Japan in Manchuria and their epidemic prevention, 1906–1945]. *Guoshiguan guankan* 45 (September 2015): 103–52.

Shen Yunlong, ed. *Jindai Zhongguo shiliao congkan: 30, Tang Jiyao* [Modern Chinese historical materials: 30, Tang Jiyao]. Taipei: Wenhai chubanshe, 1967.

Sheridan, James. *Chinese Warlord: The Career of Feng Yü-hsiang*. Stanford, CA: Stanford University Press, 1966.

Shih Chih-yu. "Ethnic Economy of Citizenship in China: Four Approaches to Identity Formation." In Goodman and Perry, *Changing Meanings of Citizenship*, 232–54.

Shinn, David H., and Joshua Eisenman. *China and Africa: A Century of Engagement*. Philadelphia: University of Pennsylvania Press, 2012.

Silverstein, Arthur. "History of Immunology: Cellular versus Humoral Immunity; Determinants and Consequences of an Epic 19th Century Battle." *Cellular Immunology* 48 (1979): 208–21.

——. *A History of Immunology*. San Diego: Academic Press, 1989.

Song Yuanmo and Lin Chunlian. *Xiandai Puxian renwu* [Modern Puxian figures]. Putian: Putian xiang xunshe, 1986.

Soon, Wayne S. "Blood, Soy Milk, and Vitality: The Wartime Origins of Blood Banking in China, 1943–45." *Bulletin of the History of Medicine* 90, no. 3 (2016): 424–54.

——. "Coming from Afar: The Overseas Chinese and the Institutionalization of Western Medicine and Science in China, 1910–1970." PhD diss., Princeton University, 2014.

Stepan, Nancy Leys. *Beginnings of Brazilian Science: Oswaldo Cruz, Medical Research and Policy, 1890–1920*. New York: Science History Publications, 1976.

Strauss, Julia C. "Morality, Coercion and State Building by Campaign in the Early PRC: Regime Consolidation and after, 1949–1956." *China Quarterly*, 188 (December 2006): 891–912.

——. "The Past in the Present: Historical and Rhetorical Lineages in China's Relations with Africa." *China Quarterly* 199 (September 2009): 777–95.

Summers, William C. *The Great Manchurian Plague of 1910–1911*. New Haven, CT: Yale University Press, 2012.

Sutton, Donald. *Provincial Militarism and the Chinese Republic: The Yunnan Army, 1905–25*. Ann Arbor: University of Michigan Press, 1980.

Tao Puqiu. "Minguo shiqi Kunming shipin weisheng yu anquan zhuangkuang yanjiu" [Research on the status of food hygiene and safety in republican Kunming]. Master's thesis, Yunnan University, 2011.

Taylor, Kim. *Chinese Medicine in Early Communist China, 1945–1963: A Medicine of Revolution*. New York: RoutledgeCurzon, 2005.

Thant Myint-U. *The Making of Modern Burma*. Cambridge: Cambridge University Press, 2001.

Thompson, C. Michele. "Mission to Macau: Smallpox, *Vaccinia*, and the Nguyễn Dynasty." *Portuguese Studies Review* 9, nos. 1–2 (2001).

——. "The Nguyễn Initiative to Acquire *Vaccinia*, 1820–1821." In *Global Movements, Local Concerns: Medicine and Health in Southeast Asia*, edited by Laurence Monnais and Harold J. Cook, 24–42. Singapore: National University of Singapore Press, 2012.

——. "Setting the Stage: Ancient Medical History of the Geographic Space That Is Now Vietnam." In *Southern Medicine for Southern People: Vietnamese Medicine in the Making*, edited by Laurence Monnais, C. Michele Thompson, and Ayo Wahlberg, 21–60. Newcastle upon Tyne, UK: Cambridge Scholars, 2012.

Thompson, Malcolm. "'Living Capital' (Shengming Ziben), Vital Statistics, and National Economics in China, 1912–1937." *Positions* 26, no. 3 (August 2018): 351–87.

Tian Jingguo. *Yunnan yiyao weisheng jianshi* [A survey of the history of medicine and public health in Yunnan]. Kunming: Yunnan keji chubanshe, 1987.

Tomes, Nancy. *The Gospel of Germs: Men, Women, and the Microbe in American Life*. Cambridge, MA: Harvard University Press, 1998.

van de Ven, Hans. *Breaking with the Past: The Maritime Customs Service and the Global Origins of Modernity in China*. New York: Columbia University Press, 2014.

——. *China at War: Triumph and Tragedy in the Emergence of the New China*. Cambridge, MA: Harvard University Press, 2018.

van Dongen, Jeroen, ed. *Cold War Science and the Transatlantic Circulation of Knowledge*. Leiden, Netherlands: Brill, 2015.

Vargha, Dora. "Between East and West: Polio Vaccination across the Iron Curtain in Cold War Hungary." *Bulletin for the History of Medicine* 88, no. 2 (2014): 319–42.

Volland, Nicolai. "Translating the Socialist State: Cultural Exchange, National Identity, and the Socialist World in the Early PRC." *Twentieth-Century China* 33, no. 2 (2008): 51–72.

Walker, Brett. "The Early Modern Japanese State and Ainu Vaccinations: Redefining the Body Politic, 1799–1868." *Past and Present* 163, no. 1 (1999): 121–60.

Wang Fei-ling. *Organizing through Division and Exclusion: China's Hukou System*. Stanford, CA: Stanford University Press, 2005.

Wang Kangjiu, ed. *Beijing weisheng zhi* [Gazetteer of public health in Beijing]. Beijing: Beijing kexue jishu chubanshe, 2001.

Wang, Zuoyue. "Transnational Science during the Cold War: The Case of Chinese/American Scientists." *Isis* 101 (2010): 367–77.

Watt, John Robertson. *A Friend in Deed: ABMAC and the Republic of China, 1937–1987*. New York: American Bureau for Medical Aid to China, 1992.

———. "Public Medicine in Wartime China: Biomedicine, State Medicine, and the Rise of China's National Medical Colleges, 1931–1945." Rosenberg Institute Occasional Paper no. 1, Rosenberg Institute for East Asian Studies, Suffolk University, Boston, 2012.

———. *Saving Lives in Wartime China: How Medical Reformers Built Modern Healthcare Systems amid War and Epidemics, 1928–1945*. Leiden, Netherlands: Brill, 2014.

Weathersby, Kathryn. "Deceiving the Deceivers: Moscow, Beijing, Pyongyang, and the Allegations of Bacteriological Weapons Use in Korea." *Cold War International History Project Bulletin 11* (1998): 176–85.

Webster, Anthony. *Gentlemen Capitalists: British Imperialism in South East Asia, 1770–1890*. London: Tauris Academic Studies, 1998.

Wei, Chunjuan Nancy. "Barefoot Doctors: The Legacy of Chairman Mao's Healthcare." In *Mr. Science and Chairman Mao's Cultural Revolution: Science and Technology in Modern China*, edited by Chunjuan Nancy Wei and Darryl E. Brock, 251–80. Lanham, MD: Lexington Books, 2013.

"Wei Xi." In *Dalian yingmo pu* [Heroic models of Dalian], edited by Dalian shi shi zhi bangongshi, 91. Dalian: Dalian chubanshe, 2001.

"Wei Xi (1903–1989)." In *Dongnan daxue xiaoyou yexu congshu, di 1 juan* [Dongnan University Alumni Association Continuing Collection, vol. 1], edited by Sun Wenzhi, 402–3. Nanjing: Dongnan daxue chubanshe, 2002.

Westad, Odd Arne. *Decisive Encounters: The Chinese Civil War, 1946–1950*. Stanford, CA: Stanford University Press, 2003.

Winckler, Edwin, and Susan Greenhalgh. *Governing China's Population: From Leninist to Neoliberal Biopolitics*. Stanford, CA: Stanford University Press, 2005.

Wolfe, Audra. *Competing with the Soviets: Science, Technology, and the State in Cold War America*. Baltimore: Johns Hopkins University Press, 2013.

Woo, Margaret Y. K. "Law and the Gendered Citizen." In Goodman and Perry, *Changing Meanings of Citizenship*, 308–29.

World Health Organization. *Bugs, Drugs, and Smoke: Stories from Public Health*. New York: World Health Organization, 2011.

———. "WHO Vaccine-Preventable Diseases: Monitoring System. 2018 Global Summary." http://apps.who.int/immunization_monitoring/globalsummary/schedules.

Wu Anran and Xie Shaowen. "In Memory of Professor Tang Fei-fan." *Chinese Medical Journal* 100, no. 6 (1987): 512–13.

Wu Chongqi. *Zhongguo xiehe yike daxue renwu huicui* [A distinguished assembly of personages at China Union Medical University]. Beijing: Beijing yike daxue, Zhongguo xiehe yike daxue lianhe chubanshe, 1992.

Wu, Qiyan, Jianquan Cheng, Dan Liu, Li Han, and Yuhong Yang. "Kunming: A Regional International Mega City in Southwest China." In *Urban Development Challenges, Risks and Resilience in Asian Mega Cities*, edited by R. B. Singh, 323–47. Tokyo: Springer Japan, 2015.

Wusheng de jiaoliang: Mie tianhua [Silent contest: The eradication of smallpox]. Documentary aired on CCTV-1, December 11, 2003. Transcript available at http://www.cntv.cn/program/jzql/20040317/101742_2.shtml; film at www.youtube.com/watch?v=PRFCuSBY97M.

"Xie Shaowen." In *Zhongguo kexueyuan yuan shi gongzuo ju Kexue de daolu (shangjuan)* [The path of science, first volume], edited by Zhongguo kexue yuan yuanshi gongzuo ju, 916–17. Shanghai: Shanghai jiaoyu chubanshe, 2005.

Xu Hui and Jiang Yutu. "The Eradication of Smallpox in Shanghai, China, October 1950–July 1951." *Bulletin of the World Health Organization* 59, no. 6 (1981): 913–17. http://apps.who.int/iris/handle/10665/262204.

Xu Lanjun. "Translation and Internationalism." In *Mao's Little Red Book: A Global History*, edited by Alexander Cook, 76–95. Cambridge: Cambridge University Press, 2014.

Xue Pangao. "'Tang shi bingdu' qidi sikao: Tang Feifan chenggong fenli shayan bingyuan du 35 zhounian jinian" ['Tang Virus' Inspiration and Consideration: Tang Feifan Succeeds in Isolating Trachoma Virus, a 35-Year Retrospective]. *Shengwu kexue xinxi* 2, no. 3 (1990): 128–30.

Yan Xuetong. *Zhongguo yu zhoubian zhongdeng guojia guanxi* [The relations between China and its bordering states]. Beijing: Shehui kexue wenxian chubanshe, 2015.

Yang Bin. *Between Wind and Clouds: The Making of Yunnan, Second Century BCE to Twentieth Century CE*. New York: Columbia University Press, 2008.

——. "The Zhang on Chinese Southern Frontiers: Disease Constructions, Environmental Changes, and Imperial Colonization." *Bulletin of the History of Medicine* 84, no. 2 (2010): 163–92.

Yang, Gonghuan, Yu Wang, Yixin Zeng, George F. Gao, Xiaofeng Liang, Maigeng Zhou, Xia Wan, et al. "Rapid Health Transition in China, 1990–2010: Findings from the Global Burden of Disease Study 2010." *Lancet* 381, no. 9882 (June 8–14, 2013): 1987–2015.

Yang Jisheng. *Tombstone: The Great Chinese Famine, 1958–1962*. Translated by Stacy Mosher and Guo Jian. New York: Farrar, Straus and Giroux, 2012.

Yang Rujian, Zhang Yingqin, and Francis Ng, eds. *Historical Treasures of China: A Collection of Rare Manuscripts from the Archives of Yunnan Province*. Hong Kong: Zero to One, 2002.

Yang Xishou. "Kangri zhanzheng shiqi de Guoli Zhongzheng Yixueyuan" [The wartime National Zhongzheng Medical College]. In *Guizhou wenshi ziliao xuanji, di 26 ji, kangri zhanzheng shiqi de Guizhou yuanxiao* [Selected historical accounts of the past in Guizhou, vol. 26: Guizhou educational institutions in the War of Resistance], edited by Zhongguo renmin zhengzhi xieshang huiyi Guizhou sheng weiyuanhui wenshi ziliao yanjiu weiyuanhui, 133–40. Guiyang: Guizhou sheng wenshi shudian, 1987.

Ye Weili. *Seeking Modernity in China's Name*. Stanford, CA: Stanford University Press, 2002.

Yeung, Hans W. Y. "Yunnan Province." In *Southeast Asia: A Historical Encyclopedia, from Angkor Wat to East Timor*, edited by Ooi Keat Gin, 1439–41. Santa Barbara, CA: ABC-CLIO, 2004.

Yip Ka-che. "Disease and the Fighting Men: Nationalist Anti-Epidemic Efforts in Wartime China, 1937–1945." In *China in the Anti-Japanese War, 1937–1945*, edited by David P. Barrett and Larry N. Shyu, 171–88. New York: Peter Lang, 2001.

——. "Health and Nationalist Reconstruction: Rural Health in Nationalist China, 1928–1937." *Modern Asian Studies* 26, no. 2 (May 1992): 395–415.

——. *Health and National Reconstruction in Nationalist China*. Ann Arbor, MI: Association for Asian Studies, 1995.

Youde, Jeremy. "China's Health Diplomacy in Africa." *China: An International Journal* 8, no. 1 (March 2010): 151–63.

Yu Xingzhong. "Citizenship, Ideology, and the PRC Constitution." In Goodman and Perry, *Changing Meanings of Citizenship*, 288–307.

Yu Xinzhong. "Epidemics and Public Health in Twentieth-Century China." In Andrews and Bullock, *Medical Transitions in 20th Century China*, 91–105.

Yuan Baohua and Zhai Taifeng. *Zhongguo gaige da cidian* [China reform dictionary]. Haikou: Hainan chubanshe, 1992.

Yunnan sheng difang zhi bianzuan weiyuanhui, ed. *Yunnan shengzhi, juan liu shi jiu: Weisheng zhi* [Yunnan provincial gazetteer: Vol. 69, Public Health]. Kunming: Yunnan renmin chubanshe, 2002.

Yunnan sheng zhi bian zuan weiyuanhui, ed. *Xu Yunnan tongzhi changbian zhongce* [The extended Yunnan gazetteer, vol. 2]. Kunming: Yunnan sheng zhi bianzuan weiyuanhui bangongshi, 1986.

Zhan Mei. "Human Oriented? Angels and Monsters in China's Health Care Reform." *East Asian Science, Technology, and Society* 5, no. 3 (2011): 291–311.

Zhang Bin, ed. *Lishi shang de weisheng bu 1949–2013* [The Ministry of Health in History, 1949–2013]. Beijing: Hongqi chubanshe, 2014.

Zhang Li. *In Search of Paradise: Middle-Class Living in a Chinese Metropolis*. Ithaca, NY: Cornell University Press, 2010.

Zhang Taishan. *Minguo shiqi de chuanranbing yu shehui: Yi chuanranbing fangzhi yu gonggong weisheng jianshe wei zhongxin* [Republican-era infectious diseases and society: The treatment and prevention of infectious diseases and public health establishment as the focus]. Beijing: Shehui kexue wenxian chubanshe, 2008.

Zhao Chun, ed. *Tang Jiyao yanjiu wenji* [Research materials on Tang Jiyao]. Kunming: Yunnan renmin chubanshe, 2011.

Zhongguo kexue jishu xiehui, ed. *Zhongguo kexue jishu xiehui nianjian 2007* [2007 yearbook of the China Association of Science and Technology]. Beijing: Zhongguo kexue jishu chubanshe, 2007.

Zhongguo renmin zhengzhi xieshang huiyi Lanzhou shi weiyuanhui wenshi ziliao weiyuanhui, ed. *Lanzhou wenshi ziliao xuanji* [Selected cultural and historical materials from Lanzhou]. Lanzhou: Lanzhou daxue chubanshe, 1992.

"Wei Xi." In *Zhongguo jinxiandai gaodeng jiaoyu renwu cidian* [Biographical dictionary of figures in modern Chinese higher education], edited by Zhou Chuan, 664. Fuzhou: Fujian jiaoyu chubanshe, 2012.

"Yu He." In *Zhongguo ershi shiji jishi benmo, fujuan renwu* [Major events in twentieth-century China: Appendix volume, personages], edited by Zhou Hong and Zhu Hanguo, 333. Jinan: Shandong renmin chubanshe, 2000.

Zhou Xun. "From China's 'Barefoot Doctor' to Alma Ata: The Primary Health Care Movement in the Long 1970s." In *China, Hong Kong and the Long 1970s: Global Perspectives*, edited by Priscilla Roberts and Odd Arne Westad, 135–57. Cham, Switzerland: Palgrave Macmillan, 2017.

Zhu Kewen, Gao Enxian, and Gong Chun. *Zhongguo junshi yixue shi* [A history of military medicine in China]. Beijing: Renmin junyi chubanshe, 1996.

Index

Studies of the Weatherhead East Asian Institute
Columbia University

Selected Titles

(Complete list at http://weai.columbia.edu/publications/studies-weai/)

Fighting for Virtue: Justice and Politics in Thailand, by Duncan McCargo. Cornell University Press, 2019.

Down and Out in Saigon: Stories of the Poor in a Colonial City, by Haydon Cherry. Yale University Press, 2019.

Beauty in the Age of Empire: Japan, Egypt, and the Global History of Aesthetic Education, by Raja Adal. Columbia University Press, 2019.

Mass Vaccination: Citizens' Bodies and State Power in Modern China, by Mary Augusta Brazelton. Cornell University Press, 2019.

Residual Futures: The Urban Ecologies of Literary and Visual Media of 1960s and 1970s Japan, by Franz Prichard. Columbia University Press, 2019.

The Making of Japanese Settler Colonialism: Malthusianism and Trans-Pacific Migration, 1868–1961, by Sidney Xu Lu. Cambridge University Press, 2019.

The Power of Print in Modern China: Intellectuals and Industrial Publishing from the end of Empire to Maoist State Socialism, by Robert Culp. Columbia University Press, 2019.

Beyond the Asylum: Mental Illness in French Colonial Vietnam, by Claire E. Edington. Cornell University Press, 2019.

Borderland Memories: Searching for Historical Identity in Post-Mao China, by Martin Fromm. Cambridge University Press, 2019.

Sovereignty Experiments: Korean Migrants and the Building of Borders in Northeast Asia, 1860–1949, by Alyssa M. Park. Cornell University Press, 2019.

The Greater East Asia Co-Prosperity Sphere: When Total Empire Met Total War, by Jeremy A. Yellen. Cornell University Press, 2019.

Thought Crime: Ideology and State Power in Interwar Japan, by Max Ward. Duke University Press, 2019.

Statebuilding by Imposition: Resistance and Control in Colonial Taiwan and the Philippines, by Reo Matsuzaki. Cornell University Press, 2019.

Nation-Empire: Ideology and Rural Youth Mobilization in Japan and Its Colonies, by Sayaka Chatani. Cornell University Press, 2019.

The Invention of Madness: State, Society, and the Insane in Modern China, by Emily Baum. University of Chicago Press, 2018.

Fixing Landscape: A Techno-Poetic History of China's Three Gorges, by Corey Byrnes. Columbia University Press, 2018.

Japan's Imperial Underworlds: Intimate Encounters at the Borders of Empire, by David Ambaras. Cambridge University Press, 2018.

Heroes and Toilers: Work as Life in Postwar North Korea, 1953–1961, by Cheehyung Harrison Kim. Columbia University Press, 2018.

Electrified Voices: How the Telephone, Phonograph, and Radio Shaped Modern Japan, 1868–1945, by Kerim Yasar. Columbia University Press, 2018.

Making Two Vietnams: War and Youth Identities, 1965–1975, by Olga Dror. Cambridge University Press, 2018.

A Misunderstood Friendship: Mao Zedong, Kim Il-sung, and Sino–North Korean Relations, 1949–1976, by Zhihua Shen and Yafeng Xia. Columbia University Press, 2018.

Playing by the Informal Rules: Why the Chinese Regime Remains Stable Despite Rising Protests, by Yao Li. Cambridge University Press, 2018.

Raising China's Revolutionaries: Modernizing Childhood for Cosmopolitan Nationalists and Liberated Comrades, by Margaret Mih Tillman. Columbia University Press, 2018.

Buddhas and Ancestors: Religion and Wealth in Fourteenth-Century Korea, by Juhn Y. Ahn. University of Washington Press, 2018.

Idly Scribbling Rhymers: Poetry, Print, and Community in Nineteenth Century Japan, by Robert Tuck. Columbia University Press, 2018.

China's War on Smuggling: Law, Economic Life, and the Making of the Modern State, 1842–1965, by Philip Thai. Columbia University Press, 2018.

Forging the Golden Urn: The Qing Empire and the Politics of Reincarnation in Tibet, by Max Oidtmann. Columbia University Press, 2018.

The Battle for Fortune: State-Led Development, Personhood, and Power among Tibetans in China, by Charlene Makley. Cornell University Press, 2018.

Aesthetic Life: Beauty and Art in Modern Japan, by Miya Elise Mizuta Lippit. Harvard University Asia Center, 2018.

Where the Party Rules: The Rank and File of China's Communist State, by Daniel Koss. Cambridge University Press, 2018.

Resurrecting Nagasaki: Reconstruction and the Formation of Atomic Narratives, by Chad R. Diehl. Cornell University Press, 2018.

China's Philological Turn: Scholars, Textualism, and the Dao in the Eighteenth Century, by Ori Sela. Columbia University Press, 2018.

Making Time: Astronomical Time Measurement in Tokugawa Japan, by Yulia Frumer. University of Chicago Press, 2018.

Mobilizing Without the Masses: Control and Contention in China, by Diana Fu. Cambridge University Press, 2018.

Post-Fascist Japan: Political Culture in Kamakura after the Second World War, by Laura Hein. Bloomsbury, 2018.

China's Conservative Revolution: The Quest for a New Order, 1927–1949, by Brian Tsui. Cambridge University Press, 2018.

Promiscuous Media: Film and Visual Culture in Imperial Japan, 1926–1945, by Hikari Hori. Cornell University Press, 2018.

The End of Japanese Cinema: Industrial Genres, National Times, and Media Ecologies, by Alexander Zahlten. Duke University Press, 2017.

The Chinese Typewriter: A History, by Thomas S. Mullaney. The MIT Press, 2017.

Forgotten Disease: Illnesses Transformed in Chinese Medicine, by Hilary A. Smith. Stanford University Press, 2017.

Borrowing Together: Microfinance and Cultivating Social Ties, by Becky Yang Hsu. Cambridge University Press, 2017.

Food of Sinful Demons: Meat, Vegetarianism, and the Limits of Buddhism in Tibet, by Geoffrey Barstow. Columbia University Press, 2017.

Youth For Nation: Culture and Protest in Cold War South Korea, by Charles R. Kim. University of Hawaii Press, 2017.

Socialist Cosmopolitanism: The Chinese Literary Universe, 1945–1965, by Nicolai Volland. Columbia University Press, 2017.

The Social Life of Inkstones: Artisans and Scholars in Early Qing China, by Dorothy Ko. University of Washington Press, 2017.

Darwin, Dharma, and the Divine: Evolutionary Theory and Religion in Modern Japan, by G. Clinton Godart. University of Hawaii Press, 2017.

Dictators and Their Secret Police: Coercive Institutions and State Violence, by Sheena Chestnut Greitens. Cambridge University Press, 2016.

The Cultural Revolution on Trial: Mao and the Gang of Four, by Alexander C. Cook. Cambridge University Press, 2016.

Inheritance of Loss: China, Japan, and the Political Economy of Redemption After Empire, by Yukiko Koga. University of Chicago Press, 2016.

Homecomings: The Belated Return of Japan's Lost Soldiers, by Yoshikuni Igarashi. Columbia University Press, 2016.

Samurai to Soldier: Remaking Military Service in Nineteenth-Century Japan, by D. Colin Jaundrill. Cornell University Press, 2016.